IAC-IARC-WHO Cytopathology Reporting Systems • 1st Edition

WHO Reporting System for Lung Cytopathology

International Academy of Cytology – International Agency for Research on Cancer – World Health Organization
Joint Editorial Board

THE INTERNATIONAL ACADEMY OF CYTOLOGY • 1957 •

International Agency for Research on Cancer

World Health Organization

Suggested citation
International Academy of Cytology – International Agency for Research on Cancer – World Health Organization Joint Editorial Board. WHO Reporting System for Lung Cytopathology. Lyon (France): International Agency for Research on Cancer; 2022. (IAC-IARC-WHO cytopathology reporting systems series, 1st ed.; vol. 1). https://publications.iarc.fr/620.

Sales, rights, and permissions
Print copies are distributed by WHO Press, World Health Organization, 20 Avenue Appia, 1211 Geneva 27, Switzerland
Tel.: +41 22 791 3264; Fax: +41 22 791 4857; email: bookorders@who.int; website: https://whobluebooks.iarc.fr

To purchase IARC publications in electronic format, see the IARC Publications website (https://publications.iarc.fr).

First print run (5000 copies)

Updated corrigenda can be found at https://publications.iarc.fr

IARC Library Cataloguing-in-Publication Data
Names: International Academy of Cytology – International Agency for Research on Cancer – World Health Organization Joint Editorial Board.
Title: WHO reporting system for lung cytopathology / edited by International Academy of Cytology – International Agency for Research on Cancer – World Health Organization Joint Editorial Board.
Description: First edition. | Lyon: International Agency for Research on Cancer, 2022. | Series: IAC-IARC-WHO cytopathology reporting systems. | Includes bibliographical references and index.
Identifiers: ISBN 9789283245162 (pbk.) | ISBN 9789283245179 (ebook)
Subjects: MESH: Respiratory System--pathology. | Respiratory Tract Neoplasms--pathology. | Respiratory Tract Diseases--diagnosis. | Cytodiagnosis--classification.
Classification: NLM WF 100

The WHO Reporting System for Lung Cytopathology presented in this book reflects the views of the International Academy of Cytology (IAC) – International Agency for Research on Cancer (IARC) – World Health Organization (WHO) Joint Editorial Board that convened via video conference 21–23 September 2021.

The IAC-IARC-WHO Joint Editorial Board

For the complete list of all contributors and their affiliations, see pages 185–186.

WHO Reporting System for Lung Cytopathology

Edited by — The IAC-IARC-WHO Joint Editorial Board

IAC-IARC Pathology Editors — Andrew S. Field, Fernando Schmitt, Ian A. Cree

Additional IARC Editing — Gabrielle Goldman-Lévy

Project Assistant — Asiedua Asante

Assistants — Anne-Sophie Bres, Laura Brispot, Nandini Deleu, Nicole Suty

Production Editor — Jessica Cox
Copy Editing — Julia Slone-Murphy

Principal Information Assistant — Alberto Machado
Information Assistant — Catarina Marques

Layout — Catarina Marques

Printed by — Omnibook
74370 Argonay, France

Publisher — International Agency for Research on Cancer (IARC)
25 Av. Tony Garnier, CS 90627
69366 Lyon, CEDEX 07, France

Contents

List of abbreviations

2D	two-dimensional
3D	three-dimensional
BAL	bronchoalveolar lavage
BB	bronchial brushing
BW	bronchial washing
CMV	cytomegalovirus
CNS	central nervous system
CT	computed tomography
CXR	chest X-ray
DNA	deoxyribonucleic acid
EBUS	endobronchial ultrasound
EBUS-TBFNAB	endobronchial ultrasound–guided transbronchial fine-needle aspiration biopsy
ER	estrogen receptor
EUS	endoscopic ultrasound, endoscopic ultrasonography
FDG	18F-fluorodeoxyglucose
FDG PET	18F-fluorodeoxyglucose positron emission tomography
FISH	fluorescence in situ hybridization
FNAB	fine-needle aspiration biopsy
GFAP	glial fibrillary acidic protein
H&E	haematoxylin and eosin stain
HPV	human papillomavirus
IAC	International Academy of Cytology
IARC	International Agency for Research on Cancer
ICC	immunocytochemistry
LBC	liquid-based cytopathology
MALT lymphoma	extranodal marginal zone lymphoma of mucosa-associated lymphoid tissue
MRI	magnetic resonance imaging
NGS	next-generation sequencing
NOS	not otherwise specified
NSE	neuron-specific enolase
Pap	Papanicolaou stain
PAS	periodic acid–Schiff
PASD	periodic acid–Schiff with diastase
PCR	polymerase chain reaction
PET	positron emission tomography
PET-CT	positron emission tomography–computed tomography
PR	progesterone receptor
PSC	Papanicolaou Society of Cytopathology
RNA	ribonucleic acid
ROM	risk of malignancy
ROSE	rapid onsite evaluation
SNV	single-nucleotide variant
TKI	tyrosine kinase inhibitor

Foreword

The classification of tumours can be viewed from many perspectives. To a histopathologist it is all about the histological patterns, to a molecular pathologist or geneticist it is all about which genes are affected, and to an epidemiologist it is about the tumours' incidence. The WHO Classification of Tumours series started in the 1960s as a result of the histopathologist's need to make diagnoses by grouping tumours according to their microscopic appearance. The programme now includes contributions from many specialties, including, of course, cytopathology. However, the cytopathologist looks at tumours slightly differently than other specialists do, and although the main classification is helpful, it has become clear that reporting systems based on the key diagnostic cytopathological features are needed, tailored to the diagnostic categories in widespread use. There is also a need for these reporting systems to be truly international, serving the needs of patients worldwide.

The International Academy of Cytology (IAC), a scientific, non-profit organization with members from 49 other cytopathology-affiliated societies, therefore approached the International Agency for Research on Cancer (IARC) – home to the WHO Classification of Tumours Programme – to see whether it would be possible to produce a complementary series of WHO Reporting Systems, particularly for the areas of diagnostic cytopathology that did not already have agreed systems published by others. The two organizations signed a memorandum of understanding in early 2020 and, despite the problems of the COVID-19 pandemic, have now produced this – the first WHO Reporting System for Lung Cytopathology. Reporting systems for pancreaticobiliary, lymph node, and soft tissue cytopathology are reaching completion, and further systems are planned.

Cytopathology plays a critical role in the diagnosis of many lung conditions, including tumours. With recent developments in sampling technology, there now remain only a few lesions that cannot be sampled for cytopathological examination. Sputum cytopathology, bronchial washing and brushing, transthoracic fine-needle aspiration biopsy (FNAB), and endobronchial ultrasound–guided transbronchial fine-needle aspiration biopsy (EBUS-TBFNAB) all have a role to play under various clinical circumstances. Imaging detection of ever-smaller lesions, combined with the ability to obtain tissue from all but a few, facilitates cytopathological and often histopathological diagnosis. Ancillary methods such as immunocytochemistry and in situ hybridization are applicable to smears and cell blocks, which also provide material for next-generation sequencing. The avoidance of formalin in cytopathological preparations allows molecular methods to be applied, whether simple PCR or next-generation sequencing, for diagnosis and predictive testing.

Just as the WHO Classification of Tumours series (also known as the WHO Blue Books), published in print volumes and as a website (https://tumourclassification.iarc.who.int), is an essential tool for standardizing diagnostic practice worldwide and serves as a vehicle for the translation of cancer research into practice, we hope that these first-edition WHO Reporting Systems will fulfil the same role for cytopathology. The key diagnostic cytopathological features listed for each tumour type under the diagnostic categories represent the first international consensus and are described in precise, uniform language. These diagnostic criteria are underpinned by evidence that has been evaluated and debated by experts in the field. Each lesion-specific section includes a dedicated subsection discussing the differential diagnosis of the lesion's cytopathological features that can be used worldwide, including in low-resource settings, followed by a subsection describing the current best-practice application of ancillary testing (including next-generation sequencing) on cytopathology material. About 60 authors and editors participated in the production of this volume, and gave their time freely to this task. We are very grateful for their help; it is a remarkable team effort.

This volume, like those of the WHO Classification of Tumours series, has been led by an editorial board composed of standing and expert members. The standing members include the chair of the WHO Classification of Tumours Editorial Board and others nominated by the IAC. The expert members, selected on the basis of informed bibliometric analysis and advice from the standing members, represent a broad international expertise, as does the authorship group. The diagnostic process is increasingly multidisciplinary, and we are delighted that several radiology and clinical experts have joined us to address specific needs.

In addition to using the International System of Units (SI) for all measurements, we have standardized the genomic nomenclature by using Human Genome Variation Society (HGVS) notation. We have also further standardized our use of units of length, adopting the convention used by the International Collaboration on Cancer Reporting (https://www.iccr-cancer.org) and the UK Royal College of Pathologists (https://www.rcpath.org/), so that the size of tumours is now given exclusively in millimetres (mm) rather than centimetres (cm). This is clearer, in our view, and avoids the use of decimal points – a common source of medical errors.

We hope this is the start of a long-term solution to meeting the needs of the cytopathology community. Like the WHO Classification of Tumours, the WHO Reporting Systems (books and website) are published on a non-profit basis, with proceeds ploughed directly back into the series to support the costs involved, including production, printing, and distribution. There are substantial discounts available for residents of low- and middle-income countries and trainees. It is of vital importance that cancers continue to be classified and diagnosed according to the same standards internationally so that patients can benefit from multicentre clinical trials and studies, as well as from the results of local research conducted on different continents.

Ian A. Cree, Fernando Schmitt, Martha Bishop Pitman, Ravi Mehrotra, Andrew S. Field

International Agency for Research on Cancer
International Academy of Cytology

December 2022

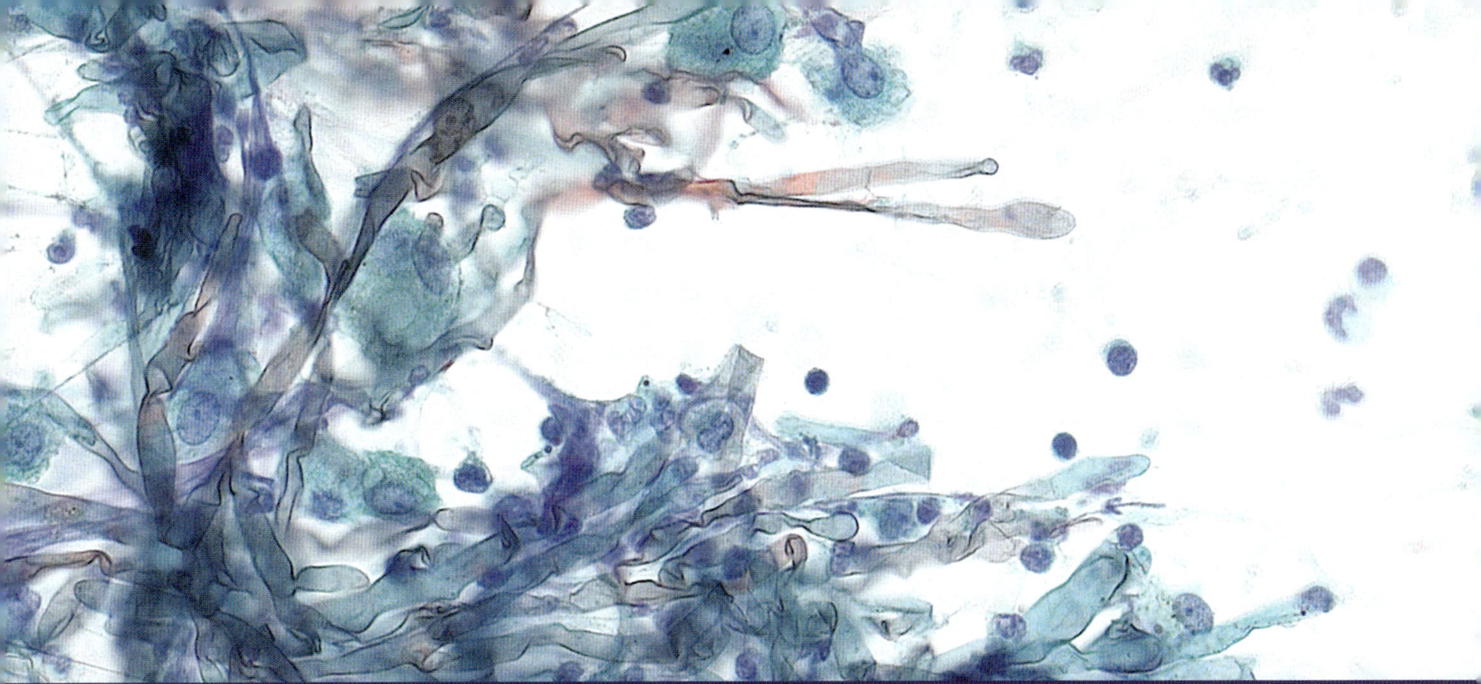

1

Introduction to the WHO Reporting System for Lung Cytopathology

Edited by: Bubendorf L, Canberk S, Field AS, Pitman MB, Schmitt F

Background
The role of lung cytopathology
Diagnostic categories and report structure
Risk of malignancy and management recommendations

Background

Michael CW
Heine R

Lung cytopathology has experienced tremendous progress since 1860 when Dr L.S. Beale published the first case report describing detection of malignant cells in a sputum sample from a patient with cancer of the pharynx, followed by Dr Papanicolaou's publications on the detection of cancer cells from the lung {673,674,672}. A pilot study for the early detection of lung cancer using sputum samples was initiated in 1945 by the American Cancer Society {181}.

The introduction of flexible bronchoscopy with fluoroscopy in the 1970s was a significant leap forward in medical practice. The technique offered the ability to reliably and safely visualize the airways down to the segmental level and to sample peripheral lesions, and specimens could be obtained with multiple minimally invasive tools including bronchial brushings, bronchial washings, bronchoalveolar lavage (BAL), transbronchial FNAB, and forceps biopsies. These techniques contributed greatly to the diagnosis of both benign and malignant lung diseases. Transthoracic CT-guided FNAB was also frequently performed, especially for the diagnosis of peripheral lung nodules. Endobronchial ultrasound, first described in 2006, uses ultrasound technology to visualize structures in the airway wall, peribronchial lung, mediastinum, and hila. Later, radial endobronchial ultrasound and transbronchial FNAB resulted in another major step forward in the practice of lung cytopathology, allowing both the diagnosis and staging of the disease to be done in one setting.

The utility of transbronchial FNAB is further maximized when rapid onsite evaluation (ROSE) of the sample can be offered by a cytopathologist or cytotechnologist, thus increasing accuracy,

Table 1.01 Terminology in small biopsy and cytopathology versus resection specimens for adenocarcinoma and squamous cell carcinoma (WHO tumour classification)

Morphology/stains	Terminology for small biopsies and cytopathology specimens	Terminology for resection specimens
Morphological squamous cell patterns clearly present	Squamous cell carcinoma	Squamous cell carcinoma
Morphological adenocarcinoma patterns clearly present	Adenocarcinoma (list the patterns in the diagnosis) • Lepidic • Acinar • Papillary • Solid • Micropapillary • Other (complex glandular pattern)	Adenocarcinoma Predominant pattern: • Lepidic • Acinar • Papillary • Solid • Micropapillary • Other (complex glandular pattern)
	Adenocarcinoma with lepidic pattern (if pure, list the differential diagnosis on the right and add a comment that an invasive component cannot be excluded)	Minimally invasive adenocarcinoma, adenocarcinoma in situ, or an invasive adenocarcinoma with a lepidic component
	Invasive mucinous adenocarcinoma (list the patterns; use the term "mucinous adenocarcinoma with lepidic pattern" if pure lepidic pattern and mention the differential diagnosis listed on the right)	Invasive mucinous adenocarcinoma Minimally invasive adenocarcinoma or adenocarcinoma in situ, mucinous type
	Adenocarcinoma with colloid features	Colloid adenocarcinoma
	Adenocarcinoma with fetal features	Fetal adenocarcinoma
	Adenocarcinoma with enteric features[a]	Enteric adenocarcinoma
Morphological squamous cell patterns not present, but supported by stains (i.e. p40+)	Non-small cell carcinoma, favour squamous cell carcinoma[b]	Squamous cell carcinoma (non-keratinizing pattern may be a component of the tumour)[b]
Morphological adenocarcinoma patterns not present, but supported by special stains (i.e. TTF1+)	Non-small cell carcinoma, favour adenocarcinoma[b]	Adenocarcinoma (solid pattern may be just one component of the tumour)[b]
No clear adenocarcinoma, squamous, or neuroendocrine morphology or staining pattern	Non-small cell carcinoma NOS[a,c]	Large cell carcinoma

TTF1, thyroid transcription factor 1.
[a]Metastatic carcinomas should be carefully excluded with clinical and appropriate but judicious immunohistochemical examination. [b]The categories do not always correspond to solid-predominant adenocarcinoma or non-keratinizing squamous cell carcinoma, respectively. Poorly differentiated components in adenocarcinoma or squamous cell carcinoma may be sampled. [c]The non-small cell carcinoma NOS pattern can be seen not only in large cell carcinomas but also when the solid, poorly differentiated component of adenocarcinomas or squamous cell carcinomas is sampled but does not express immunohistochemical markers or mucin.

reducing the "Inadequate" rate of the technique, and facilitating efficient and cost-effective triage for ancillary testing {568}. In addition, the concept of the clinical cytopathology laboratory emerged, where the interventionalist can be trained to smear and assess the sample, offering a cost-effective alternative to ROSE that is practised in many countries and is especially well suited to low-resource settings. The integration of molecular testing for targeted therapy further enhanced the utility of lung cytopathology. Currently, approximately 70% of lung cancers are diagnosed by cytopathology or small biopsies {916}.

Cytopathology plays a crucial role in the management of patients with pulmonary nodules. This is particularly important considering that the majority of patients with lung cancer present with advanced disease and surgery is not a therapeutic option {849}. Thus, cytopathological samples and, where necessary, core needle biopsies or forceps biopsies are frequently the only source of tissue for diagnosis and for the determination of predictive markers. Cytopathology offers a variety of sampling techniques that are complementary to each other and that are often used in combination for the evaluation of lung nodules {736,850}. In addition, cytopathological evaluation of intrathoracic lymph nodes utilizing endobronchial ultrasound guidance during bronchoscopy at the same time as FNAB and diagnosis of the mass lesion in the lung is an efficient and safe method for staging of the disease, which in turn determines clinical management and prognosis. Evaluation of pleural effusions is also used for determining stage IV in lung cancer.

The emergence of prognostic markers and targeted therapies required more specific classification of lung carcinomas and a multidisciplinary approach to patient management. Consequently, there is a pressing need to develop a standardized diagnostic terminology that allows clear communication of the diagnosis and critical information relevant to patient management and to enrolment in trial studies.

Small biopsies and FNAB are sampling techniques and may not demonstrate the architectural pattern of a tumour (particularly FNAB). The diagnosis by FNAB and small biopsy, which in most cases is a core needle biopsy, and the terminology used by cytopathologists and those reporting core needle biopsy and resection specimens, will vary to a minor extent (see Table 1.01 and Table 1.02). Classification and subclassification of cancers are possible in many cases by integrating the histopathology, cytopathology, and cell block findings with immunohistochemistry, but the subclassification into adenocarcinoma subtypes may not be possible and requires an intact and good-quality small biopsy or excision. In some cases where good FNAB smears are available with or without cell block material, lepidic, papillary, micropapillary, or solid subtypes can be described and mentioned as a component of the tumour (see Box 1.01, p. 4) {976}.

Practical considerations

In practical terms, decisions in this volume were made to use commonly used abbreviations, which are listed at the front of the book. Of note, immunochemistry of cytopathological specimens including cell blocks, direct scrapes of direct smears, and liquid-based cytopathology, is designated "immunocytochemistry" (ICC). The term "non-small cell lung carcinoma" (NSCLC) is used, although it is recognized that the term "non-small cell carcinoma" (NSCC) should be used for NSCCs diagnosed in cytopathology and small biopsy specimens in which the type of carcinoma cannot be determined by morphology or ICC or in which even a metastasis cannot be excluded.

Wherever cytopathology features are listed that may show different features in the alcohol-fixed Papanicolaou (Pap) or haematoxylin and eosin (H&E) and the air-dried Romanowsky–Giemsa stain (Giemsa), then the stain is noted; for example, keratinized squamous cells are eosinophilic in the Pap and light-blue in the Giemsa. Similarly, described nuclear features may differ in the air-dried and alcohol-fixed stains; for example, vesicular nuclei, which usually represent prominent perinucleolar chromatin clearing, are seen in Pap, but not in Giemsa. The term "Giemsa" has been used throughout this volume for the many variants of it (e.g. Romanowsky, Wright–Giemsa, May–Grünwald–Giemsa, and commercial products) as a shortened form, because practice varies widely. All figure descriptions include the specific stain type and, unless otherwise stated, represent FNAB rather than bronchial brushing, bronchial washing, or sputum sample.

This cytopathology reporting system volume is cross-referenced to the fifth-edition *Thoracic tumours* volume of the WHO

Table 1.02 Terminology for small biopsies and cytopathology versus resection specimens for small cell carcinoma, large cell neuroendocrine carcinoma, adenosquamous carcinoma, and pleomorphic carcinoma

Terminology for small biopsies and cytopathology specimens	Terminology for resection specimens
Small cell carcinoma	Small cell carcinoma
Non-small cell carcinoma with neuroendocrine morphology and positive neuroendocrine markers, possible large cell neuroendocrine carcinoma	Large cell neuroendocrine carcinoma
Morphological squamous cell and adenocarcinoma patterns both present: non-small cell carcinoma NOS Comment that adenocarcinoma and squamous components are present and that this could represent adenosquamous carcinoma	Adenosquamous carcinoma (if both components ≥ 10%)
Morphological squamous cell or adenocarcinoma patterns not present, but immunohistochemical stains favour separate squamous and adenocarcinoma components: non-small cell carcinoma NOS Specify the results of the immunohistochemical stains and their interpretation, and comment that this could represent adenosquamous carcinoma but that diagnosis requires a resection specimen	Adenocarcinoma, squamous cell carcinoma, adenosquamous carcinoma, or large cell carcinoma with unclear immunohistochemical features
Non-small cell carcinoma with spindle cells or giant cells Mention if adenocarcinoma or squamous carcinoma is present; comment that this could represent a pleomorphic carcinoma but that diagnosis requires a resection specimen	Pleomorphic, spindle cell, and/or giant cell carcinoma

Classification of Tumours series (also known as the WHO Blue Books) on the website, and it is not intended to repeat the information presented in that publication. The codes, epidemiology, etiology, pathogenesis, and staging sections of the thoracic WHO Blue Book are not included in this cytopathology volume, and readers are referred to the tumour classification volume. However, the *Definition*, *Clinical features and imaging*, and *Histopathology* subsections are designed to assist the cytopathologist or cytotechnologist in their diagnostic approach; for example, the clinical history and the site of the lesion in some cases is a determinant of the differential diagnosis. In the near future, the electronic versions of the cytopathology text will be directly linked section by section to the WHO Blue Book electronic version, and vice versa. On the website for each text, the individual references can be accessed by direct links using the PubMed reference numbers (PMIDs) in the text. The text aims at being clear, succinct, and able to cover the essential facts and differential diagnosis.

Each lesion or tumour will be presented using the following subheadings:

Definition

This is fundamentally the same as in the corresponding tumour classification WHO Blue Book, with the provision that it can be modified to suit any cytopathological nuance that is required. It is a short, succinct statement.

Clinical features and imaging

These are brief and emphasize any factors that assist in the diagnosis.

Histopathology

These subsections are brief and aimed at assisting cytopathologists in understanding features seen in cytopathology, and readers are referred to the tumour classification. Correlation between histopathology and cytopathology is a core element of teaching and reporting cytopathology.

Key diagnostic cytopathological features

These are generally presented as bullet points rather than free text, to maximize the clarity of the criteria, and features are described in both air-dried Giemsa-stained and alcohol-fixed Pap-stained direct smears and, where appropriate, in cytospin and/or liquid-based cytology. Pattern or overall low-power appearance, architecture of individual tissue fragments if present, cell features including size and cytoplasmic features, nuclear features, background components, and other features are presented.

Discussion and differential diagnosis

This subsection discusses and expands on the features and presents any variants or nuances. If a group of rare processes or tumours in the lung, such as soft tissue tumours, is grouped under one heading, different subtypes of tumours can be discussed here. Then the differential diagnosis is presented, focusing on the cytopathological details of the tumour as compared with other processes and tumours. This is a crucial part of the text for all cytopathologists and cytotechnologists, and this is particularly the case in low- and middle-income countries where there is greater reliance on just the cytomorphology. The findings of ancillary testing are constantly checked against the cytomorphology.

Box 1.01 Guidelines for good practice of small biopsies and cytological preparations

1. For small biopsies and cytopathology, non-small cell carcinoma should be further classified into a more specific type, such as adenocarcinoma or squamous cell carcinoma, whenever possible.
2. The term "non-small cell lung carcinoma NOS" should be used as little as possible, and only when a more specific diagnosis is not possible.
3. When a diagnosis is made in a small biopsy or cytopathology specimen in conjunction with special studies, it should be clarified whether the diagnosis was established on the basis of light microscopy (including mucin stains) alone or whether immunohistochemistry was diagnostic.
4. The term "non-squamous cell carcinoma" should not be used by pathologists in diagnostic reports.
5. The above classification of adenocarcinoma vs other histopathology and the terminology in Table 1.01 (p. 2) and Table 1.02 (p. 3) should be used in routine diagnosis, future research, and clinical trials, to ensure a uniform classification of disease cohorts in relation to tumour subtypes, stratified according to diagnoses made by light microscopy alone vs diagnoses requiring immunohistochemistry.
6. When paired cytopathology and biopsy specimens exist, they should be reviewed together to achieve the most specific and concordant diagnosis.
7. The terms "adenocarcinoma in situ" and "minimally invasive adenocarcinoma" should not be used for diagnosis of small biopsies or cytopathology specimens. If a non-invasive pattern is present in a small biopsy, it should be referred to as a lepidic growth pattern. Similarly, if a cytopathology specimen has the attributes of adenocarcinoma in situ, the tumour should be diagnosed as an adenocarcinoma, possibly with a comment that this may represent, at least in part, adenocarcinoma in situ with a lepidic growth pattern.
8. The term "large cell carcinoma" should not be used for diagnosis in small biopsy or cytopathology specimens and should be restricted to resection specimens where the tumour is thoroughly sampled to exclude a differentiated component.
9. Tumour biopsies that show sarcomatoid features (e.g. marked nuclear pleomorphism, malignant giant cells, or spindle cell morphology) should be initially classified as above in relation to adenocarcinoma; non-small cell carcinoma, favour adenocarcinoma; squamous cell carcinoma; or non-small cell carcinoma, favour squamous cell carcinoma. This diagnosis may influence management. An additional statement can be made that giant and/or spindle cell features are present. If such features are not present, the term "non-small cell carcinoma NOS" should be used, again with a comment on the sarcomatoid features.
10. Staining for neuroendocrine immunohistochemical markers should be performed only in cases where there is suspected neuroendocrine morphology.

Ancillary testing

This subsection is for the presentation of the flow cytometry, ICC, in situ hybridization, and next-generation sequencing that help diagnose the lesion and distinguish the lesion or tumour from other processes.

Specific ancillary testing is presented for each lesion, or potentially each group of lesions, in the diagnostic category chapters, and there is also an overview chapter of diagnostic ancillary testing. The WHO Reporting System for Lung Cytopathology aims to present current best practice in the selection of ancillary testing and recommends that when the ancillary testing results are available, these should be added to the cytopathology report as supplementary reports, producing one final integrated report. The ancillary tests will often augment and refine the cytopathology report, and they may change the category and enable a specific diagnosis.

Sample reports

At the end of each diagnostic category chapter there are sample reports to assist cytopathologists in writing standardized reports. There will be regional historical or information technology–related issues influencing the style and formatting of reports, and the recommendations relate to the components of the report rather than any rigid style.

The WHO Reporting System for Lung Cytopathology

After this first iteration, this reporting system will evolve with usage, research, and the testing of its hierarchical category and related risk-of-malignancy structure. It is a system for categorizing cytopathology cases, so that we can provide information to clinicians that is uniform nationally and internationally, assisting them in making management decisions to achieve a full diagnosis. This is a fundamental difference to the tumour classification WHO Blue Books, which define and classify tumour types. The second aim of the cytopathology series is to standardize the diagnostic cytopathological criteria of each lesion, which will improve the quality and reproducibility of cytopathology reporting. Of course ancillary testing greatly assists this diagnostic process, and best practice in the selection and interpretation of ancillary testing will be provided for all lesions. This is a more similar role to that of the WHO Blue Books.

In preparation for this initiative, an international survey of 82 questions was offered. Participants included pathologists, non-pathologists, and cytotechnologists. The survey demonstrated a diverse practice among various laboratories and countries using a wide spectrum of techniques for specimen processing and handling and various reporting systems {465, 338}, and it informed the discussions of the International Academy of Cytology (IAC) – International Agency for Research on Cancer (IARC) – World Health Organization (WHO) Joint Editorial Board.

The role of lung cytopathology

Moreira AL
Travis WD

Sputum samples

Sputum sample cytopathology is a simple, non-invasive, and economical technique for the detection of malignancy and infectious processes in the respiratory tract. Sputum sample cytopathology has been used for many years as an efficient diagnostic tool for lung carcinomas {786} and, more recently, in association with lung cancer screening programmes {991, 240,351,348}. However, as lung cancer screening shifted to the evaluation of small peripheral lesions, other diagnostic technologies became more prevalent {932}. In geographical regions with limited resources, sputum sampling is still a cost-effective diagnostic modality.

Sputum samples can be obtained spontaneously or induced. Spontaneous sputum samples can be produced by instructing the patient to cough deeply and to expel the contents into a sterile container. Induced sputum samples can be produced by the same process but after inhalation of a bronchodilator and/or saline. The latter has been reported to produce more adequate and better-quality samples for cytopathological evaluation in comparison to spontaneous sputum samples, especially for the evaluation of small peripheral nodules {5}.

There is a wide range of reported sensitivity and specificity for the diagnosis of lung carcinoma in sputum samples (see Table 1.03), mostly due to variations in specimen processing, tumour location, histopathological type, and pathological stage {568,854,240}. On average, the sensitivity for the diagnosis of malignancy has been reported to be 66%, ranging from 34% for peripheral lesions to 97% for centrally located lesions, with a specificity of 99% (range: 68–100%) {568,754}. The diagnostic rate increases with the use of sequential specimens, with three to five consecutive daily collections being reported as the most effective {323}. Whether the sputum sample is collected fresh on demand or in the mornings does not appear to greatly influence the diagnostic rate {927}, although one study did show a higher yield of malignant cells with morning samples {927}. Prompt specimen fixation after collection has been shown to increase diagnostic yields, as well as facilitating cell block preparations and the use of molecular diagnostics tests {799}. Cell block preparation has been reported to increase the sensitivity and specificity of sputum sample cytopathology {245}. The use of molecular techniques such as DNA promoter methylation {348,351} and microRNA analysis {348,991} have been used with sputum sample cytopathology for the early detection of lung cancer.

Bronchoalveolar lavage

Bronchoalveolar lavage (BAL) is a commonly used procedure for the evaluation of both non-neoplastic and neoplastic diseases of the lower respiratory tract. The procedure is performed by the insertion of a bronchoscope into the bronchial tree and the instillation of 100–300 mL of sterile room-temperature saline into a segmental bronchus. At least 30% of the instilled saline should be recovered for cytopathological examination {568}. The sensitivity of BAL for the diagnosis of lung cancer varies from 15% to 65% {288,1021,815,196}. The sensitivity tends to be lower in peripheral lesions smaller than 20 mm {815}. Because of its low sensitivity, BAL is rarely used as a sole diagnostic procedure for the diagnosis of lung cancer. It is often used in association with other cytopathological sampling techniques or small forceps biopsies {288,1021}. BAL is more commonly used in the evaluation of inflammatory cell counts and composition in interstitial lung diseases and infections {196}. There are suggestions, however, that BAL could be used in the surveillance of lung cancer as an indicator of local recurrence and response to therapy, local immune response, and tumour microenvironment {216}.

Bronchial washing and brushing

Bronchial washings and bronchial brushings are obtained during bronchoscopy in a similar manner to BAL. For these procedures, the lesion is sampled under direct visualization. In bronchial brushings, the entrapped cells on the bristles can be used for direct smears or collected in saline or other carrier liquids such as cell culture medium or fixative, according to the laboratory protocol {568}. In bronchial washings, 5–20 mL of fluid is instilled directly onto the lesion and the recovered fluid is then processed for diagnosis. The sensitivity for these modalities varies from 33% to 60% for bronchial brushings and is slightly lower for bronchial washings {815}. The combination

Table 1.03 Sensitivity and specificity of cytological sampling methods for the diagnosis of malignancy

Sampling technique	Sensitivity (%)		Specificity (%)	
	Average	Range	Average	Range
Sputum sampling	66	34–97	99	68–100
Bronchoalveolar lavage (BAL)	22.9	15–65	n/a	n/a
Bronchial wash/brush	52	33–60	n/a	n/a
Transbronchial FNAB	89	87–97	100	n/a
Transthoracic FNAB	90	88–96	97	96–98

n/a, not applicable.

with endobronchial biopsy increases the sensitivity to 88% {815}. This technique is mostly used when a central visible lesion is targeted, as opposed to submucosal or small peripheral lesions.

FNAB

Endobronchial ultrasound–guided transbronchial FNAB (EBUS-TBFNAB) and transthoracic FNAB are minimally invasive procedures used in the diagnosis and staging of lung cancer {778, 568}. EBUS-TBFNAB is the diagnostic procedure of choice for the evaluation of hilar and mediastinal lymph nodes to achieve tumour staging, and for centrally located lesions to diagnose the tumour. More peripheral lesions can also be sampled by this technique if associated with an airway that can accommodate the endoscope. EBUS-TBFNAB is often used for the evaluation of recurrence and/or disease metastatic to the mediastinal and hilar lymph nodes {778}.

Transthoracic FNAB involves the introduction of a needle through the skin and chest wall into the pulmonary lesion under CT guidance and is preferentially used for the diagnosis of peripheral nodules.

Both FNAB procedures are usually performed under moderate or general sedation. Pneumothorax and intraparenchymal bleeding are rare complications {778,656}. The diagnostic yield for both procedures is high, with an average sensitivity of 89% (range: 76–95%) and a specificity of 100% {778,936,941,656, 753}. The best diagnostic rates for EBUS-TBFNAB are seen in centrally located tumours measuring > 20 mm {753,656}. A minimum of two and as many as five passes should be performed for each procedure to ensure adequate diagnostic material {778, 568}. Rapid onsite evaluation (ROSE) is often recommended for specimen adequacy and triage {778}. Material obtained by these procedures can be prepared as direct smears for adequacy assessment and diagnosis at ROSE, and part or all of the specimen can be placed in transport medium for further cytopathological evaluation including cell block preparation. There is very good correlation of adequacy for molecular testing of samples procured by EBUS-TBFNAB and FNAB {484,736,376}.

Transbronchial core needle biopsy

Transbronchial core needle biopsy is obtained through a bronchoscope under endobronchial ultrasound guidance using a large-bore needle (usually 19–22 gauge) {936,38}. These core needles were created in response to the increased demand for core biopsy material in patients with advanced inoperable stages of lung cancer, for the determination of biomarkers for targeted therapy and inclusion in clinical trial protocols for lung cancer. The procedure produces a delicate core of tissue embedded in a blood clot. Touch preparations of the core can be used for ROSE but there is a risk of compromising the tissue for histopathology. Squash preparations can also be used for ROSE, but this sacrifices the core and the ability to perform subsequent ancillary studies {38}. The core should be placed directly into formalin and not saline for formalin-fixed, paraffin-embedded processing. The sensitivity and specificity for the diagnosis of lung cancer is high, ranging from 87% to 97%, which is similar to that of EBUS-TBFNAB {936,38,742}. There is good utilization for ancillary tests, including molecular analysis {366}. Transbronchial core needle biopsy is also used to supplement FNAB for the diagnosis of non-neoplastic lesions such as those in sarcoidosis {278,594,38} and lymphoproliferative disorders {278}.

Diagnostic categories and report structure

Field AS
Layfield LJ

Categories

Each of the categories generates a risk of malignancy (ROM) that is directly linked to a recommendation for further diagnostic testing aimed at achieving a specific diagnosis or refining a differential diagnosis. Specific processes or tumours, which have a similar ROM when diagnosed on cytopathology, are placed in the same category; for example, inflammatory and benign neoplastic entities are placed in the "Benign" category. The WHO Reporting Systems use categories to assist communication of ROM, but a specific diagnosis or differential diagnosis further refined by ancillary testing is the aim of all cytopathology reporting and is paramount in the report.

The WHO Reporting System for Lung Cytopathology applies the same five categories for all lung cytopathological specimen types:

- "Insufficient/Inadequate/Non-diagnostic"
- "Benign"
- "Atypical"
- "Suspicious for malignancy"
- "Malignant"

Currently there are limited publications defining the ROM for these categories, and there is a need for further research using the WHO Reporting System to more clearly define the ROM.

Individual cytopathologists and departments with more than one cytopathologist should choose one term from "Insufficient", "Inadequate", and "Non-diagnostic" for cases where there is no material for assessment or there are technical problems that prevent the assessment and diagnosis of the material on the slides. If sputum, bronchial washing (BW), and bronchial brushing (BB), and FNAB specimens have adequate benign material then this is described and reported as "Benign". Correlation with imaging should be carried out wherever possible with lung cytopathology specimens, and if the material on the slides shows benign material that does not correlate with or explain the imaging or clinical findings, then it is mandatory to place a caveat in the report conclusion, that the material "may not represent the lesion seen on imaging and further diagnostic workup is recommended". However, it is recognized that some cytopathologists prefer the term "Non-diagnostic" to encompass not only cases where there is insufficient or technically obscured material, but also cases where there is benign cytopathological material that does not correlate with or explain the clinical and/or imaging findings; for example, a bronchial brush may show only bronchial epithelium or an FNAB may show only benign components of lung in a patient with a solid lesion on imaging. This is the first WHO Reporting System for Lung Cytopathology, and it accepts that some cytopathologists prefer to categorize these cases as "Non-diagnostic" and place them in the "Insufficient/Inadequate/Non-diagnostic" category. Research into the impact of this approach on the ROM is required.

The "Benign" category includes normal lung components, inflammatory processes, and benign tumours such as pulmonary hamartomas. If the features are benign but a precise diagnosis cannot be made, the features should be described and a differential diagnosis provided of the findings if possible. As with all categories, correlation with clinical and (wherever possible) imaging findings is mandatory.

The "Atypical" category is expected to have a relatively low to intermediate ROM and allows for a high negative predictive value for a "Benign" categorization, while the "Suspicious for malignancy" category is expected to have a high ROM and provide for a high positive predictive value approaching 100% for a "Malignant" categorization. The categories stratify the ROM and allow for the development of management recommendations. The "Atypical" category will include cases where there is scant or poorly prepared but atypical material, and cases where mainly benign cytopathological features are present, but there are some features, such as nuclear atypia or limited necrosis, which may raise the possibility of malignancy. If any atypical features are seen in a case showing otherwise insufficient material, then the case is regarded as "Atypical" and not "Insufficient".

The "Suspicious for malignancy" category includes cases where there is scant, poorly smeared, or poorly prepared and stained material suggestive of malignancy, as well as cases where there is considerable material, some of which appears malignant, but not all features of a particular malignancy are present or there may be discrepant features.

The "Malignant" category is reserved for those cases in which there are unequivocal features of malignancy without any discrepant findings. All cytopathology specimen types are obtained by sampling techniques, and it is not always possible to make a precise diagnosis of a specific carcinoma or other malignancy, even with ancillary testing. The precise diagnosis of carcinoma subtypes usually requires assessment of the entire resected tumour, most typically for mixed tumours such as carcinosarcoma.

The presentation of tumours in this WHO Reporting System follows the order found in the fifth-edition WHO classification of thoracic tumours, but not all tumours are included in this volume, because they have not all been described in the cytopathology literature.

Spindle cell lesions with a low risk of recurrence or rare metastasis, such as inflammatory myofibroblastic tumour, are presented in Chapter 4: *Diagnostic category: Benign*, with a clear discussion of the cytopathological features and ancillary studies that often allow a specific diagnosis.

Structured reporting

Each cytopathology report on a sputum sample, BW, BB, and transthoracic or endobronchial ultrasound–directed FNAB should have a structured format, with a heading of a specific diagnostic category using the WHO Reporting System's standardized descriptive terminology and a diagnosis. Structured reporting improves the quality, clarity, and reproducibility of reports within individual pathology departments and between countries, and it will improve patient management and facilitate research and quality assurance measures. Standard guidelines for cell block preparation, ICC, in situ hybridization, and other molecular tests of prognostic and predictive markers improve diagnostic accuracy, reduce cost, and improve patient care. The establishment of key diagnostic cytopathological findings for each lesion, which will act as a checklist for the reporting cytopathologist, will also improve reporting.

There are essential or core components in a cytopathology report and these are presented here. This is not intended to make any particular format mandatory, but some components are a general requirement, namely the diagnostic category using the defined terminology of the reporting system, and a diagnosis or conclusion, which may be specific or descriptive with a differential diagnosis. Frequently, a microscopic description of the key diagnostic features can be added, particularly in cases where the diagnostic conclusion is a differential diagnosis. An addendum outlining any ancillary tests and their results is also required wherever possible. The diagnostic summary must be clearly delineated and stand out in the report so that it can be easily seen by the patient care team.

A number should not be used in place of the diagnostic category terminology or a specific diagnosis. A category number can be included in the body of the report for audit and research purposes, but it should not appear in the conclusion. Reducing a cytopathology report to a number reduces the information that can be given to the clinician and management team and increases the risk of error.

The diagnostic category states whether there is inadequate material and an "Insufficient/Inadequate/Non-diagnostic" categorization is applicable, or whether there is adequate material and a "Benign", "Atypical", "Suspicious for malignancy", or "Malignant" category can be applied. But it is recognized that some cytopathologists prefer to include a statement on specimen quality in the microscopic description of the report that "there is adequate material for assessment". Other cytopathologists require a statement to be included regarding the degree of cellularity of the material, referring to the cellularity of the material from the target lesion rather than inflammatory cells.

The microscopic description should provide a clear, concise cytopathological description, which includes the degree of cellularity and focuses on the presence or absence of key cytopathological diagnostic features. Some cytopathologists prefer a full description of these features; others may prefer only a brief comment or, in cases where there is a specific diagnosis, no description at all.

The aim of cytopathology is to provide as specific a diagnosis as possible in the vast majority of cases. The indeterminate categories of "Atypical" and "Suspicious for malignancy" establish a ROM and subsequent management recommendations as part of an algorithm to aid communication with the clinician about a particular biopsy and the further diagnostic management of the patient.

The ancillary tests should always be part of the final cytopathology report, and if flow cytometry, in situ hybridization, or molecular pathology reports are issued by a different laboratory, then it is recommended that they should be referred to in the report. Wherever possible, the ancillary results should be added as a supplementary report or addendum to the original cytopathology report, with the aim of having a final all-inclusive report for optimal patient care.

The WHO cytopathology reporting systems are based on cytomorphology for the initial categorization and reporting of the lesion, which can be applied in any well-resourced or low- and middle-income country setting, but which also incorporate the application of appropriate ancillary testing as current best practice. Subsequent ancillary testing may well change the final diagnostic category and provide a specific diagnosis of a particular case.

The standardized cytopathology report

Demographic information

- Patient's name, date of birth, address, patient identifiers / patient episode, date of request, and laboratory accession number
- Referring doctor and contact details

Type of specimen

- Sputum sample, BW, bronchoalveolar lavage (BAL), BB, FNAB (endobronchial ultrasound, transthoracic)

Clinical and imaging information

- Site, size (mm), imaging (ultrasound, CXR, tomogram, CT, MRI) features
- Previous cytopathology procedures and results and previous other biopsy results when available

Diagnostic summary

- Totally in bold, on the first page (if the laboratory information system supports this)
- Each institution should select a term for the main heading of the diagnostic summary, such as "Diagnostic summary" (as used throughout this volume), "Diagnosis", or "Final diagnosis", and use it consistently

Category

- Reporting system diagnostic category: using terminology not a number

Diagnosis

- Specific diagnosis or differential diagnosis
- Optional but recommended to include in the diagnostic summary: the specimen type and exact site of a BW/BB or FNAB (verbatim from the request form), e.g. "FNAB of right upper lobe of lung: adenocarcinoma"; this should correlate with the labelling of any specimen container, and if it does not, the clinician should be contacted

Other information included in the report

Macroscopic description

- Number of air-dried slides, number of alcohol-fixed slides
- Type (saline, RPMI medium, formalin, only specimen without diluent, liquid-based cytology) and volume of fluid received, with description of fluid (colour, presence of blood, viscosity, presence of particulate matter), including any other specimens received and specifically designated for flow cytometry, microbiology, cell block

Details of rapid onsite evaluation (ROSE) (if conducted)

- Number of passes, gauge of needle used, imaging modality used
- Names of those performing the clinical and diagnostic procedures, including the cytology biomedical scientist, pathology trainee, or cytopathologist attending ROSE
- Number of slides processed and stained at ROSE, air-dried and alcohol-fixed, and other specimen types prepared
- The specific ROSE report provided verbatim and documented, and the name of the cytopathologist or cytology biomedical scientist issuing ROSE, with further noting of subsequent ROSE cytopathological procedures

Microscopic description

- Optional but recommended to include a statement of the degree of cellularity (e.g. scant, mildly cellular, moderately cellular, highly cellular) or the specimen quality (e.g. "specimen satisfactory for assessment")
- Optional to include the key diagnostic cytopathological features whether present or absent, but if the final diagnosis is not specific and is based on a differential diagnosis, then a microscopic description is required
- Include a specific diagnosis or, if this is not possible, a discussion of the differential diagnosis, emphasizing the most likely diagnosis; cytopathologists may prefer a subheading at the end of the microscopic description to convey the diagnosis
- If the lesion is "Insufficient/Inadequate/Non-diagnostic", "Atypical", or "Suspicious for malignancy", then the report should include a clear description of what material is present on the slides, and the reason why the material is insufficient, atypical, or suspicious for malignancy should be stated; for the "Atypical" and "Suspicious for malignancy" categories, this may include a discussion of the differential diagnosis

Ancillary testing

- Depending on local practice, the cytopathology report (including its conclusion) can be issued as a final or provisional report, with supplementary reports or addenda on ancillary studies to follow and to be added to the final report, or the cytopathology report can be withheld until ancillary reports are available
- Includes all cell block H&E and special stains, ICC, in situ hybridization, molecular techniques performed on cell block or direct smear slide scrapings, and further stains; the report should state which type of specimen was used for each ancillary test to facilitate continuous quality assurance (e.g. cell blocks or direct smears)
- If flow cytometry results are issued by the same laboratory, then these results should be entered here; if flow cytometry results are issued by a different laboratory, their results should be added as a supplementary report, when available, under ancillary testing in the original report
- If a core needle biopsy or other surgical biopsy was performed at the same time as the FNAB, the supplementary report should recommend correlation with the surgical report and its accession number

Reference(s): {455,31,389,238,466,465,105,332,338,467}

Risk of malignancy and management recommendations

Layfield LJ
Satoh Y
Scagliotti GV

The WHO Reporting System for Lung Cytopathology is designed not only to provide standardized terminology for categories and key diagnostic cytopathological criteria for cytomorphological diagnosis, but also to supply clinically relevant information on the estimated risk of malignancy (ROM) of each category. The ROM for each category is linked to a set of recommendations that then assist the clinician in managing patients and making clinical decisions. Each category has a distinct ROM and the ROM shows a progressive increase from the "Benign" category to the "Malignant" category.

A summary of the recommendations for each category provided in the category chapters is presented in Chapter 8: *Management recommendations for each diagnostic category*, to assist clinicians.

The specific cytopathological diagnosis, or in some cases the differential diagnosis, remains paramount in clinical decision-making. The recommendations presented in this volume are suggestions to help standardize management, including further diagnostic procedures to make (or to make more specific) a particular diagnosis, and are not intended to impose strict management guidelines on clinicians using the WHO Reporting System. The recommendations are suggestions for diagnostic follow-up and not mandated guidelines, and they should be applied where clinically relevant. They are summarized in Table 1.04 and Table 1.05.

The performance measures and ROM for each category are dependent on the cytopathology sampling method. The ROMs for the categories "Insufficient/Inadequate/Non-diagnostic" and "Benign" are higher for sputum sample cytopathology than for FNAB, and the recommendations following these cytopathology report categorizations vary with the specimen type and ROM. In these situations, FNAB of any mass lesion is the usual key follow-up recommendation.

The FNAB ROM estimates are based on published experience at academic centres and may differ from those associated with other practice types. The ROMs represent historical

Table 1.04 The WHO Reporting System for Lung Cytopathology on sputum sample, bronchial washing (BW), and bronchial brushing (BB): implied risk of malignancy (ROM) and clinical management options by diagnostic category

Diagnostic category	Estimated ROM[a]	Clinical management options[b]
"Insufficient/Inadequate/Non-diagnostic"	Sputum sample: 0–100% BW: 38–81% BB: 0–75%	Consider repeating the sampling or use BB/BW (in case of sputum sample) and/or FNAB, depending on CLIN-IMG-MICRO
"Benign"	Sputum sample: 0–42% BW: 38–42% BB: 32–38%	Correlate with CLIN-IMG-MICRO; if these confirm a benign diagnosis, then routine follow-up at 3–6 months; if no correlation, consider new sampling
"Atypical"	Sputum sample: 86–100% BW: 62–86% BB: 79–100%	Correlate with CLIN-IMG-MICRO; if these are "Benign", repeat; if "Atypical" or "Suspicious for malignancy", perform BB/BW or FNAB with or without CNB
"Suspicious for malignancy"	Sputum sample: 100% BW: 83–100% BB: 75–100%	Correlate with CLIN-IMG-MICRO, and perform BB/BW or FNAB with or without CNB; these cases need to be discussed at MDT meetings
"Malignant"	Sputum sample: 100% BW: 98–100% BB: 94–100%	Correlate with CLIN-IMG-MICRO, and perform BB/BW or FNAB with or without CNB to confirm diagnosis before definitive treatment

CLIN-IMG-MICRO, clinical, imaging, and microbiological findings; CNB, core needle biopsy, including endobronchial biopsy; FNAB, fine-needle aspiration biopsy, including endobronchial ultrasound–guided and transthoracic FNAB; MDT, multidisciplinary team.
[a]Estimated ROMs are based on few retrospective studies {105,467}. For some types of sampling, the number of cases studied is low. Prospective studies are strongly recommended in this field. [b]Management options for patients with lung lesions may depend on a variety of factors, including clinical and imaging characteristics, the site of the lesion, the risk of carcinoma of the lung, local disease prevalence, and the local medical infrastructure available. Some clinical management suggestions are outlined above. In medically poorly resourced settings, an "Insufficient", "Atypical", or "Suspicious for malignancy" sputum sample report after correlation with imaging such as a CXR would usually be repeated and the slides reviewed if BB, BW, and endobronchial ultrasound–guided transbronchial FNAB are not available. Similarly, if BB and BW were "Insufficient", "Atypical", or "Suspicious for malignancy" a repeat BW and BB procedure would be recommended after correlation with imaging if endobronchial ultrasound–guided transbronchial FNAB is not available.

Recommendations:
1. When repeating a sputum sample, always provide clear instructions regarding the procedure or assist the patient with a physiotherapist or trained paramedic.
2. Whenever a sputum sample, BW/BB, or FNAB result is received, correlation with clinical, imaging, and microbiological findings is mandatory; in patients suspected of having a malignancy, this will ideally be carried out in a multidisciplinary meeting.
3. Whenever an "Atypical" or "Suspicious for malignancy" report is provided, or whenever there is discrepancy between the clinical, imaging, and microbiological findings and the cytopathology report, the reporting cytopathologist should, if possible, get a second expert opinion on the cytopathology.
4. Routine follow-up at 3–6 months for "Benign" and "Atypical" reports is determined by the patient's lung cancer risk.

Table 1.05 The WHO Reporting System for Lung Cytopathology on FNAB: implied risk of malignancy (ROM) and clinical management options by diagnostic category

Diagnostic category	Estimated ROM[a]	Clinical management options[b]
"Insufficient/Inadequate/Non-diagnostic"	43–53%	Correlate with CLIN-IMG-MICRO, ideally discuss at an MDT meeting, and perform repeat FNAB with or without CNB
"Benign"	19–64%	Correlate with CLIN-IMG-MICRO; if these confirm a benign diagnosis, then routine follow-up at 3–6 months; if no correlation, perform repeat FNAB with or without CNB
"Atypical"	46–55%	Correlate with CLIN-IMG-MICRO, and ideally discuss at an MDT meeting; if all show a benign diagnosis, then routine follow-up at 3–6 months; if no correlation, perform repeat FNAB with ROSE with or without CNB
"Suspicious for malignancy"	75–88%	Correlate with CLIN-IMG-MICRO, and ideally discuss at an MDT meeting; if all four support a diagnosis of malignancy, consider definitive treatment; if no correlation that lesion is malignant, perform repeat FNAB with ROSE with or without CNB
"Malignant"	87–100%	Correlate with CLIN-IMG-MICRO, and ideally discuss at an MDT meeting; if all four support a diagnosis of malignancy, provide definitive treatment; if no correlation that lesion is malignant, consider repeat FNAB with ROSE with or without CNB

CLIN-IMG-MICRO, clinical, imaging, and microbiological findings; CNB, core needle biopsy, including endobronchial biopsy; FNAB, fine-needle aspiration biopsy, including endobronchial ultrasound–guided and transthoracic FNAB; MDT, multidisciplinary team; ROSE, rapid onsite evaluation.

[a]Estimated ROMs are based on few retrospective studies {105,338,467}. Prospective studies are strongly recommended in this field. [b]Management options for patients with lung lesions may depend on a variety of factors, including clinical and imaging characteristics, the site of the lesion, the risk of carcinoma of the lung, local disease prevalence, and the local medical infrastructure available. Some clinical management suggestions are outlined above.

Recommendations:

1. Whenever an FNAB result is received, correlation with clinical, imaging, and microbiological findings is mandatory; in patients suspected of having a malignancy, this will be carried out in a multidisciplinary meeting.
2. Whenever an "Atypical" or "Suspicious for malignancy" report is provided, or whenever there is discrepancy between the clinical, imaging, and microbiological findings and the cytopathology report, the reporting cytopathologist should get a second expert opinion on the cytopathology.
3. Routine follow-up at 3–6 months for "Benign" and "Atypical" reports is determined by the patient's lung cancer risk.
4. ROSE is recommended at transthoracic FNAB and endobronchial ultrasound–guided FNAB.
5. CT or ultrasound is recommended at transthoracic FNAB.

published ranges and will be the subject of further research and subsequent modification in future editions of the WHO Reporting System {105,338,467}.

In the lung, the site of a lesion and the imaging findings (i.e. benign, indeterminate, or suspicious), the state of the patient and their comorbidities, and the availability of biopsy techniques (endobronchial ultrasound–directed transbronchial FNAB, endobronchial ultrasound–directed transbronchial core needle biopsy, and transthoracic FNAB) all form a relatively complex matrix of information along with the type of cytopathology specimen, the report category, and in many cases the specific diagnosis or differential diagnosis. This is quite different to other FNAB sites, such as thyroid and breast, where there is only one cytopathology specimen type – FNAB – and recommendations regarding further diagnostic management are relatively straightforward. The recommendations for further diagnostic management are presented in Table 1.04 and Table 1.05, and comments regarding poorly resourced situations in low- and middle-income countries are provided, because the WHO Reporting System is designed to be applicable internationally.

Correlation with clinical and imaging findings is required in the management of all categories. Apart from "Benign" cytopathology cases that are found to correlate with the imaging findings, the other categories usually require further diagnostic investigation, ideally to attain further cytopathological or histopathological material to facilitate a specific pathological diagnosis.

The ROM estimates given in Table 1.04 and Table 1.05 are derived from those cited in studies utilizing the Papanicolaou Society of Cytopathology (PSC) system {465}, other classification systems {338}, and studies applying categories similar to those used in the present system to their own data {105,466, 405,17,622,878}.

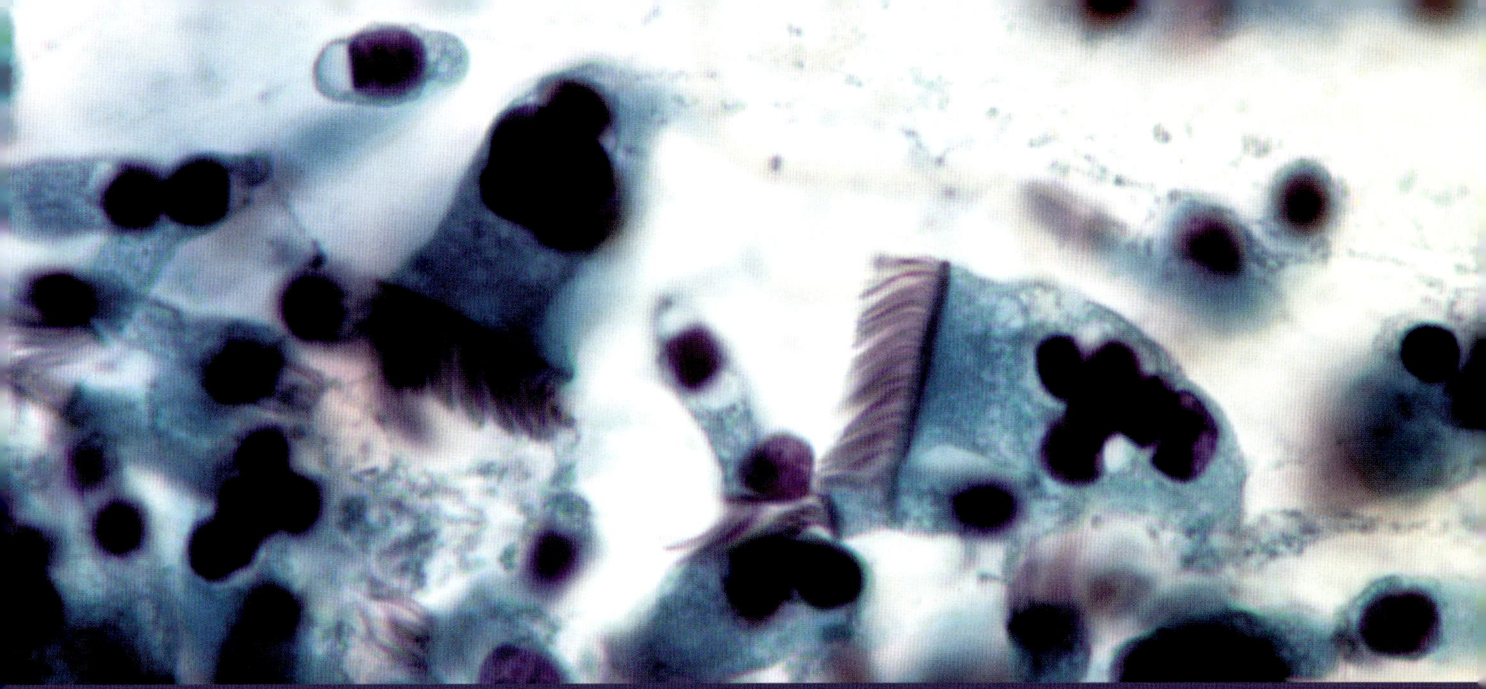

2

Lung cytopathology techniques

Edited by: Bubendorf L, Field AS, Roy-Chowdhuri S, Schmitt F

FNAB techniques and specimen management

Jain D
Heine R
Kholova I

FNAB is a frequently used and indispensable diagnostic technique in the current practice of pulmonary medicine (see Table 2.01). Broadly, there are two approaches: the percutaneous transthoracic biopsy and the transbronchial (or transtracheal) biopsy performed at bronchoscopy. The former is done under ultrasound guidance in case of subpleural lesions or usually under CT guidance if the lesion is deeply situated {528,817A}. The transbronchial or endobronchial FNAB are performed through a flexible bronchoscope using fluoroscopic or ultrasound guidance, the latter known as endobronchial ultrasound–guided transbronchial FNAB (EBUS-TBFNAB) {754,628,303}. In addition to endobronchial and peribronchial lesions, EBUS-TBFNAB can also access enlarged mediastinal and hilar lymph nodes or mass lesions {231,948}. Furthermore, electromagnetic navigation, ultrathin bronchoscopy, and radial probe endobronchial ultrasound are other technologies that assist in the sampling of small and peripherally placed lung lesions {215,520,634}. To further increase the diagnostic yield of sampling, the most recent technological advancement is robotic bronchoscopy, which enables better acquisition of the target and hence a potentially improved diagnostic yield of the procedure {129,260,598}. FNAB samples a broader area of the lesion, because the needle can be directed in multiple directions into the lesion, in contrast to the unidirectional sampling of core needle biopsy procedures.

Processing of FNAB samples

All pulmonary FNABs are carried out by either a radiologist or an interventional physician, under imaging guidance. It is preferable if a cytopathology biomedical scientist or a cytopathologist is also present on site to provide rapid onsite evaluation (ROSE) and liaise with the physician, including viewing imaging. After FNAB, the material is expelled onto a glass slide and smeared. The material can be split between several slides. Air-dried smears can be used for ROSE using Giemsa staining, while other smears for Pap staining should be immediately and rapidly immersed in 95% ethyl alcohol as soon as they are prepared, to avoid air-drying artefact. A rapid Pap or H&E can also be used for ROSE. The needles and syringes, if they contain material or blood, should

Table 2.01 Different types of FNAB techniques and indications

Type of FNAB	Indications	Advantages	Limitations
Percutaneous transthoracic FNAB	New or enlarging solitary lung nodules on CXR or CT that are not amenable to diagnosis by bronchoscopy	High diagnostic yield Avoids open lung biopsy	Risk of pneumothorax
Ultrasound-guided	Sonographically visible subpleural or superficial lesions that are in contact with the chest wall	Quick and easy to perform	Only for superficial lesions
CT-guided	For deep parenchymal lesions	Deep lesions can be sampled	Time-consuming
Transbronchial/endobronchial FNAB without imaging guidance (blind/conventional TBFNAB)	Endobronchial lesions Peribronchial parenchymal lesions Bronchial submucosal lesions Mediastinal, hilar, and subcarinal lymph nodes or hilar mass lesions for staging lung cancer, diagnosis of granulomatous diseases, lymphoma, extrapulmonary metastasis, or workup of nonspecific mediastinal lymphadenopathy	High sensitivity	Limited accessibility of mediastinum
EBUS-TBFNAB (lung)	Same as conventional TBFNAB	Can also access peripheral pulmonary lesions with the help of radial probe (radial EBUS) Can access nodal stations 10 (hilar), 11 (interlobar), and partial 12 (lobar)	Cannot access posteroinferior mediastinum and upper lobe lesions Costly; limited availability
EBUS-TBFNAB (lymph nodes)	Mediastinal lymphadenopathy of stations 8 (para-oesophageal, below carina) and 9 (pulmonary ligament)	Can be done safely alongside EBUS in a single session	n/a

EBUS, endobronchial ultrasound; EBUS-TBFNAB, endobronchial ultrasound–guided transbronchial FNAB; n/a, not applicable; TBFNAB, transbronchial FNAB.

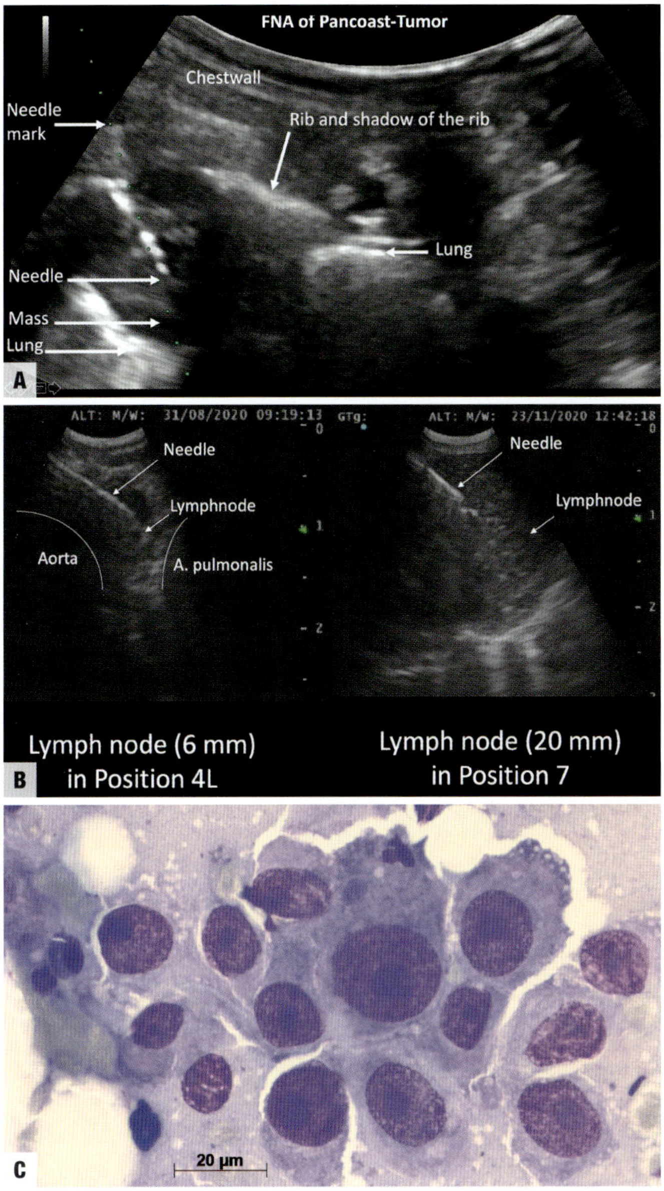

Fig. 2.01 **A** Pancoast tumour. Endobronchial ultrasound–guided transbronchial FNAB of a Pancoast tumour, showing the needle within the mass. **B** Mediastinal lymph nodes in a case of lung carcinoma. Endobronchial ultrasound–guided transbronchial FNAB of lymph node stations 4L and 7, with the fine needle in the lymph node. The lymph node in position 4L is small (6 mm) and located between the aorta and the pulmonary artery. **C** Adenocarcinoma. A small, discohesive tissue fragment of large cells with round to oval nuclei and considerable eccentric cytoplasm of adenocarcinoma (Giemsa).

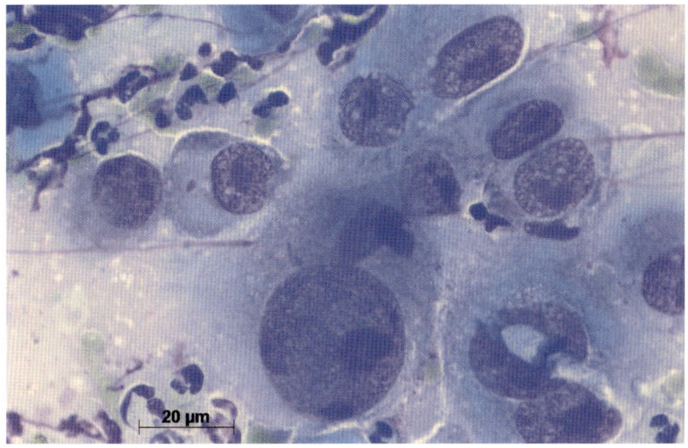

Fig. 2.02 Squamous cell carcinoma. Direct smear of large cells with dense, well-defined, and in some cases dense, light-blue keratinized cytoplasm and large pleomorphic nuclei (Giemsa).

be immediately rinsed (along with any repeat FNAB) into an appropriate collecting medium for cell blocks. The cell blocks can be made as per individual laboratory-based standardized protocols. Additional FNAB passes can be requested if a satisfactory specimen has not been obtained or to provide more material for ancillary studies based on the ROSE {372, 1007,610,373}.

Complications

The most common complication of percutaneous FNAB is pneumothorax, which has been reported to occur in 0–61% of cases (varying with the study definition of pneumothorax and other factors), and this has required intervention in 3–15% of cases. Other potential complications include pulmonary haemorrhage (in ~5–15% of cases) and haemoptysis (in ~1–5%) {528}. The use of a large-diameter needle (i.e. > 22 gauge) rather than a finer-gauge needle that defines FNAB, as well as obtaining FNABs of small and deeply located lesions, increases the risk of postprocedure complications {324} including bleeding and the small risk of neoplastic cell implantation {546}. Complications related to endobronchial ultrasound procedures are very low. In a systematic review and meta-analysis of 1299 patients, major complications due to EBUS-TBFNAB occurred in 0.07% patients in the form of pneumothorax and hypoxaemia {303}.

Bronchial wash and bronchial brush techniques and specimen management

Jain D
Heine R
Kholova I

Flexible fibre-optic bronchoscopy is the basic procedure for the diagnosis of diseases of the lung and mediastinum, and it enables a large number of investigations including bronchial washing (BW) and bronchial brushing (BB), which are simple methods for sampling mucosal surfaces of the bronchial tree and collecting samples to assist in the diagnoses of tumours and infections (see Table 2.02). In BW, 3–5 mL of balanced salt solution is instilled through the working channel of the bronchoscope into the bronchial system and then aspirated back into a container. The BB technique is a targeted method in which the brush is guided under fluoroscopy to the endobronchial lesion or lesions beyond the visual segmental bronchi. BBs are obtained by the use of a small circular stiff-bristle brush, which is moved back and forth after positioning in the target lesion {152}. BB samples must be obtained before transbronchial biopsies to avoid an excessive and obscuring haemorrhagic background, whereas BW samples obtained after abrading the bronchial surface with a brush give optimum results {488}.

The diagnostic accuracy of BW and BB cytopathology is comparable to that of transbronchial biopsy. In central lesions, the sensitivities from BW and BB alone, which are 48% and 59% respectively, can be improved by combining them with FNAB and/or forceps biopsies. In peripheral lesions, transbronchial biopsies provide the highest sensitivity (57%), followed by BB (54%) and BW and bronchoalveolar lavage (BAL) (43%) {754}. Multiple brushings increase the sensitivity to 90% and decrease the need for repeated bronchoscopy {707}. Very peripheral lesions, pleural lesions, submucosal masses, and mediastinal masses cannot be directly sampled using these techniques.

Processing of samples

In BW the sediment of the recovered fluid subsequent to centrifugation is used for the preparation of smears, which can either be immediately fixed in alcohol for Pap staining, or rapidly air-dried using a warm plate or hairdryer for Giemsa staining. The remaining material should be used for cell block preparation and microbiological examination.

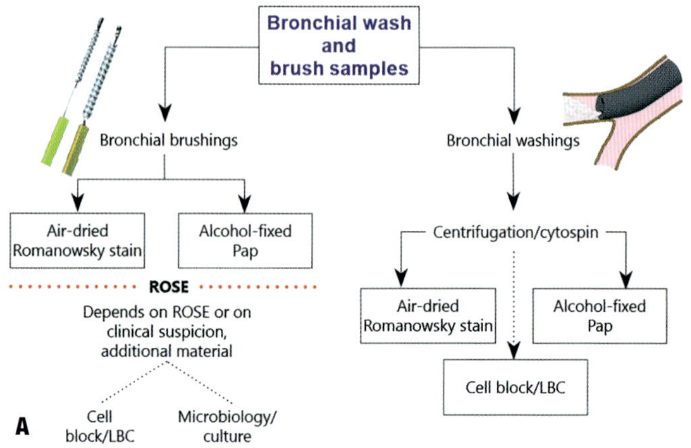

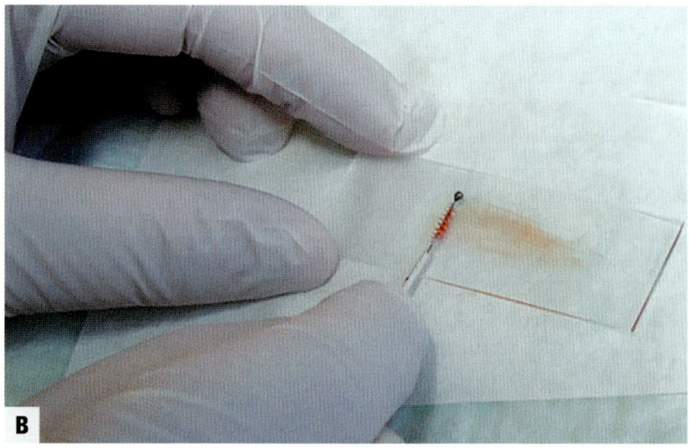

Fig. 2.04 **A** Bronchial wash/brush. Processing of bronchial wash/brush specimens. **B** Bronchial brush preparation technique. Preparation of a brush sample by rapidly rolling or quickly moving the brush across the slide and immediately (without any pause) placing the slide in alcohol.

In the endoscopy suite, brushes can be rapidly and directly smeared onto the glass slides by rolling the end of the brush and immediately fixing in alcohol. If necessary for rapid onsite evaluation (ROSE), air-dried slides can be prepared. Alternatively,

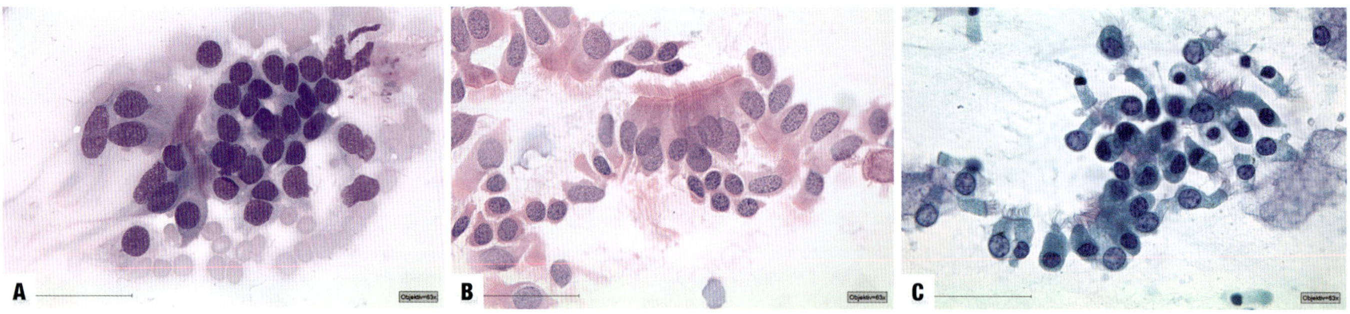

Fig. 2.03 **A** Normal ciliated bronchial cells. Tissue fragment of ciliated respiratory epithelium at the left, basal epithelial cells at the right (bronchial brushing, Giemsa). **B** Normal bronchial epithelium. Tissue fragment of bronchial epithelium showing the terminal bar and cilia and the underlying basal cells (bronchial brushing, H&E). **C** Bronchial epithelial cells. Tissue fragment of bronchial cells with cilia (bronchial washing, Pap).

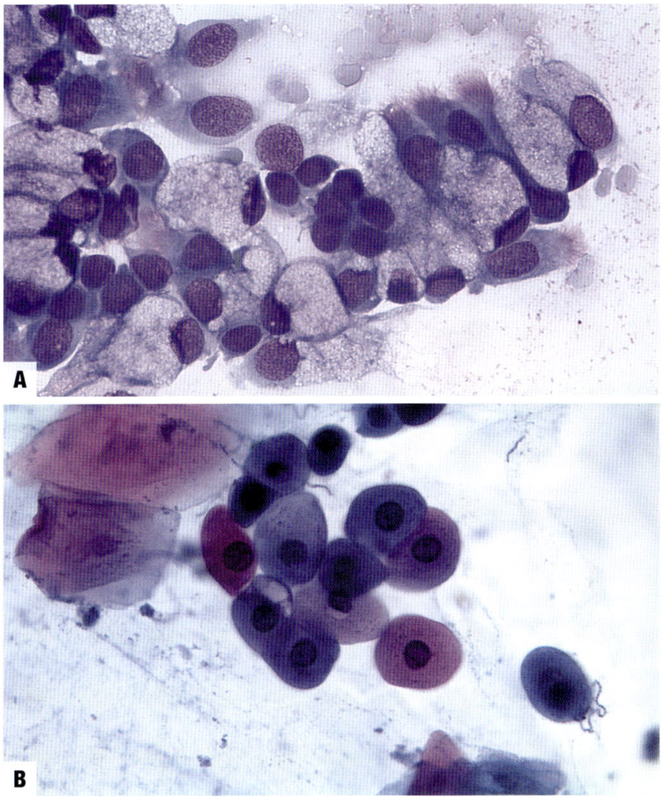

Fig. 2.05 **A** Goblet cell hyperplasia. Tissue fragment of ciliated bronchial cells and goblet cells (bronchial brushing, Giemsa). **B** Squamous cell metaplasia. Several metaplastic cells of small or medium size with dense cytoplasm and contaminant upper airway squamous cells at 9 to 10 o'clock (bronchial washing, Pap).

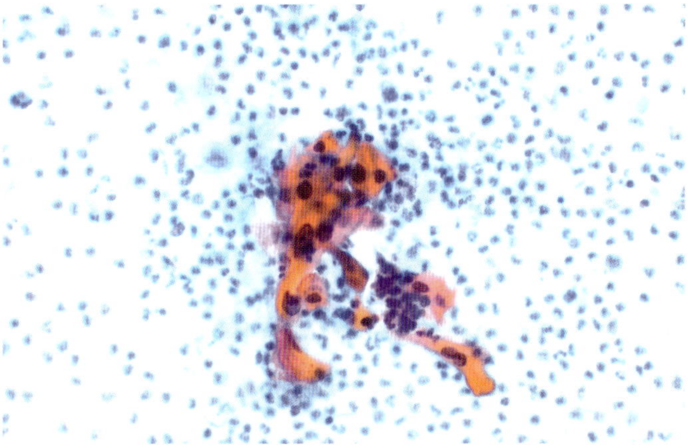

Fig. 2.06 Squamous cell carcinoma. A Pap-stained bronchial brushing.

Table 2.02 Indications, advantages, and limitations of bronchial wash and bronchial brush

Type of examination	Indications	Advantages	Limitations
Bronchial wash	Visible central lesions in combination with FNAB or forceps biopsy Bronchial infections	Easy and inexpensive No risk for the patient	Low sensitivity (47.6%) and specificity (71.4%) {152}
Bronchial brush	Peripheral tumours and peripheral infiltrates, visible on X-ray or CT Central lesions in combination with FNAB and forceps biopsy	High diagnostic yield {289} Low rate of complications Avoidance of more-invasive diagnostic procedures	Need for fluoroscopy and examination table suitable for fluoroscopy in the endoscopy suite

brushes can be rinsed in saline solution or alcohol-based fixatives and sent to the laboratory for further processing.

In general, a satisfactory specimen should contain cells or microorganisms diagnostic of a pathological process. Although adequacy criteria are poorly developed for BW and BB samples, specimens with few bronchial cells or macrophages and those heavily contaminated and obscured by blood, inflammation, or large numbers of oral squamous cells or oral saprophytes are considered unsatisfactory {676,465}.

Complications

Flexible fibre-optic bronchoscopy is a safe procedure with rare complications {401,285}.

Bronchoalveolar lavage techniques and specimen management

Jain D
Heine R
Kholova I

Bronchoalveolar lavage (BAL) is fluid collection from lung parenchyma through a bronchoscope positioned tightly into a subsegmental bronchus. BAL was initially a therapeutic procedure to clear the alveolar spaces of accumulated secretions blocking gaseous exchange. Routine analysis of cell-type counts of BAL samples is recommended in clinically suspected cases of interstitial lung diseases and asthma {565,601,429}. Creola bodies (crowded, cohesive tissue fragments of bronchial epithelial cells) and eosinophils are indicators of allergic asthma in paediatric patients as well as in adult patients {429,601}. BAL plays an important role in the diagnosis of infectious diseases in immunocompetent patients, as well as in patients who are immunocompromised due to organ transplant and other treatments {541}. In lung transplantation patients, BAL is routinely used for monitoring the lung allograft and detecting infections {541}. In addition, it is used to identify lipid-laden macrophages after aspiration mostly in paediatric patients {166,7,908}. In clinically suspected cases, lipid-laden macrophages in BAL fluid may potentially be a marker of vaping-related lung injury {517, 98}. BAL has been shown to be useful in diagnosing peripheral primary lung lesions of > 20–30 mm in size, with a detection rate ranging from 30% to > 60% {200}.

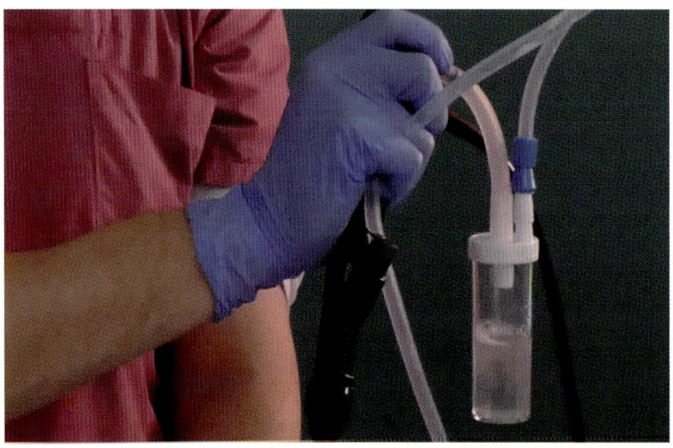

Fig. 2.07 Bronchoalveolar lavage (BAL) technique. Recovery of the instilled fluid. Slightly cloudy liquid is expected in a good-quality BAL.

Processing of samples

The procedure is performed under local anaesthesia in cooperative adult patients, and under general anaesthesia or conscious sedation in most paediatric patients and many disabled adults {164,833}.

The bronchoscope is passed to the lung segment of interest into (usually) a secondary or tertiary bronchus, and then wedged to occlude the bronchial lumen. Sterile normal saline is instilled in 20–50 mL aliquots to a total amount of 100–300 mL. At least 5–30% of the instilled fluid should be retrieved to get a diagnostic BAL. An optimum volume of 10–20 mL (minimum 5 mL) of pooled aliquots of retrieved BAL should be immediately sent to the laboratory for processing. In case of delay, the sample is stored and transported at 4 °C for up to 24 hours {164}.

A differential count of inflammatory cells is performed on air-dried Giemsa-stained cytospin smears with the help of a haemocytometer. Wet-fixed Pap-stained slides are used for screening for malignant cells. A fresh BAL sample can be sent for microbiological culture and flow cytometric analysis, if clinically indicated {676}. Methenamine silver, PASD, and Ziehl–Neelsen or related mycobacterial stains are used to detect infectious agents, especially in the workup of immunosuppressed transplant recipients. Oil Red O staining is performed to identify and quantify lipid-laden macrophages, but it is challenging to interpret and calculate the lipid-laden macrophage index {908}.

If the BAL procedure is properly performed, the sample should mainly contain alveolar macrophages and inflammatory cells within their designated cut-off values {565}. Excess

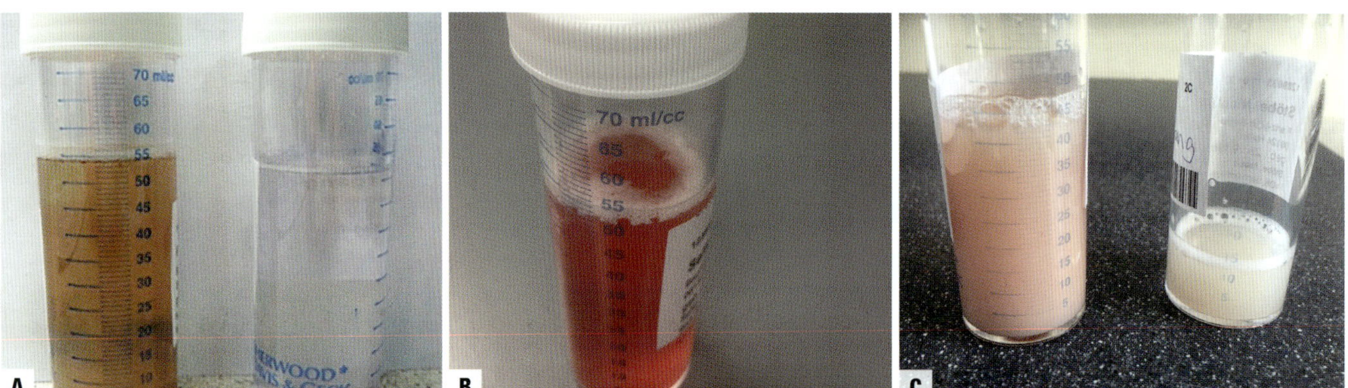

Fig. 2.08 Bronchoalveolar lavage (BAL) technique. **A** BAL of a smoker: brown-coloured fluid (left). BAL of a non-smoker: slightly cloudy fluid (right). **B** Haemorrhagic BAL specimen. **C** Milky BAL fluid from a patient with alveolar proteinosis.

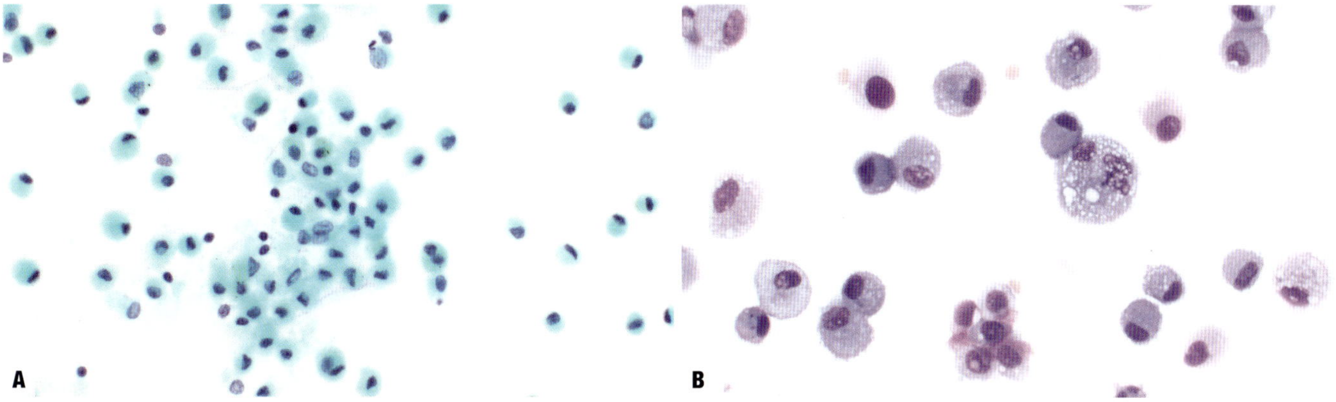

Fig. 2.09 Bronchoalveolar lavage (BAL) macrophages. **A** A Pap-stained preparation. **B** A Giemsa-stained preparation.

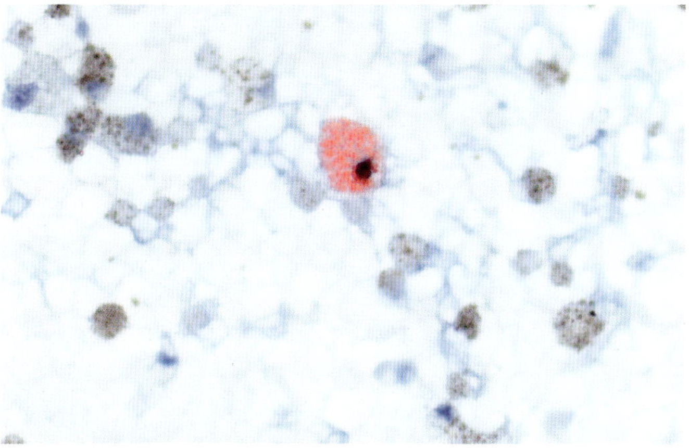

Fig. 2.10 Macrophages stained positive with Oil Red O. Cells staining positive are easily distinguished from the background macrophages with their carbon pigment.

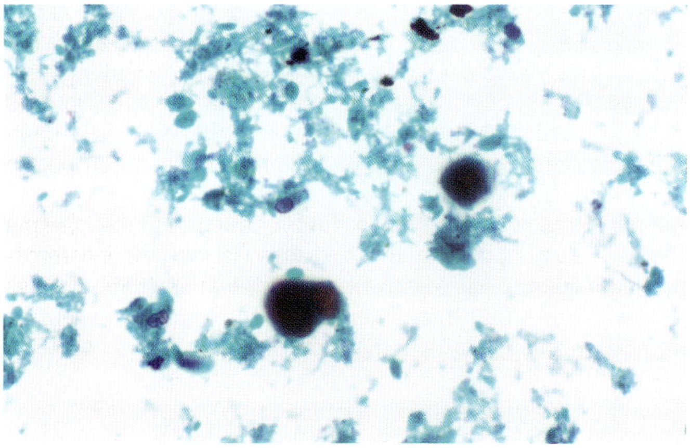

Fig. 2.11 Alveolar proteinosis. Cytospin smear from the bronchoalveolar lavage (BAL) specimen shows abundant granular material along with round, amorphous globules of surfactant-related material (Pap).

squamous and ciliated columnar cells indicate upper and lower airway contamination, respectively, and these should not be taken into consideration in the differential counting of inflammatory cells {48,565}.

Complications

BAL is a safe procedure, and the complications relate to the bronchoscopy procedure.

Sputum sampling techniques and specimen management

Jain D
Heine R
Kholova I

Sputum sample cytopathology is a simple, non-invasive, and inexpensive tool for sampling the airways for the analysis of cellular components and infectious agents and for diagnosing malignant lung diseases. However, with the development of less invasive flexible bronchoscopic procedures, bronchoscopic diagnostic methods including bronchial washings and brushings, bronchoalveolar lavage (BAL), forceps biopsy, and transbronchial FNAB when available, are more effective and preferred to sputum sampling.

Sputum samples can be collected spontaneously or can be aerosol-induced. Early morning samples on three consecutive days of spontaneous sputum samples produced by deep cough reportedly give better diagnostic yields than isolated samples. After thoroughly rinsing the mouth with water, the patient must be encouraged to cough from the deep airways {752}. In patients who are unable to spontaneously expectorate an adequate sputum sample, sputum production is induced by inhalation of nebulized sterile isotonic or hypertonic saline solution. An adequate amount of sample is usually obtained after 15–20 min, during which the patient is asked to cough and expectorate at 5 min intervals. Induced specimens, especially with hypertonic saline, reportedly produce better-quality specimens and better diagnostic yield for peripheral smaller lesions than spontaneous sputum samples {413,5}.

Sputum sample cytopathology is used in diagnosing malignant lung tumours in individuals suspected of having lung cancer. It is used in resource-limited settings where bronchoscopy or FNAB are not easily available, or if there are any contraindications for the use of invasive bronchoscopy-related methods. The efficiency of the technique depends on the location, size, and exfoliative tendency of the tumour, as well as the number of sputum samples, with 3–5 being preferable {71}. The diagnostic yield is highest for large, centrally placed, and airway-communicating lesions, with better sensitivity for 3-day pooled sputum samples or an increased number of sputum samples. The sensitivity ranges from 27% to > 80%, and specificity is about 99%. The diagnostic accuracy is > 80% with ≥ 3 samples {626}. The sensitivity is higher in central tumours (71%) than in peripheral lesions (49%) {815}. Because a sputum sample result does not localize the lesion, bronchoscopy is required after a positive sputum sample. Although molecular biomarker-based studies have been performed to detect early lung cancer from sputum samples, it

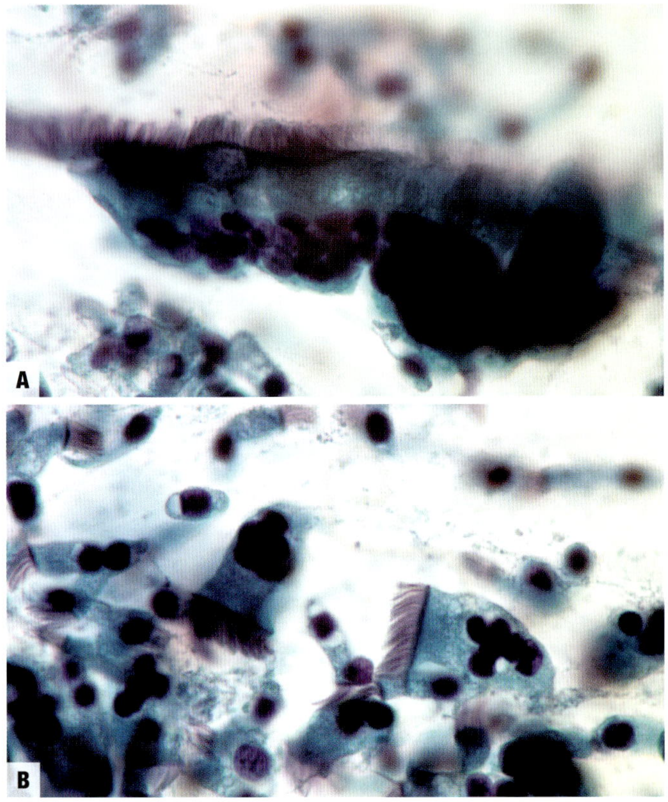

Fig. 2.13 Postbronchoscopy sputum sample. **A** Strip tissue fragment of ciliated bronchial epithelium with basal nuclei and columnar cytoplasm (sputum sample, Pap). **B** Dispersed columnar multinucleated bronchial cells with terminal bars and cilia (sputum sample, Pap).

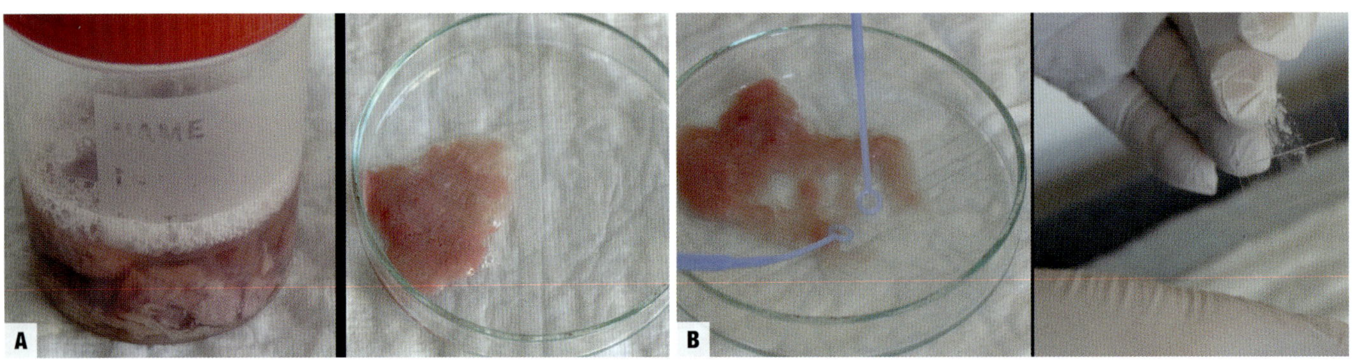

Fig. 2.12 **A** Sputum sample of a patient with central lung cancer and severe pulmonary infection. Haemorrhagic and purulent sputum sample. **B** Preparation of sputum sample. Two eyelets are used to select suspicious areas, which are picked out and placed on the glass slide, which is then smeared, fixed, and stained.

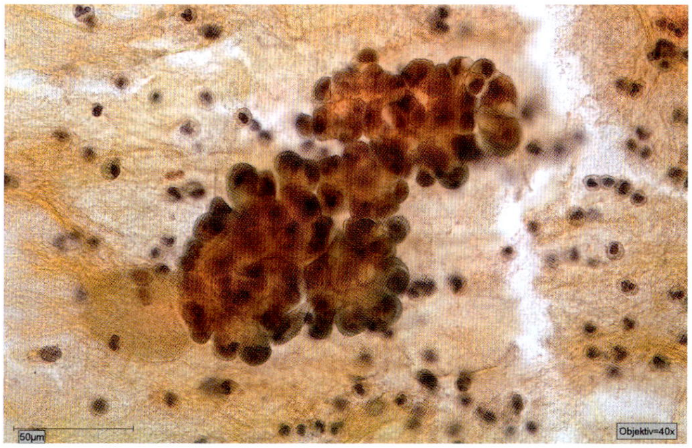

Fig. 2.14 Pulmonary adenocarcinoma. Tissue fragment showing an acinar architecture, with crowded cells with eccentric cytoplasm towards the gland centres, occasionally containing a vacuole and moderately pleomorphic nuclei. Mucus and inflammatory cells are present in the background (sputum sample, Pap).

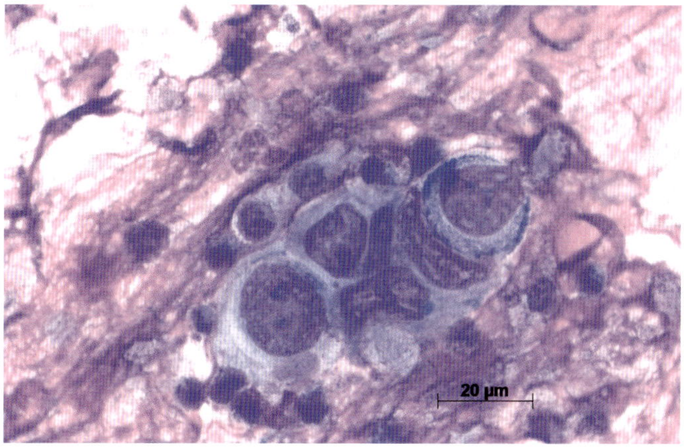

Fig. 2.15 Poorly differentiated squamous cell carcinoma. Minute crowded tissue fragment of squamous cell cancer, showing defined cytoplasm with minimal evidence of keratinization and with moderately pleomorphic nuclei, in a background of magenta mucus (sputum sample, Giemsa).

has no role in lung cancer screening programmes because of its low sensitivity {932}.

Sputum sample cytopathology can be also used for the assessment of airway inflammation in obstructive pulmonary diseases, the diagnosis of tuberculosis and opportunistic infections in immunocompromised hosts, and in some lung transplant protocols {377,85,458}.

Processing of samples

All samples should be regarded as potentially infectious and processed with standard precautions for aerosol-generating procedures. The sputum specimens should be collected in a clean, shallow, wide-mouthed, sterile glass bottle or plastic container and sent to the laboratory unfixed, if no significant delay is expected. In case of delay in transportation, Saccomanno fixative (50% ethyl alcohol and 2% carbowax) has been recommended for collection, transport, and fixation {787}. Alternatively, sputum samples can also be collected in 70% ethyl alcohol.

The sample is decanted into a Petri dish and checked grossly against a dark background for tissue fragments and blood-tinged areas using a pick-and-smear method. Smears are prepared from these areas and fixed in 95% alcohol for Pap staining {819}.

In the Saccomanno technique, the specimen is blended with the fixative in a high-speed laboratory blender or homogenizer for effective fixation, mechanical liquefaction, and mixing of the specimen; this is followed by centrifugation and smear formation from the cell button {787}. Mucolytic agents such as dithiothreitol (DTT) and acetylcysteine (also called *N*-acetylcysteine [NAC]) can also be used for chemical liquefaction {799}. Liquid-based cytopathology, with or without mucolytic agents, reduces the unsatisfactory rate and increases the diagnostic yield of sputum sample cytopathology significantly by eliminating mucus and blood from the background, but it is more costly {567}.

Pap staining is recommended for sputum specimens to better delineate nuclear characteristics in the mucoid background. Squamous differentiation and keratinization are well demonstrated, and squamous cell carcinoma is the most commonly detected malignant neoplasm in sputum sample cytopathology. Giemsa staining can also be used, preferably in tandem with the Pap.

In general, sputum is composed of a variable number of inflammatory cells and squamous epithelial cells. Changes in inflammatory cell composition, pigmentation in alveolar macrophages, Curschmann spirals and cytomorphological atypia in epithelial cells signify an underlying pathological process. An adequate sputum sample must contain alveolar macrophages, although no numerical cut-off value has been established {676}.

Complications

Induction of sputum production can cause bronchoconstriction {33}.

Rapid onsite evaluation

Jain D
Heine R
Kholova I

Rapid onsite evaluation (ROSE) refers to quick onsite evaluation of the FNAB sample obtained by a radiologist, interventional pulmonologist, or thoracic surgeon to check for adequacy of the specimen, ensure sufficient material has been obtained for cytopathological diagnosis and ancillary testing, triage the material for cost-effective and efficient ancillary testing, and provide a preliminary diagnosis {372}. It requires some basic facilities (see Box 2.01).

ROSE can be performed either by a cytopathologist or by a trained cytotechnologist, whereas provisional diagnoses at ROSE can only be provided by the cytopathologist. However, pulmonologists, once trained, can be competent in assessing the adequacy of the specimen if onsite cytopathologists are not available {930,681}. Alternatively, to minimize the time taken by cytopathology staff to reach the bronchoscopy suite and the downtime between passes, telecytopathology has been adopted by some centres to improve the efficiency of ROSE as the cytopathologist remains in the laboratory and interprets images remotely on slides prepared by a cytotechnologist at the ROSE suite {491}. The advantages and limitations of ROSE are given in Box 2.02.

Processing of samples

ROSE is widely used in interventional pulmonology during thoracoscopy for pleural lesions, and transthoracic or transbronchial FNAB of lung, mediastinal, or hilar lesions {974,778,306}, and it can also be used on imprints from forceps and core needle biopsies, bronchial brush material {444}, transbronchial catheter aspirations {271}, and intraoperative imprints and FNAB {602,603}.

ROSE includes four steps: (1) preparation of smears, (2) staining, (3) interpretation, and (4) triaging the sample.

1. The material is quickly expressed over labelled glass slides for direct smear preparation.
2. The prepared smears are stained by rapid stains, usually with an air-dried Giemsa but some institutions use toluidine blue or a Leishman stain on air-dried slides or a rapid Pap or H&E on alcohol-fixed smears. The air-drying should be rapid for the Giemsa using a warm plate or hairdryer, and, similarly, alcohol-fixed stains should be immediately placed in alcohol, although some may use an alcohol spray fixative. The choice of stain depends on laboratory infrastructure and set-up, available resources, and trained personnel for staining {3,508}.
3. The material is evaluated under a light microscope, usually without coverslipping. A sample is considered adequate if it contains diagnostic material – such as granulomas, an infectious agent, or tumour cells – that correlates with the clinical and imaging findings. If the sample contains only normal components of lung, then correlation with the clinical and imaging findings is required, and in most cases at ROSE, repeat FNAB is recommended to gain further material. An adequate transbronchial FNAB sample from a hilar lymph node should

Box 2.01 Requirements for rapid onsite evaluation (ROSE)

1. Sufficient space in the procedure room for the microscope, spreading out slides, and staining; there must be clear access for the proceduralist to rapidly deliver the material expelled from the FNAB on to slides
2. Light microscope
3. 95% ethyl alcohol jars for wet fixation of slides
4. Rack for air-dried slides
5. Jars containing reagents for rapid staining
6. 10% formalin jars for cell blocks or obvious tissue fragments/clots
7. Other tubes containing media, saline, etc. for ancillary testing
8. Glass slides
9. Pencil for labelling slides
10. Personnel for ROSE

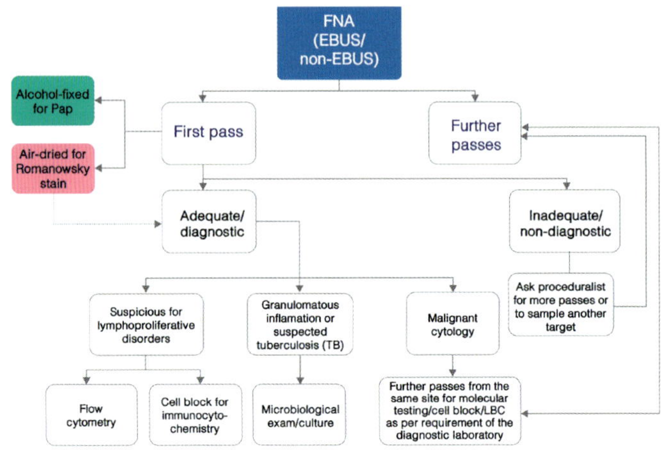

Fig. 2.16 Rapid onsite evaluation (ROSE). Algorithmic workflow. EBUS, endobronchial ultrasound;

Box 2.02 Advantages and limitations of rapid onsite evaluation (ROSE)

Advantages of ROSE:
- Adequacy assessment with real-time guidance to the physician performing the FNAB procedure
- Increased diagnostic yield
- Appropriate guided termination of the procedure after obtaining the appropriate material
- Reduction in number of unnecessary passes and slides
- Triage of sample and ancillary testing possible
- Careful control of preanalytical factors with a possibility of sampling/testing at different sites
- Possible benefits to sample and patient management

Limitations of ROSE:
- Staff requirement – either a cytopathologist or a trained cytotechnologist must be in attendance
- Time-consuming process for which cost reimbursement is an issue in some countries {491}

possess lymphoid cells and/or anthracotic pigment-laden macrophages in the absence of any specific diagnosis {148}.

4. Subsequent to acquisition of adequate diagnostic material, the procedure can either be terminated or additional passes can be requested for ancillary testing on the basis of the preliminary diagnosis on ROSE. ROSE triaging allows for a timely and efficient decision to be made as to how to handle the material. Needle and syringe rinses and any clots from the prior passes can be collected for making cell blocks. If the material is lymphoid, it can be collected into RPMI medium or Hanks solution or sterile buffered saline for flow cytometry, clonality assays, or gene rearrangement analysis and cell block; or, if the material suggests an infectious or granulomatous process, it can be collected into sterile saline and sent for microbiological examination. If ROSE suggests carcinoma or a metastasis such as melanoma, extra samples should be obtained for cell block and molecular testing, and placement directly into formalin is generally recommended, although some institutions place the material into RPMI medium or saline at ROSE and then in the laboratory prepare the cell block before placement into formalin.

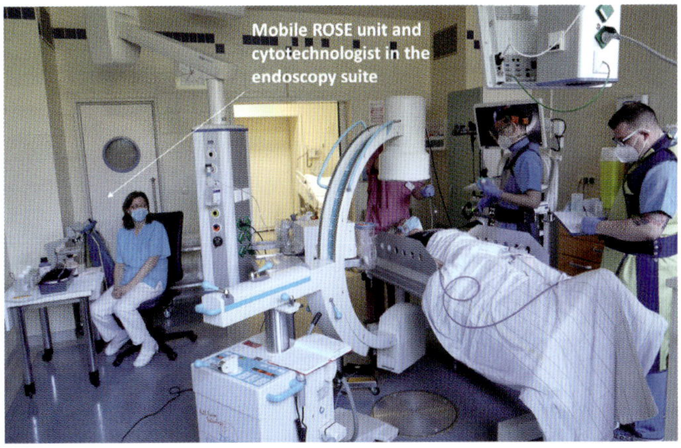

Fig. 2.17 Mobile rapid onsite evaluation (ROSE) unit. Mobile ROSE unit in endoscopy suite and cytotechnologist during bronchoscopy with peripheral biopsy and endobronchial ultrasound–guided transbronchial FNAB.

Chapter 2

Cell preparation methods

Jain D
Heine R
Kholova I

The samples should be optimally collected, transported, and kept according to guidelines issued or supervised by the cytopathology laboratory. The preanalytical steps have a critical role in specimen processing. The processing in the laboratory should be carried out according to the standard operating procedure of the cytopathology laboratory, validated and audited for quality assurance and quality control at designated regular intervals to enable the ideal diagnostic workup and interpretation.

Processing of samples

Cell collection, transportation, and storage

Bronchial washing (BW) and bronchoalveolar lavage (BAL) specimens can be directly fixed in 50% ethanol, and liquid-based cytopathology (LBC) specimens are fixed in their commercial media. LBC offers transportation in a stable collecting medium {567}. The volume of fixation fluid should be sufficient and at least the same volume as the sample itself. In an institutional setting, BW specimens may be directly and rapidly transported to the laboratory, centrifuged, and then handled by cytospin or direct smearing using appropriate biohazard cabinets, before actual fixation in alcohol; but since the COVID-19 pandemic, direct fixation of respiratory specimens has been recommended {130,667}. Direct smears from FNAB and bronchial brushing (BB) can be either air-dried or fixed by spraying with ethanol or by immersing immediately in 96% ethanol for 15 min. Some institutions process BB immediately into LBC medium. Referral to laboratory should be accompanied by a request form that includes the patient's demographics, the proceduralist and referring clinician information, the specimen type and site, the sampling technique, indications, disease-related clinical data, and treatment history. The specimens can be transported at room temperature but should be stored at +4 °C. Longer storage at room temperature can cause bacterial or fungal contaminant growth in a poorly preserved specimen.

Adequacy assessment and triage of material

On arrival in the laboratory, visual inspection and the nature of the clinical information guide the triaging of sample material. Haemorrhagic, mucinous, and sparse specimens may need pretreatment with various haemolytic and mucolytic agents. Cell concentration methods may be applicable in sparse specimens. In cases of possible lymphoproliferative lesions, fresh material for flow cytometry should be submitted in Hanks solution, RPMI medium, or sterile buffered saline. If an infectious agent is considered, material should be placed in a sterile container for microbial culture, and this may be routine in some settings, such as the assessment of sputa in areas of the world where mycobacterial infections are endemic, or the evaluation of BW or BAL specimens in heart, lung, renal, bone marrow, and other transplant patients.

Preparation methods

Direct smears

Smears can be prepared by spreading material into a thin, even layer on a glass slide. The slides can be rapidly air-dried using a heating plate or hairdryer or immediately fixed by immersing the slides in 96% ethanol for 15 min or using an alcohol spray. Some institutions place FNAB and other smears for a short period into modified Carnoy fixative to lyse red cells in place of ethanol, and then transfer to ethanol.

Table 2.03 Comparison of cell block preparatory methods

Type of method	Practical use	Advantages	Shortcomings
Clot and scrape	Where there is no provision for other cell block methods Highly cellular FNAB material	Inexpensive No set-up or equipment required	Not applicable to all types of samples No uniform cellularity Scraping induces crushing of cells
Simple sedimentation	Highly cellular exudative fluids	Inexpensive No expertise required Easy to perform	Not applicable to all types of samples Breakage of frail sediment during processing Variable cellularity
Plasma thrombin	Any type of FNAB and fluid	Simple Low cost, high user satisfaction Compatible with ICC and molecular testing	Cross-contamination from donor plasma and thromboplastin, which interferes in molecular testing
Agar-based and collodion bag	Any type of FNAB and fluid	Compatible with ICC and molecular testing	Agar and collodion handling is a cumbersome process and needs technical expertise for correct proportion and temperature for satisfactory cell block making
Automated (Cellient)	Scant / sparsely cellular specimens	Fully automated Free from cross-contamination of manual methods Good-quality nucleic acid yield for molecular testing	High cost Only specimens collected in methanol-based fixatives can be used Technical expertise needed for cutting thin sections from cell blocks Some antibodies do not work because of alcohol fixation

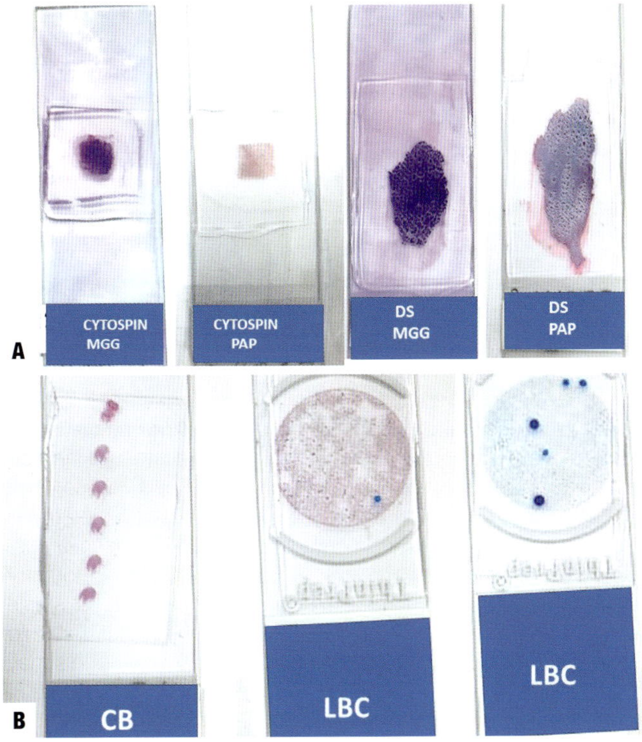

Fig. 2.18 Cell preparations. **A** Cytospin and direct smear (DS) cell preparations. MGG, Giemsa staining; PAP, Pap staining. **B** CB, cell block; LBC, liquid-based cytopathology.

Cytospins of ethanol-fixed material and fluids

Fluid cytopathological material including BW and FNAB rinses or brushed material fixed in ethanol can be spun down using a centrifuge to make a cytospin preparation. This technique is well established but may be more sensitive to technical variables than LBC. Because of biosafety issues in the COVID-19 pandemic era, fixation is preferable in potentially infected samples {130,667}.

Liquid-based preparation

Various commercial systems are widely available. LBC has been reported to reduce the unsatisfactory rate of specimens. It offers certain advantages over conventional methods, such as elimination of obscuring elements, ease of screening, excellent preservation, and easy application of ancillary techniques {567}, but it may reduce the diagnostic cytopathological information by eluting the background elements and rounding up all epithelial tissue fragments and components, making assessment more difficult. LBC may be more expensive in many laboratory settings.

Cell blocks

A cell block involves the collection of any type of cytopathological material derived from FNAB, BB, or BW, which is concentrated and processed as a formalin-fixed, paraffin-embedded biopsy by embedding a centrifuged compacted cell pellet into a paraffin block (see Table 2.03). As with surgical biopsies, the paraffin block material can be stained with H&E, potentially offering diagnostic architectural features, and it can then be used for ancillary techniques including ICC, special stains, FISH, and molecular techniques. Cell blocks greatly enhance the use of cytopathology in the assessment of lung lesions.

Optimum cell block cellularity depends on the intrinsic nature of the lesion, with fibrotic and cystic lesions often providing limited material; the collection and triage of the sample; the expertise of the cytotechnologists; and the type of preparation method. Cell blocks can be prepared by a variety of techniques, which include simple clot and scrape, plasma thrombin, agar, colloidal bag, and automated methods. The methods also vary as to whether formalin or alcohol-based fixatives are used, and as to the method of concentration, which can include centrifugation, filtration, or scraping. Different adjuvants, such as thrombin clot, agar, or albumin, are used to bind cells into the compact button. The majority of the methods are modified in-house techniques (which depend on the availability of resources, funding, laboratory infrastructure, and the historical preference of cytopathologists) and are not standardized across laboratories {441A,610,373,839,784}. In general, the methods using simple sedimentation with formalin fixation of the cell pellet and the use of plasma thrombin are the most popular and widely used {174}.

Cell culture

FNAB material and malignant pleural effusions have been used to produce different types of cancer cell cultures {25,766,526}. Subsequently to determining the adequacy of the specimen and tumour typing, samples are used to establish cell cultures. In brief, density gradient centrifugation and hypotonic lysis are used to purify tumour cells before plating them in culture Petri dishes or flasks. Finally, cultures are checked by in vitro growth kinetic and in vivo xenograft experiments.

Alternatively, commercially available cell lines of different tumours can be prepared as cytospins after fixation for their use as ICC positive controls {449}.

Recently, cultured tumour cells have been used to study chemotherapeutic and immunotherapeutic drug responses, enabling better and personalized treatment approaches by testing for individual drug sensitivity and resistance. Technical limitations due to patient sample acquisition, cellular variability, and culture conditions are the main reasons for the limited use of these techniques in clinical practice, as well as cost {986,886,766,783}.

Staining methods

A wide variety of Romanowsky (Giemsa) stains, including the May–Grünwald–Giemsa, Wright–Giemsa, and others, can be used on air-dried slides. They are quick and easy to perform, cost-effective, and useful in rapid onsite evaluation (ROSE). The stain enhances cytoplasmic features, the background elements, and the stroma including the extracellular matrix. Pap and H&E require immediate fixation in ethanol and offer excellent nuclear detail and enhanced evaluation of squamous lesions. LBC primarily uses commercial variants of ethanol fixation. Ideally for FNAB, both Giemsa and Pap are used routinely to optimize the diagnostic cytopathological features. Pap staining is routinely used for sputum, BW, BB, and BAL specimens. Special stains for bacteria (e.g. Gram and Warthin–Starry stains), mycobacteria (including the Ziehl–Neelsen and related stains), and fungi (e.g. the methenamine silver stain) can be applied to direct smears and cytospin preparations. Various mucin stains such as the PASD can assist in the diagnosis of adenocarcinomas and adenosquamous carcinomas.

Quality assurance

The laboratory process should be validated and audited internally and externally on a regular basis. The preanalytical component of processing should be included in any quality assurance programme.

Introduction: The role of ancillary testing

Roy-Chowdhuri S
Bubendorf L

With advances in minimally invasive sampling techniques, lung carcinoma is frequently diagnosed by cytopathology alone. The ability to perform reliable and accurate immunostaining in cytopathological specimens to confirm the diagnosis, subtype primary lung carcinoma, and differentiate it from metastases from other sites is crucial {1000,999}. In addition, owing to the rapid growth in therapeutic options for patients with advanced-stage non-small cell lung carcinoma, predictive biomarker testing to identify targetable oncogenic driver alterations is the cornerstone for determining the best therapeutic option in these patients {701,618}. Molecular profiling with matched targeted therapy has led to unprecedented outcome improvements in a significant subset of patients with non-small cell lung carcinoma {343,848}.

Cytopathology specimens are highly relevant as a tissue source for ancillary testing, because they may often be the only source of tumour material available from a patient. Frequently, cytopathology provides complementary tumour material to small biopsies, which may have a limited number of tumour cells that may fall short of adequate material for molecular testing {776, 134}. Current clinical practice guidelines indicate that any cytopathology preparation (direct smears, cytospins, liquid-based preparations, or cell block), can be used for molecular testing {494}. A wide variety of ancillary tests, including ICC, FISH, and molecular techniques, can be successfully employed in cytopathology specimens, provided the assays have been adequately validated for cytopathological substrates and a robust and rigorous quality assurance is in place {778}.

Immunocytochemistry

Bubendorf L
Lozano MD
Michael CW

Introduction

Immunocytochemistry (ICC) is an excellent ancillary technique for confirming and subtyping primary lung carcinoma and for differentiating it from pulmonary metastases {1000,999}. The ability to perform highly accurate ICC in cytopathological specimens is crucial, given that as many as 40% of all lung cancer diagnoses are made by cytopathology alone. The major differences and challenges in cytopathology compared with immunohistochemistry of surgical specimens relate to the greater variability of preanalytical conditions and the lack of tissue architecture that provides context, which together may necessitate different protocols and scoring strategies.

Technical requirements

ICC plays a significant role in the workup of lung cytopathology (see Box 2.03, p. 28) and can be successfully performed on various types of cytopathological preparations (see Box 2.04, p. 30). Regardless of the preparation used, a uniform, well-spread sample with minimal obscuring material is a prerequisite for reliable ICC staining {233,883}. The protocol used should be validated for each marker to confirm that the results are reproducible when compared with a known gold standard. The College of American Pathologists (CAP) guidelines mandate a concordance level of 90%. An adequate number of positive and negative controls should be used as determined by the cytopathology laboratory protocols. Suggested gold standards include data from published literature; a corresponding assay validated on formalin-fixed, paraffin-embedded biopsies; protocols from other laboratories; or results of previously validated non-ICC assays (e.g. FISH). The staining protocols used for formalin-fixed, paraffin-embedded tissue sections should be optimized for the cytopathology preparation to avoid false negative or positive results {813,269}.

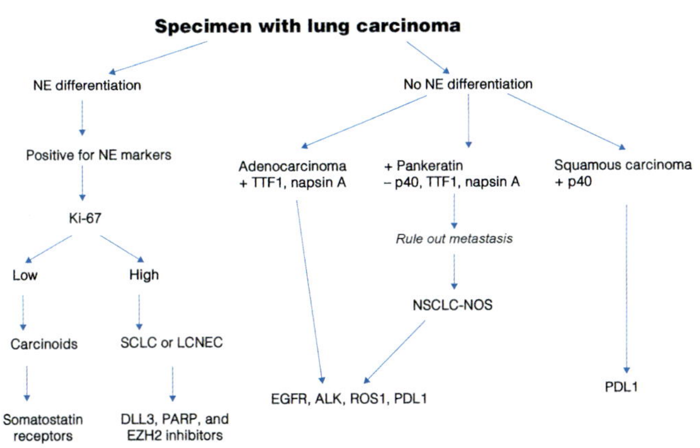

Fig. 2.19 Immunocytochemistry (ICC) algorithm for subtyping lung cancer. LCNEC, large cell neuroendocrine carcinoma; NE, neuroendocrine; NSCLC, non-small cell lung carcinoma; PARP, poly (ADP-ribose) polymerase; SCLC, small cell lung carcinoma; TTF1, thyroid transcription factor 1.

Management of types of cytopathological specimens

In addition to the cell block, other cytopathology preparations that can be used for ICC include direct smears, cytospins, and liquid-based cytopathology (LBC) (see Table 2.04, p. 30). The

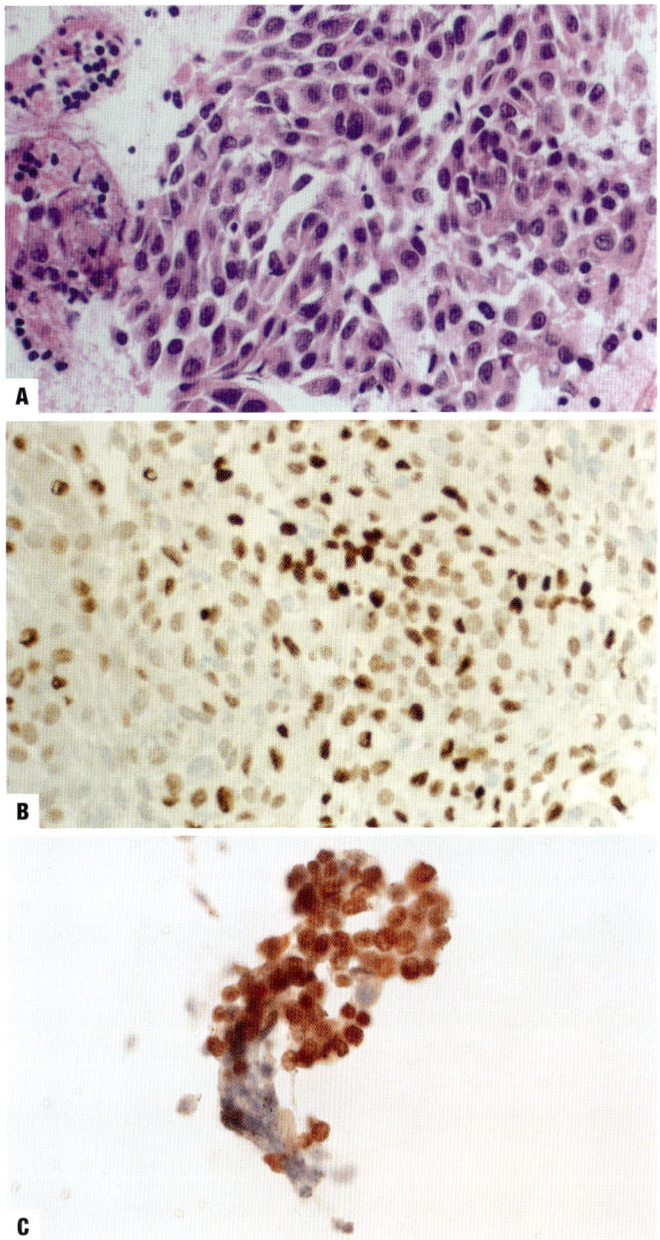

Fig. 2.20 Adenocarcinoma. **A** Tissue fragment of large cells with large, highly pleomorphic nuclei and eccentric cytoplasm (cell block, H&E). **B** Positive nuclear staining (cell block, thyroid transcription factor 1 [TTF1] ICC). **C** Positive nuclear TTF1 staining in a previously Pap-stained smear (bronchial brushing, ICC).

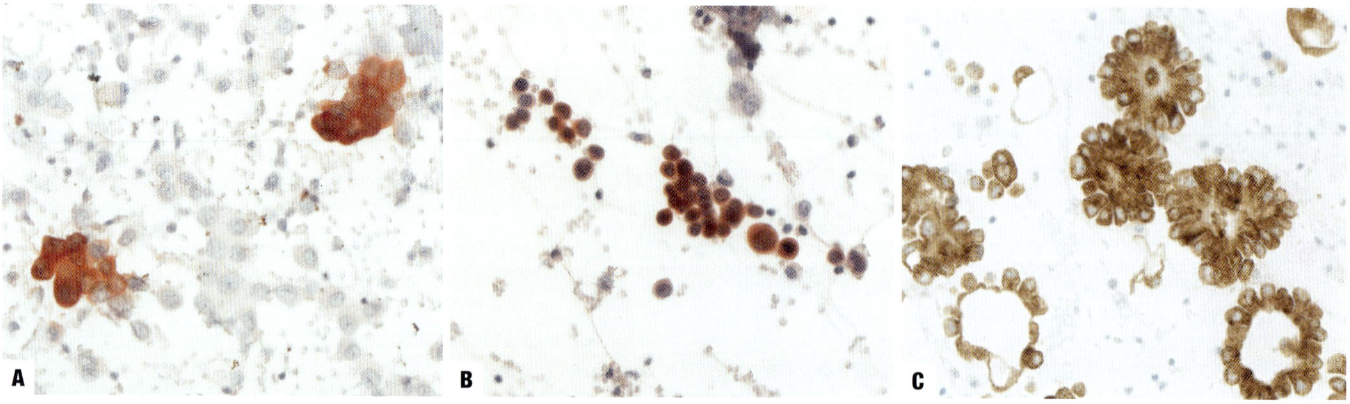

Fig. 2.21 Non-small cell lung carcinoma (NSCLC). **A** ALK-positive NSCLC on a previously Pap-stained smear of a pleural effusion, in a background of ALK-negative mesothelial cells and macrophages (5A4 ICC). **B** ROS1-positive NSCLC on a previously Pap-stained (bronchoalveolar lavage [BAL], Cell Signaling Technology D4D6 antibody). **C** ROS1-positive NSCLC on a cell block of a malignant effusion (D4D6 ICC).

choice of method is based on the laboratory preferences as long as the selected method undergoes the required validation {374,269}. Although the majority of antigens have been validated on LBC, some antibodies, particularly nuclear ones, were reported to have either reduced expression or false negative results {804,316,296,952,294,522,302}. Cell blocks are the most commonly used preparation. ICC on cell blocks can be easily optimized using similar protocols and controls to those used for histopathology. Diligent validation of markers is needed, as with LBC {804}.

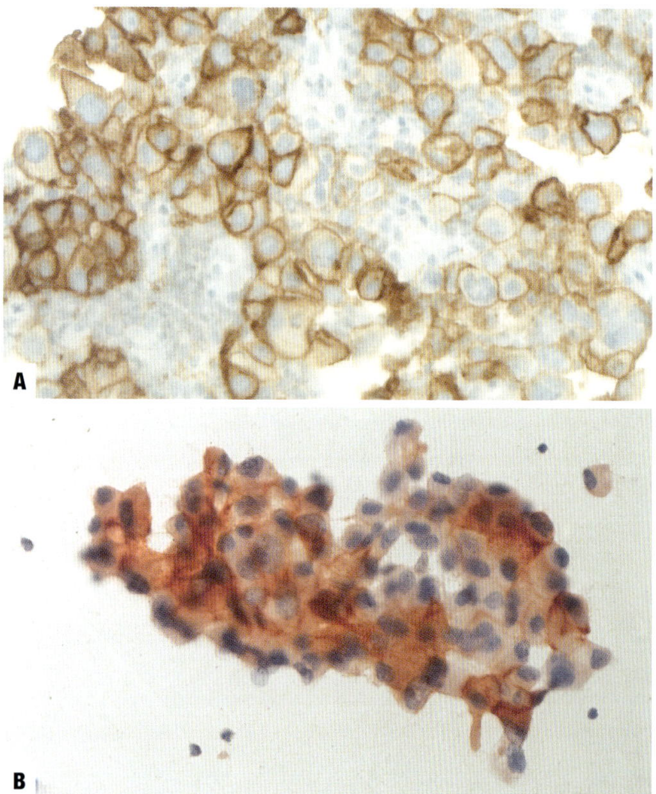

Fig. 2.22 **A** PDL1 on cell block. Distinct circumferential membranous PDL1 staining of all non-small cell lung carcinoma cells (cell block, 22C3 ICC). **B** Positive PDL1 on direct smear. PDL1 on an ethanol-fixed and previously Pap-stained direct smear: the majority of non-small cell lung carcinoma cells show membranous and/or diffuse cytoplasmic-like staining (direct smear, SP263 ICC).

Fixation

Cell blocks fixed in formalin and embedded in paraffin are considered the optimal specimen preparation and fixation for ICC because of the ease of standardization and optimization of staining protocols with those used in histopathology. For non–cell block cytopathology, most fixatives can be used after diligent validation. The following results have been reported {883}:

- Both immediate fixation in alcohol and postfixation in alcohol after material has been placed in formal saline provide good antigen preservation but may produce high background staining
- Air-dried smears fixed in 0.1% formal saline and postfixed in 100% ethanol produce the best and most consistent results
- Acetone gives inconsistent results
- Saline-rehydrated air-dried smears fixed in 95% alcohol plus 5% acetic acid are unsatisfactory {256,483,840}
- Air-dried smears fixed in 4–10% formalin are well suited for nuclear antigens
- Certain antigens are leached in alcohol fixative, for example S100, ER, BAP1, and MTAP

Controls

A positive and negative control should be used for each case. The controls can be collected from smears, cytospins, or direct imprints obtained from surgical bench macroscopic specimens, whereas discarded surplus material from effusions can be used, or well-characterized in vitro cell lines can be utilized {813}. The control slides can be coverslipped and/or refrigerated or stored

Box 2.03 Contributions of immunostains in the workup of lung cytopathology

1. Identifying cell lineage (e.g. epithelial, mesenchymal, or haematopoietic)
2. Confirming cell origin (i.e. lung primary vs metastasis)
3. Identifying cell type (e.g. adenocarcinoma, squamous carcinoma, etc.)
4. Identifying infectious organisms (e.g. fungus, virus, etc.)
5. Tumour grading (e.g. using Ki-67 to separate low-grade and high-grade neuroendocrine tumours [NETs])
6. Serving as prognostic and predictive biomarkers for targeted therapy

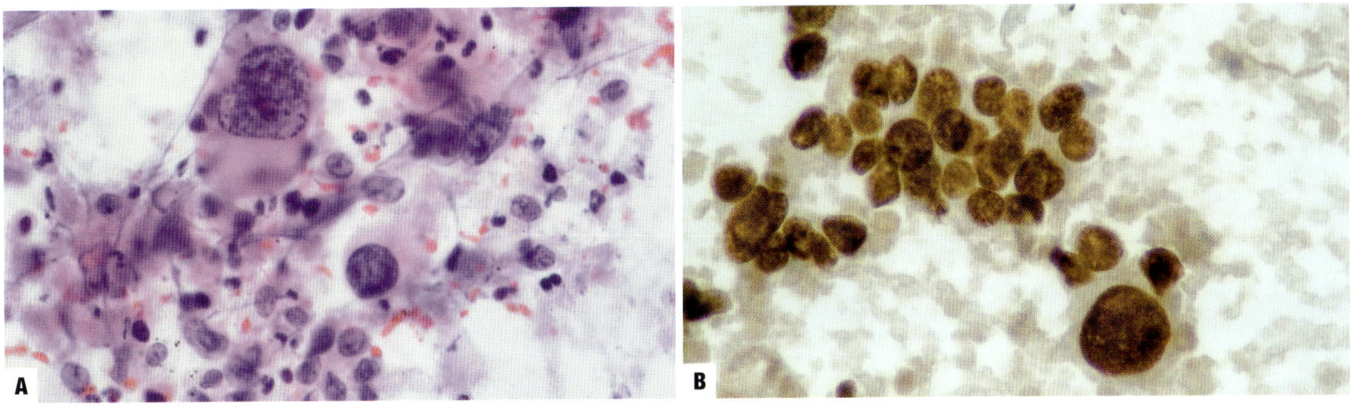

Fig. 2.23 Poorly differentiated squamous cell carcinoma. **A** Poorly differentiated non-small cell carcinoma in a direct smear, requiring ICC for specific diagnosis (direct smear, H&E). **B** Positive nuclear staining with p40 ICC (direct smear).

at −20 °C or −70 °C to preserve the antigens {961}. LBC is best stored in its original suspension {887}.

Procedures

Immunostaining can be performed either manually or using automated immunostainers. Manual staining is less standardized and operator-dependent. Therefore, the number of technologists involved in the manual staining should be limited to allow adequate experience and reproducibility {374,855}.

Both Pap-stained and Giemsa-stained slides (coverslipped) can be used within 1–2 years without the need to destain the slide. Soaking in xylene to remove the mounting medium does not have a negative effect. Slides should always be fixed before ICC and can lose antigenicity rapidly if stored as air-dried slides without postfixation {374,951}.

The majority of cytoplasmic and membranous antigens do not require antigen retrieval in alcohol-fixed preparations {207,294, 361}. A short period of heat-induced antigen retrieval is recommended for uncovering epitope reactivity for most nuclear and some membranous antigens in alcohol-fixed preparations and all formalin-fixed preparations, and for selected antigens in LBC {207, 208}. Protease antigen retrieval should be avoided {319,207,269}.

Diagnostic applications

Non-small cell lung carcinoma should be confirmed by ICC if the cytomorphological features are equivocal. Non-small cell carcinoma not classified by cytomorphology alone should be subtyped as favouring adenocarcinoma, favouring squamous, or NOS by using ICC. When non-small cell lung carcinoma is confirmed, the specimen should be further evaluated for predictive markers (see flow chart in Fig. 2.19) {374,563}.

For subtyping non-small cell lung carcinoma, thyroid transcription factor 1 (TTF1) and p40 are the gold standards. TTF1 is positive in the majority (~75–80%) of adenocarcinoma cases {962,735}. The TTF1 clone 8G7G3/1 is the most specific for lung adenocarcinoma but is less sensitive than SPT24 {1000}. Focal TTF1 staining can be considered positive. Napsin A can serve as a second marker for adenocarcinoma. As a squamous marker, p40 is preferred over p63, and > 50% of cells should stain for a positive interpretation. When evaluating tumours, a positive immunoreaction for TTF1 in pneumocytes contaminating the sample must be carefully excluded. Several tumours other than lung adenocarcinomas can also express TTF1, for example neuroendocrine tumours (NETs) and thyroid tumours {1019,1000}, and napsin A can stain renal cell carcinomas {650}. CK7 is not specific for pulmonary adenocarcinomas {1000}. In bronchial cytopathology, bronchial basal cells positive for p40 must not be mistaken for squamous cell carcinoma {1000}. Neuroendocrine markers should only be used if NET differentiation is suspected.

Predictive ICC markers on cytopathology material have good reproducibly for both cell block and non–cell block techniques

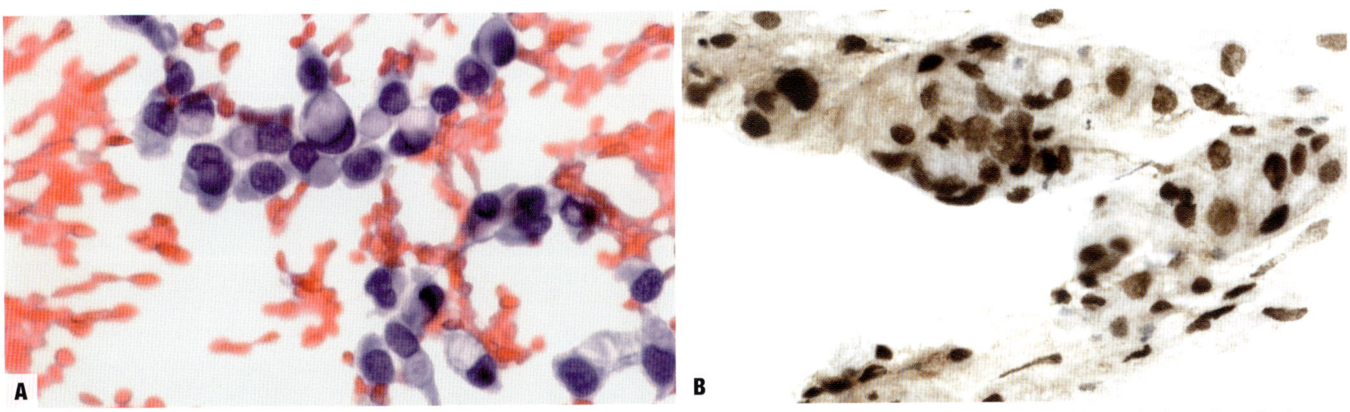

Fig. 2.24 Metastatic lung adenocarcinoma. **A** Signet-ring cell adenocarcinoma metastatic to mediastinal lymph node (direct smear, Pap). **B** Metastatic signet-ring cell adenocarcinoma of the lung showing thyroid transcription factor 1 (TTF1) nuclear positivity (direct smear).

Box 2.04 Various cytology preparations used in immunostaining

Immunohistochemistry
Formalin-fixed, paraffin-embedded cell blocks
Methanol-fixed, paraffin-embedded Cellient cell blocks (Hologic)

Immunocytochemistry
Direct smears: air-dried or fixed
Cytospins: air-dried or fixed
Imprints
Liquid-based cytology
- ThinPrep (Hologic) – collected in CytoLyt and PreservCyt (methanol-based and contain mucolytic and haemolytic agents)
- SurePath (BD) – collected in CytoRich Red (ethanol-based)

and can be used primarily for screening cases before molecular testing for ALK, ROS1, and NTRK {374,548}. ICC is not recommended for EGFR or RET {1000,55}.

ICC on cytopathology specimens can be performed for PDL1 with good reproducibly but may be more challenging to interpret {374,563}. PDL1 ICC in cytopathology is most commonly performed on cell blocks using the assays and protocols developed for histopathological specimens. There is a high concordance between cell block and matched histopathology {297}. Emerging evidence suggests that PDL1 ICC can also be applied to ethanol-fixed non–cell block specimens such as direct smears, cytospins, or liquid-based preparations {374, 637,509}. However, this is currently not yet recommended for broad use, because of the limited number of studies and lack of standardization. As in histopathology, a minimum number of 100 viable tumour cells is considered a requisite for PDL1 ICC. In histopathological specimens and cell blocks, PDL1 staining is defined by complete circumferential or partial linear membrane staining of tumour cells, irrespective of the intensity. In non–cell block specimens, membranous staining is less distinct, because the cell membranes are intact and not cut through by microtome sectioning {374}. Therefore, PDL1 staining of the horizontal cell membrane mostly appears as diffuse surface staining, mimicking cytoplasmic staining. Admixed macrophages showing membranous and cytoplasmic staining can be particularly challenging in samples with predominantly single dispersed tumour cells, because they may lead to an overestimation of PDL1 positivity. Immunostaining a corresponding section for TTF1 and/or a panleukocyte marker (e.g. CD45) will aid in identifying tumour cells for PDL1 scoring {637}.

Table 2.04 Different cytology preparations

Feature	Direct smears	Cytospin	Liquid-based preparation
Ease of technique	Easiest, minimal labour	Easy, requires some labour	Automated, requires some training
Cost	Minimal expense	Some expense	Greater expense
Air-dried slides	Yes	Yes	No
Fixed slides	Yes	Yes	Yes
Fixative used	Any fixative	Any fixative	Methanol (Hologic) Ethanol (SurePath)
Need for pretreatment	Haemolytic and mucolytic agents recommended Peroxidase block for inflammatory smears	Haemolytic or mucolytic agents recommended Peroxidase block for inflammatory smears	Not required Not required
Reagents	Large amount to cover slide	Minimal amount	Intermediate amount
Disposables	None	Minimal	More
Background staining	Can be high	Can be high	Clean
Stain interpretation	Easier for nuclear than cytoplasmic stains	Easier for nuclear than cytoplasmic stains Difficulty with 3D tissue fragments	Reduced or false negative results reported for nuclear stains
Storage	Prior coverslipping and fixation required to preserve antigenicity	Prior coverslipping and fixation required to preserve antigenicity	Best to store as cell suspension

In situ hybridization

Bubendorf L
Lozano MD
Michael CW

Chapter 2

Introduction

FISH is a well-established method for visualizing and diagnosing numerical and structural abnormalities in chromosomal DNA. It is widely used in clinical laboratories as a gold standard to identify deletions, amplifications, and rearrangements of selected genes {806,548}. The advantage of FISH lies in the low number of tumour cells needed and the fact that alterations can be detected specifically within the neoplastic cells of interest.

Technical requirements

FISH is a robust method that is applicable to almost all types of cytopathological specimens. Targeted evaluation of cells of interest is a prerequisite for reliable FISH results. FISH requires as few as 50–100 tumour cells and permits direct correlation with cytomorphology {806}. Internal validation of FISH assays is needed and external quality assurance is recommended {495, 531,412}. Using national regulatory body–approved probes, all steps of the procedure should be followed according to the manufacturer's specifications, with some adjustments appropriate to smaller biopsy specimens and preparations {698,778}. Any deviation requires separate validation. The use of adhesive slides with electrostatic positive charge is recommended to prevent cell loss during pretreatment and DNA denaturation {510}. FISH analysis requires a fluorescence microscope with appropriate filters, ideally equipped with an automated stage for precise relocalization of cells of interest. Scoring of FISH signals can be done at the fluorescence microscope or be based on high-quality compressed 2D images from z-stacks at the computer screen {805}. Probes for chromogenic in situ hybridization for ALK gene rearrangement detections have been designed but are not widely used {811}.

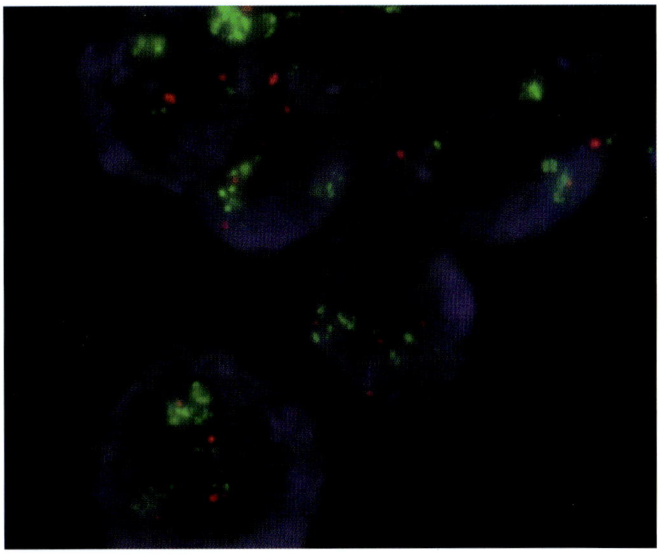

Fig. 2.25 Adenocarcinoma with high-level *MET* amplification. Pap-stained specimen used for FISH to demonstrate *MET* amplification (green, *MET*; red, CEP17; mean number of *MET* signals/cell: 222; *MET*:CEP17 ratio: 23).

Table 2.05 Advantages and disadvantages of different cytopathological samples for FISH analysis

Type of cytopathological sample	Advantages	Disadvantages
Formalin-fixed, paraffin-embedded cell block	Preservation of tissue architecture No overlapping cells Cell blocks made from FNAB may be enriched in tumour cells	Formalin fixation Probe signal loss due to nuclear truncation from sectioning Some cell blocks are poorly cellular May have autofluorescent background that obscures signals
Smears	No nuclear truncation artefact Allows rapid onsite evaluation (ROSE) of specimen adequacy at time of procedure No alterations related to formalin fixation Smears made from FNAB may be enriched in tumour cells	Cell overlapping May have autofluorescent background Legal issues due to loss of diagnostic smears
Cytospins	No nuclear truncation artefact Cells are concentrated in a smaller area	May have inadequate cellularity
Liquid-based cytopathology	No nuclear truncation artefact Monolayer preparation minimizes nuclear overlap, although tissue fragments tend to round up and become denser Less background Cells are concentrated in a smaller area	More expensive than other cytopathological preparations Special instrumentation needed for slide preparation May have inadequate cellularity

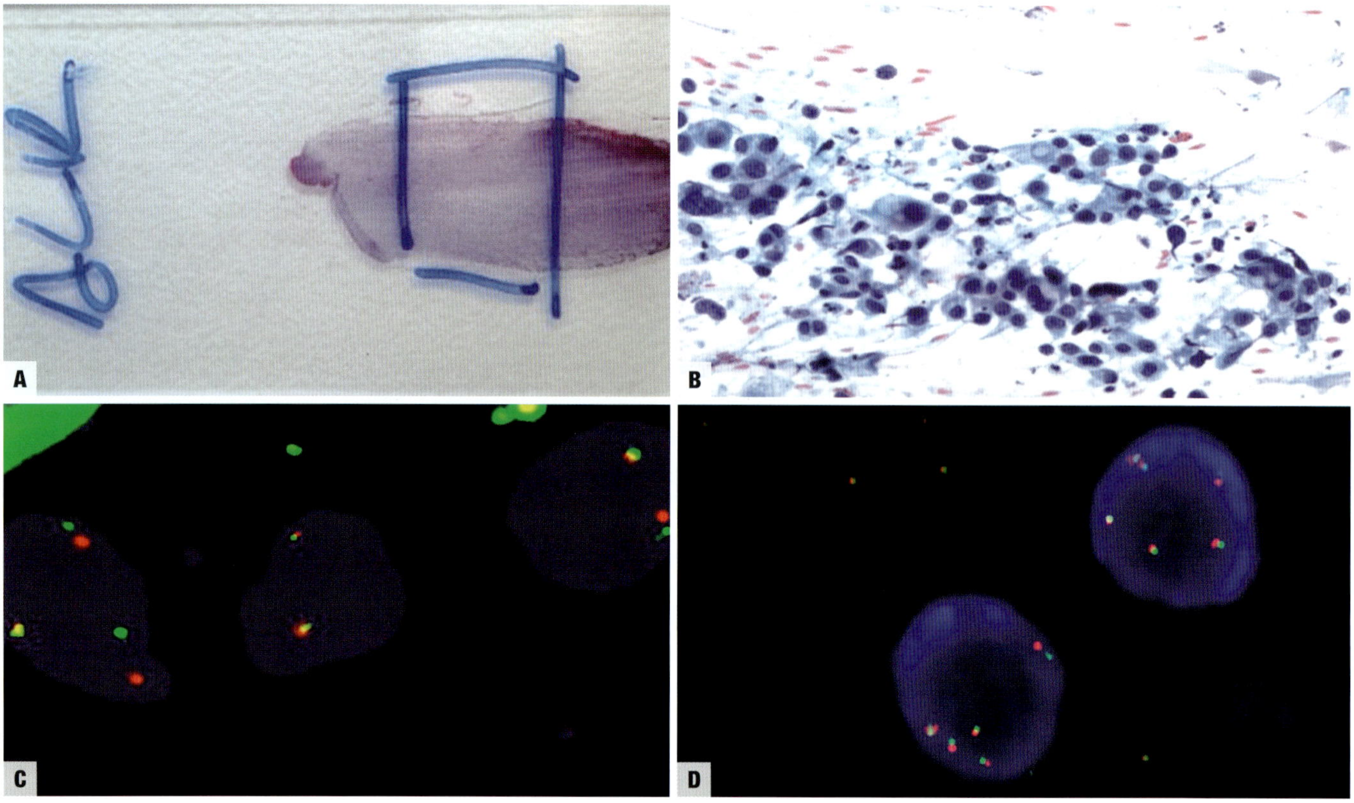

Fig. 2.26 A,B *ALK* assessment on a direct smear. Selection of tumour-rich areas located under the microscope is used to avoid overlapping and other artefacts (Pap). This approach allows the *ALK* probe to be used efficiently for FISH, improves the cost-effectiveness of the technique, and shows separation of the red and green signals. **C** *ALK* assessment on a direct smear. FISH of *ALK* shows separation of the red and green signals. **D** *ALK* FISH. An example of negative and polysomal *ALK* in a FISH study carried out on a direct smear.

Management of types of cytopathological specimens

A wide range of cytopathological preparations have been used for FISH, including unstained smears; Pap-, Giemsa-, or H&E-stained smears; cytospins; liquid-based cytopathology preparations; and unstained formalin-fixed, paraffin-embedded cell blocks {806,698,761,60}. The major advantages and disadvantages of different cytopathological samples for FISH analysis are shown in Table 2.05 (p. 31). Cell blocks are usually preferred for FISH analysis because they can be handled like surgical pathology specimens. However, the quality of DNA is compromised by formaldehyde fixation due to cross-linking and chemical modifications of nucleotides {761,510,60}. The wide variety of cell block processing protocols introduces an additional factor of variability {778,761}.

Besides the lack of formalin fixation, the main advantage of performing FISH on non–cell block cytopathology specimens is that the tumour cells are complete rather than sectioned, and so they have intact, non-truncated nuclei containing the true number of signals {806,510,60,713}. FISH is also feasible on previously immunostained ethanol-fixed cytopathological slides, for example thyroid transcription factor 1 (TTF1)-stained slides, as long as autofluorescent DAB is avoided as a chromogen {809}.

Validation is needed in each laboratory to control for potentially interfering factors due to variability in staining and fixation protocols. At least 50 tumour cells should be evaluated, avoiding 3D tissue fragments with overlapping nuclei and areas with necrosis. The best suited area for FISH analysis should be selected on the stained smears allowing for efficient use of the probe {806,510,60,259}. To avoid potential legal issues when using the only diagnostic slide in a particular case, capturing images of selected areas or digitally scanning the whole slide before the procedure is recommended. When testing for rearrangements, a positive result is considered when > 15% of tumour cells have either isolated 3′ signals in the deletion pattern or break-apart patterns. However, results should be interpreted with caution when within the borderline range (15–20% of cells) because of possible false positive results due to technical factors {807,921}.

Fixation

Although formalin fixation is standard for surgical pathology specimens, alcohol fixatives are mostly used for non–cell block cytopathological preparations. The quality of DNA in air-dried or alcohol-fixed cytopathological samples is actually better than that after formaldehyde fixation {806,698,510,60,713}. Fixatives containing acidic components, such as Bouin or acidic decalcification solutions, have been shown to yield suboptimal FISH results {816}.

Controls

Running external or on-slide control specimens is not required for FISH. The presence of signals in all cell nuclei in a specimen serves as the internal control for good hybridization efficiency.

Procedures

The steps involved in FISH include slide pretreatment, denaturation of the probe and the slide to obtain single-stranded DNA,

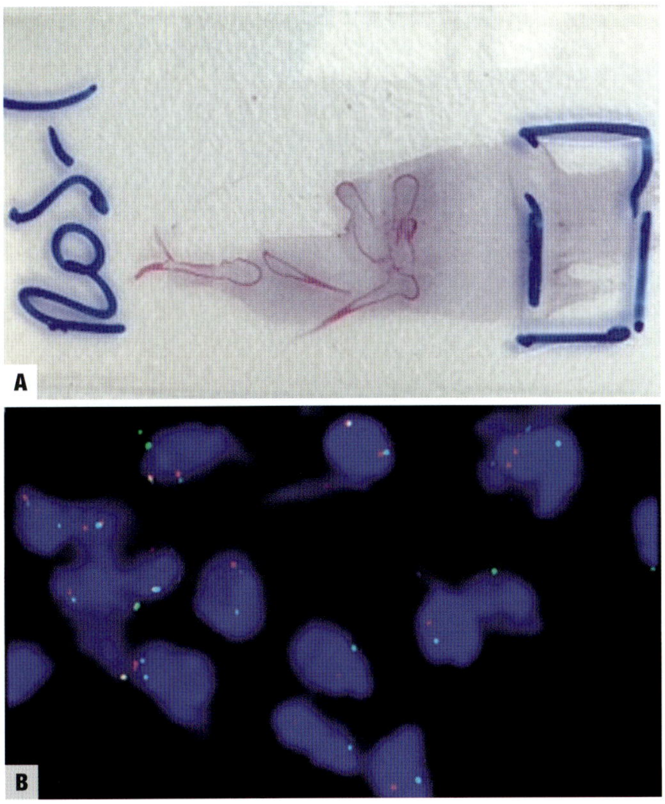

Fig. 2.27 *ROS1* translocation. **A,B** Presence of *ROS1* translocation in FISH performed on a Pap-stained direct smear. The direct smear has been assessed under microscopy to select the best area for the FISH.

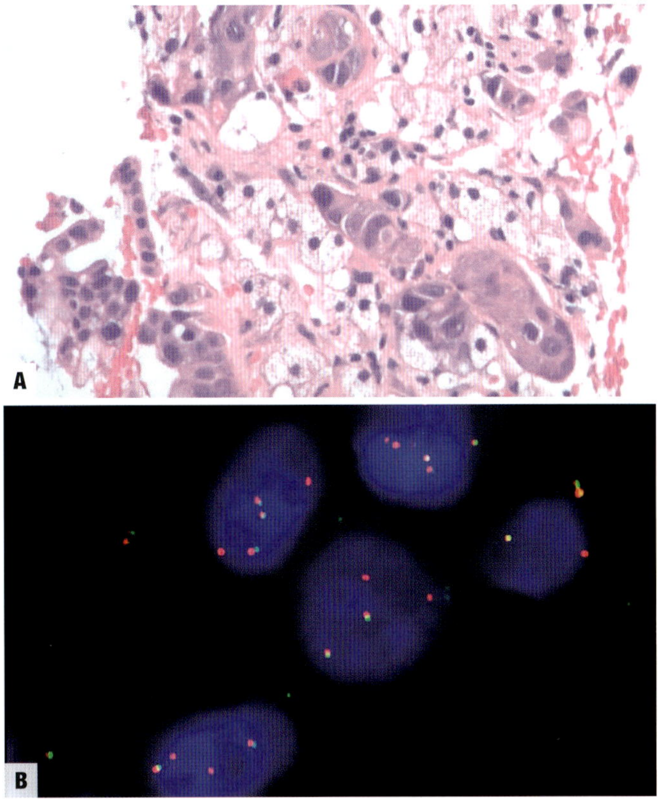

Fig. 2.28 ALK-positive carcinoma. **A** Appearances suggestive of squamous cell carcinoma (cell block, H&E). **B** ALK-positive carcinoma demonstrated by loss of green signals and retention of red signals in positive cells on this direct smear (*ALK* FISH).

hybridization, post-hybridization washes, nuclear DNA counterstaining, and examination and scoring {806,746}. There are different protocols for FISH analysis in different types of cytopathological specimens. If smears or cytospins are used, adhesive-coated slides are recommended to avoid tumour cells floating off during the procedure. In cytopathological specimens, the target cells for FISH evaluation may be sparse and strongly intermixed with benign cells, and therefore, in some cases, it may be difficult to differentiate benign from malignant cells on the DAPI-counterstained slide after hybridization. This can be resolved by using relocation software coupled with an automated stage and photodocumentation of the cells before uncovering and hybridizing the specimen. This approach improves the sensitivity and specificity of FISH analyses {806,698}. There are also fully automated FISH systems for the scanning and computer-assisted interpretation of FISH images {167,489}.

Diagnostic applications

FISH is widely used to test for predictive gene rearrangements (including *ALK*, *ROS1*, and *RET*) in non-small cell lung carcinoma (NSCLC) and thus identify patients for targeted treatments {548,921}. FISH testing for *NTRK1/2/3* rearrangements is more laborious and expensive because it requires three different break-apart probes to assess for the three rearrangements. According to current recommendations, a next-generation sequencing–based approach is preferred over individual FISH testing to comprehensively cover gene rearrangements {534,55}. However, FISH for rearrangement testing in NSCLC is indicated when the material is insufficient for next-generation sequencing or if next-generation sequencing is not available.

Testing for *MET* amplification is another common FISH analysis applied in NSCLC. *MET* amplification, which can be targeted with c-Met (MET) inhibitors, occurs rarely in treatment-naïve NSCLC but is one of the most common mechanisms of acquired resistance to EGFR tyrosine kinase inhibitors {103}. However, different cut-off points for defining *MET* positivity have been proposed, and no clear consensus has been reached regarding the definition of *MET* amplification {224,1002}.

Molecular testing

Roy-Chowdhuri S
Engels M
Lozano MD
Savic Prince S
Troncone G

Introduction

With recent progress in treatment options for patients with advanced, inoperable non-small cell lung cancer (NSCLC), predictive biomarkers – including morphological subtype, PDL1 status, and the results of targetable oncogenic driver molecular alterations – are a prerequisite for deciding on the best possible therapy {701,617}. In particular, adenocarcinoma represents a group of distinct molecular subtypes defined by oncogenic driver alterations, comprising gene mutations, rearrangements, and amplifications {920}. Molecular subtyping with matched targeted therapy has led to unprecedented improvements in outcomes in a significant subset of patients with NSCLC {343,848}.

Metastatic non-squamous NSCLC should be tested for targetable oncogenic driver alterations {701,494,617}. The primary tumour or a metastasis can be investigated {494}. As treatment options are rapidly evolving, broad molecular profiling is encouraged as the best standard of care, and, when available, this will enable enrolment in clinical trials and access to the off-label use of drugs. Routine molecular testing is not recommended for pure squamous cell carcinoma, except in select patients with a history of never smoking or light smoking, those of a young age, and those whose malignancies have been diagnosed by small biopsy or cytopathology samples, where the glandular component of an underlying adenosquamous carcinoma may not have been sampled {494}. In the case of acquired resistance while under targeted therapy, molecular reanalysis of metastases at the time of progression enables optimal adjustment of treatment.

Advances in minimally invasive sampling techniques have made cytopathology specimens highly relevant as a source of material for predictive biomarker testing. Often lung cancer is diagnosed by cytopathology alone. Frequently cytopathology may provide complementary tumour material to small biopsies, which may have a limited number of tumour cells and fall short of adequate material for molecular testing {776,134}. Assessment of all available tumour material with optimal triage and processing is the key to obtaining all treatment-relevant information. Current guidelines acknowledge that any cytopathology preparation, including direct smears, cytospins, liquid-based preparations, or cell block, can be used for predictive molecular testing {494}. As discussed below, a wide range of molecular techniques, with varying requirements on tumour cell fraction and quantity, are applicable to cytopathology specimens, provided the assays have been validated for cytopathological substrates and a robust and rigorous quality assurance is in place {778}.

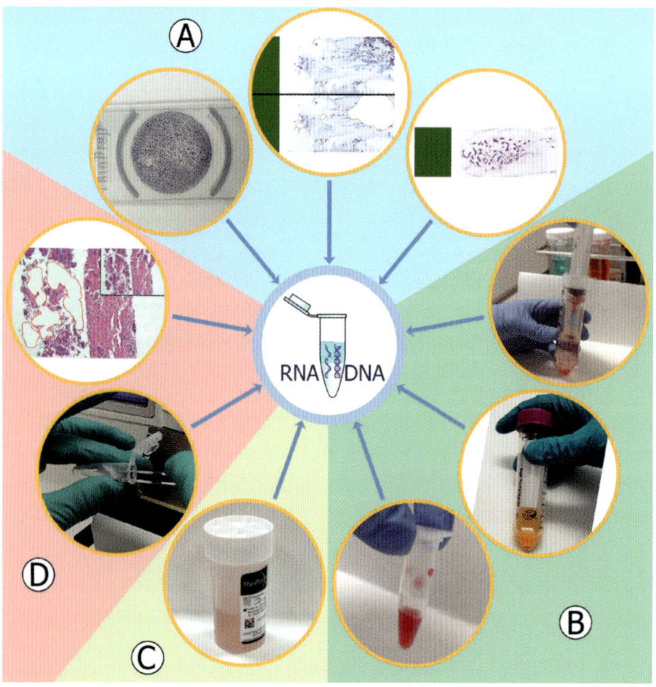

Fig. 2.29 Different types of cytological samples. **A** Direct smears (with/without microdissection/macrodissection). Pap-stained and Giemsa-stained and/or unstained slides. Cell scraping preferred. **B** Needle-rinse, supernatant, and fresh samples. **A** and **B** give high-quality DNA/RNA. **C** Optimal quality for extraction of DNA/RNA. **D** Cell blocks; long formalin fixation can lead to C>T or G>A artefacts.

Technical requirements

Successful molecular testing of lung cancer cytopathology samples is directly dependent on specimen adequacy {259, 510}. Sequencing-based molecular testing has two basic input requirements: the amount of nucleic acid yield, which is based on the overall cellularity of the specimen; and the tumour to neoplastic cell or neoplastic nuclear fraction {780,54}. A minimal amount of amplifiable DNA/RNA is required to obtain a result, and a minimum neoplastic cell fraction corresponding to the analytical sensitivity of the assay is essential to detect a mutation in a background of wildtype signal {780,54,761}. When DNA/RNA is insufficient, no result is obtained, and this is regarded as "uninformative", whereas an insufficient neoplastic cell fraction can lead to false negative results, regarded as "misinformative". The minimum requirement for the neoplastic cell fraction depends on the molecular assay used and the analytical sensitivity of the assay. Enrichment of neoplastic cells by macrodissection or microdissection may be necessary to avoid false negative results due to contaminating DNA from admixed benign cells.

Rapid onsite evaluation (ROSE) by a cytopathologist or trained cytology biomedical scientist can improve the adequacy of cytopathology samples for molecular studies. Cytopathologists are pivotal in the preanalytical evaluation of cytopathological samples for molecular analysis. In this setting, their role is to review the adequacy of the cytopathological material in terms of the neoplastic cell content and the presence of contaminants, which may either lead to false negative results due to non-neoplastic cells or necrosis, or inhibit the amplification process because of mucus.

Table 2.06 Commonly used testing methodologies for guideline-recommended molecular targets in non-small cell lung carcinoma

Molecular alteration	Commonly used testing methodology
EGFR mutations • Most common (~90%) *EGFR* sensitizing mutations include exon 19 deletion and p.L858R point mutation in exon 21; predictive of response to EGFR TKIs • Exon 20 mutations (usually insertions) are heterogeneous, with a subset that respond to TKI therapy and therefore require knowledge of specific mutation • *EGFR* p.T790M mutation is the most common resistance mechanism to first- and second-generation TKI therapy, detection of which warrants switching to third-generation TKIs	• Sanger sequencing with tumour enrichment • Real-time PCR • Next-generation sequencing
ALK rearrangements • Most common fusion partner is *EML4*, but variety of fusion partners identified • Predictive of response to ALK TKIs	• FISH using break-apart probes • Immunochemistry (D5F3 clone; 5A4 clone); may be used as a standalone test without confirmation • Next-generation sequencing
ROS1 rearrangements • Variety of fusion partners identified including *CD74*, *SLC34A2*, *CCDC6*, *GOPC* (*FIG*) • Predictive of response to ROS1 TKIs	• FISH using break-apart probes • Immunochemistry (D4D6 clone); can be used as screening, but if positive requires confirmation by molecular test • Next-generation sequencing
BRAF p.V600E mutations • Activating mutations result in unregulated MAPK/ERK signalling • Predictive of response to combined therapy using BRAF and MEK inhibitors	• Real-time PCR • Sanger sequencing with tumour enrichment • Next-generation sequencing • BRAF p.V600E antibody for immunochemistry not extensively validated
MET exon 14–skipping mutations • Predictive of response to MET TKIs	• Next-generation sequencing
KRAS p.G12C mutations • Most commonly involving mutations in codon 12 • Previously prognostic, but recently p.G12C mutations targetable	• Real-time PCR • Sanger sequencing with tumour enrichment • Next-generation sequencing
RET rearrangements • Variety of fusion partners identified, including *KIF5B*, *CCDC6*, *NCOA4* • Predictive of response to oral RET TKIs	• FISH using break-apart probes; sensitivity dependent on fusion partner (low sensitivity for *NCOA4::RET*) • Targeted real-time reverse transcriptase PCR; may not detect novel partners • Next-generation sequencing
NTRK1/2/3 fusions • Variety of fusion partners identified	• FISH: requires three separate probe sets • Immunochemistry: high sensitivity, but may have underlying baseline expression in some tissues • Next-generation sequencing
PDL1 • Expressed in tumour cells and inhibits T cell–mediated cell death • High PDL1 expression predictive of response to checkpoint inhibitor therapy	• Immunohistochemistry using PDL1 antibody clones (please refer to *Immunocytochemistry*, p. 27)

TKI, tyrosine kinase inhibitor.

Besides specific analytical considerations that are dependent on the given molecular technique, standardized protocols for appropriate test request, specimen collection, fixation, processing, staining, storage conditions, tumour fraction enrichment, nucleic acid quality/quantity assessment, and quality assurance / quality control metrics are also crucial {203,725,91}. In particular, assessment of the quantity and quality of nucleic acids requires several techniques to be used in a complementary manner {54}. Routine lung cancer cytopathological samples may yield only very limited amounts of nucleic acid. Lowering the input DNA concentration below the manufacturer's recommended threshold may be feasible in cytopathological samples, but the DNA input requirements vary between different sequencing platforms {510,699}. Although the exponential increase of target DNA via PCR usually leads to technically adequate results, the total mutation burden may drop below the lower threshold of detection for the assay. Therefore, assay validation with low-input DNA levels is crucial to reliably process cytopathological samples {54}. Indeed, a number of factors can affect the yield and quality of DNA. Fully frosted slides yield lower amounts of DNA, partly because of their high cellular adhesion capability, which poses difficulty when dislodging cellular material during tissue extraction {777}. Significantly higher DNA yield has been reported from slides using a low-hazard, organic, polymer-based mounting medium when compared with the xylene-based mounting medium {54}.

Management of types of cytopathological specimens

DNA and RNA can be extracted from different types of routine cytopathological specimens. Different approaches are used for processing the specimens depending on individual laboratory preferences. Any of the resulting cytopathology specimen preparations and stains are suitable for molecular testing {185,376}.

As previously mentioned, cytomorphological assessment of adequacy and careful selection of specimens are crucial for reliable results. A cytopathological slide or an area on a slide with adequate tumour cell fraction and quantity is selected. The coverslip is removed using xylene and the selected cells on the slide are transferred into buffer medium for nucleic acid extraction without destaining the cells. The most common method for transfer of tumour cells is macrodissection by scraping off the selected area of tumour cells with a scalpel blade. Laser capture microdissection has the benefit of enabling the harvesting of tumour cells from specimens with a very low tumour cell fraction {93,185,54}. In cases where only a single diagnostic slide is available for molecular testing, whole slide image scanning and digital archiving of the slide for cytomorphological evidence of malignancy, before sacrificing the slide for molecular testing, will avoid medicolegal issues {54}. Cell blocks can be processed according to biopsy protocols, using an H&E-stained section for the assessment of adequacy.

In addition to the analysis of intact tumour cells, the analysis of cell-free tumour DNA or liquid biopsy from peripheral blood, residual liquid-based cytopathology fluid, supernatants of FNAB, and effusion or cerebrospinal fluid material has become an option for molecular testing in selected patients. Because the sensitivity of liquid biopsy is still lower than that of tumour samples, a negative liquid biopsy cannot exclude a false negative result and requires molecular testing of a tumour sample for confirmation {996,706,762}.

Fixation

Among preanalytical factors affecting the quality of molecular assays, fixation is key. As a general rule, non-cross-linking fixation using alcoholic reagents (such as wet or spray fixatives) or air-drying provides higher-quality nucleic acids than fixation in formalin. In fact, a prolonged fixation time in formalin leads to C>T sequence artefact, a potential pitfall of cell block–based molecular assays {532}. In general, air-dried and ethanol-fixed slides provide high-quality nucleic acids and similar results in terms of DNA quality {54,780}. Assessment of nucleic acid quantity and quality to assure successful sequencing-based molecular testing requires several techniques to be used in a complementary manner, including spectrophotometer analysis, fluorescence assays, capillary electrophoresis, and quantitative PCR assays {54}.

Controls

Several single-institution studies have shown that the quality of next-generation sequencing (NGS) multigene mutation assays on lung cancer cytopathological specimens is high. However, multi-institutional studies are needed to exclude potential sources of inconsistent results due to differences in gene panels, target enrichment strategies, and platforms across institutions. Because the cell material from routine cytopathological samples is limited, the availability of control specimens is an issue. To get around this limitation, genetically engineered cell lines can be used to mimic actual clinical cytopathological samples in routine practice. However, genetically engineered cell lines have traditionally been only available as artificial formalin-fixed, paraffin-embedded histopathological sections or scrolls. More recently, to fill this gap, the Molecular Cytopathology Meeting Group has developed molecular reference slides harbouring concurrent mutations in the *EGFR*, *KRAS*, *NRAS*, *BRAF*, and *PIK3CA* genes at various allelic ratios, including low allele frequencies (1%), to mimic actual direct smears {521,699}. In multicentre international studies, all participating laboratories successfully detected the mutations in the study set, with minimal variations despite the use of different sequencing platforms. Therefore, quantitative molecular reference slides are a useful tool for monitoring the performance of different multigene mutation assays, and this could lead to better standardization of molecular cytopathology procedures.

Procedures

A variety of molecular testing methodologies are used for interrogating NSCLC specimens (see Table 2.06). These include mutation analysis methods ranging from single-gene-based assays, such as Sanger sequencing, real-time PCR, or multiplexed PCR assays, to broad and expanded molecular profiling approaches such as NGS, as well as testing for gene rearrangements using FISH, ICC, targeted real-time PCR, and NGS assays {845,496}. In general, testing using a broad, expanded panel-based approach is recommended over single-gene-based testing approaches to ensure the adequacy of small thoracic specimens for the evaluation of all the clinically relevant molecular targets required for therapeutic decision-making {619}.

NGS is a massively parallel sequencing platform that can simultaneously screen (depending on the design of the assay)

Table 2.07 Molecular testing of cytological specimens

Basic terminology	Definition	Testing recommendation
Analytical threshold	Minimal input requirement for successful testing as determined by laboratory validation (LOD)	Analytical performance of an assay is measured by its accuracy, precision, analytical specificity, and analytical sensitivity (LOD); establishment of the LOD is critical for sequencing assays used to detect the presence of low-frequency variants (SNVs, indels) and is defined as the lowest allelic frequency at which the mutant alleles can be consistently detected in ≥ 95% of the test cases
Preanalytics	Collection, processing, and handling of specimens	Specimens must be of sufficient quality to be successfully analysed by molecular testing methods
Tumour fraction (T%) or neoplastic cell fraction	Percentage of tumour/neoplastic cell nuclei in a sample (total number of tumour/neoplastic cell nuclei relative to total number of all nucleated cells)	For NGS: 1. T% ≥ 20: reliable NGS readout 2. T% < 20: use one of the following: a. single-target mutation analysis of high sensitivity (PCR-based methods such as Droplet Digital PCR) b. NGS testing with enrichment of tumour cells (laser microdissection) c. NGS with molecular barcodes that label each original DNA fragment within the sample and thereby increase analytical sensitivity and specificity
Input DNA/RNA	Minimum amount of DNA/RNA to obtain valid results	Nucleic acid input for NGS testing depends on the assay and platform used, gene panel size, target enrichment method, and DNA quality

LOD, lowest limit of detection; NGS, next-generation sequencing.

for a variety of genetic alterations, including single-nucleotide variations, indels, copy-number changes, gene fusions (including the ability to detect novel fusion partners), tumour mutation burden, and microsatellite instability. In general, RNA-based testing is superior to DNA-based testing for fusion detection using NGS.

Molecular targets for NSCLC are a rapidly evolving field, with nine biomarkers currently recommended by the National Comprehensive Cancer Network (NCCN) guidelines, several of which are also recommended by the College of American Pathologists / International Association for the Study of Lung Cancer / Association for Molecular Pathology (CAP/IASLC/AMP) guidelines and endorsed by the American Society of Clinical Oncology (ASCO) {620,397,493}. Table 2.07 summarizes some of the guideline-recommended molecular targets in NSCLC and the commonly used testing methodologies.

Other emerging molecular targets have been identified, including high-level *MET* amplification, *ERBB2* (*HER2*) mutations, and tumour mutation burden, and they may potentially benefit some patients with NSCLC {619}. Testing for these rare driver variants is recommended as part of a broader molecular profiling to identify patients who may benefit from a specific targeted therapy or may be eligible for clinical trials for these targeted agents.

Current guidelines recommend tissue-based testing for patients with NSCLC, with cell-free tumour DNA liquid biopsy testing considered in situations where there is insufficient material for testing or the patient is medically unfit for more-invasive tissue sampling {493}.

Diagnostic applications

Testing for predictive markers in NSCLC is performed as a standard of care to identify patients eligible for targeted therapy or immunotherapy, and it is based on studies showing improvements in overall survival when compared with conventional chemotherapy regimens {493,620}.

The presence of sensitizing mutations in *EGFR* (exons 18–21) predicts the response to *EGFR* tyrosine kinase inhibitor (TKI) therapy {513,663,670}. Sensitizing *EGFR* mutations are detected in approximately 10% of White patients with NSCLC but can be found at a much higher prevalence (as high as 50%) in Asian patients. Patients with *EGFR* exon 20 insertion mutations are usually resistant to *EGFR* TKI, although a subset of exon 20 alterations confer TKI sensitivity {659}. Therefore, knowledge of the specific *EGFR* exon 20 mutation is critical for guiding therapeutic decisions.

BRAF p.V600E mutations are seen in a very small subset (1–2%) of patients with lung adenocarcinoma and respond to combination therapy using dabrafenib and trametinib {700,620}. Although non-p.V600E mutations in *BRAF* are seen in patients with NSCLC, these are currently not targeted by specific therapeutic agents.

ALK and *ROS1* fusions have been identified in a small subset of patients with NSCLC (5% and 2%, respectively) and show various fusion partners, with all fusion variants predictive of a response to appropriately targeted therapy {450,197}.

NTRK1/2/3 fusions are seen in a wide range of solid tumours, including in 0.2% of patients with lung cancer. Patients with NSCLC harbouring NTRK gene fusions are eligible for treatment with NTRK inhibitors as a first-line or subsequent therapy option {225,620}.

The presence of *MET* exon 14–skipping mutations, seen in 3–4% of patients with NSCLC, predicts responsiveness to selective c-Met (MET) inhibitors {983,620}.

RET rearrangements are found in 1–2% of patients with NSCLC, and testing is recommended to determine eligibility for targeted therapy with selective RET inhibitors {226,620}.

Unfortunately, the development of secondary resistance to first-line targeted treatment is inevitable. Molecular resistance mechanisms in general include on-target secondary mutations and off-target pathway activations; for example, *EGFR* TKI therapy can lead to acquired resistance mechanisms including an *EGFR* exon 20 p.T790M mutation in 60% of patients under first- or second-generation EGFR TKI therapy, and the acquisition of *MET* or *ERBB2* amplifications accompanied by histopathological transformation to small cell carcinoma {241,671}.

PDL1 testing and implications for therapy are covered elsewhere in this volume.

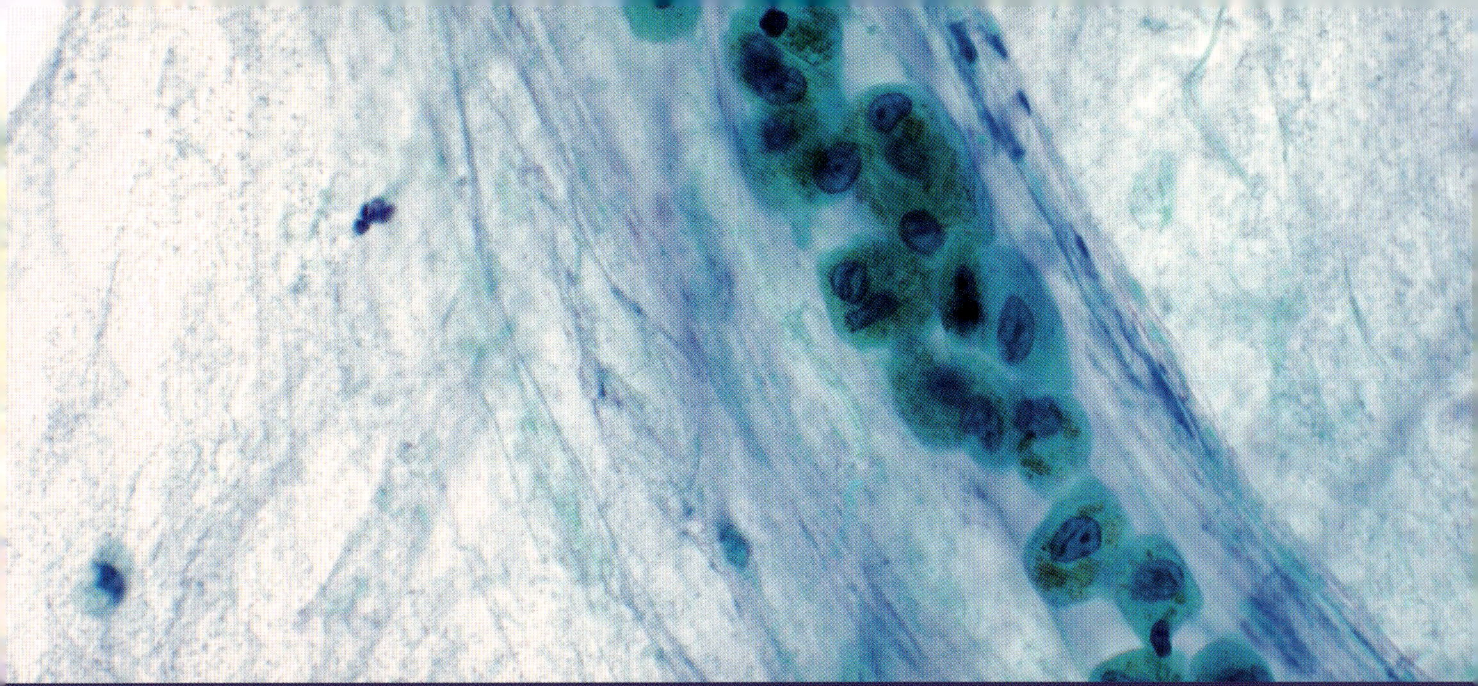

3

Diagnostic category: Insufficient/Inadequate/Non-diagnostic

Edited by: Field AS, Kholova I

Introduction

Canberk S
Bellevicine C
Bongiovanni M
Maleki Z
Savic Prince S
Vigliar E

In respiratory cytopathology, specimen adequacy plays a pivotal role in the interpretation and rendering of a diagnosis, the application of ancillary studies, and clinical decision-making. Specimen adequacy is defined in relation to the specimen type, medical history, clinical symptoms, and imaging findings using the triple-test approach {465,895}. Terms such as "Insufficient", "Inadequate", and "Non-diagnostic" have been used interchangeably to describe this category of specimens. A specimen is categorized as "Insufficient/Inadequate/Non-diagnostic" when the cytopathology material does not contain any diagnostic material that could explain the imaging findings or clinical symptoms. A cytopathologist or institution should select one term and use it consistently. The report should always state that "correlation with clinical and imaging findings is required".

Until recently, sputum specimens have been the only respiratory specimen with a relatively well-defined adequacy criterion {300,149}. More recently, there have been several published definitions of an inadequate sample, by the Papanicolaou Society of Cytopathology (PSC) in 2016 {465,676}, and by the Japan Lung Cancer Society (JLCS) and the Japanese Society of Clinical Cytology (JSCC) in 2020 in a revised cytology reporting system for lung cancer {338}. These reflect the different modalities available for the cytopathological diagnosis of pulmonary lesions, each of which strictly requires a different definition of what is "Satisfactory" or "Adequate". The PSC guidelines include the category "Non-diagnostic" for a "specimen [...] which provides no useful diagnostic information about the pulmonary nodule, cyst, or mass lesion identified by imaging findings". The Japanese system uses a stepwise approach, with an initial assessment of "Adequate", which is defined as adequate for cytopathological evaluation and clarified as the presence of abundant cellular material, or "Inadequate", where there is no abundant cellular material or where obscuring artefact is present, but both of these can have limitations in interpretation and may not diagnose the lesion identified on imaging {106}.

Definition

Raymond WA
Canberk S
Maleki Z

A specimen categorized as "Insufficient/Inadequate/Non-diagnostic" lacks sufficient material in quantity or quality for a reliable diagnosis (see Box 3.01).

Discussion and background

Canberk S
Bellevicine C
Vigliar E

The causes of "Insufficient/Inadequate/Non-diagnostic" cytopathology include a paucity of cellular material; extensive necrosis; poor preparation, fixation, or staining; and obscuring of potentially diagnostic material by blood, inflammatory cells, mucus, or other material. The reasons for an "Insufficient" specimen should be documented in the report. If there is any atypical material, however scant, in a cytopathology specimen, even if the slides are otherwise insufficient, the case is immediately categorized as "Atypical" rather than "Insufficient".

Adequacy assessment in lung cytopathology is critical to rendering an accurate diagnosis and allowing triage for the selection of cost-effective ancillary testing if needed for timely management. However, such assessments are challenging, primarily because of poorly defined adequacy criteria for both exfoliative and FNAB samples. In this context, integration with clinical and imaging findings is required in a triple-test approach, wherever possible. It is recognized that in some low- and middle-income country settings there may not be any imaging available with which to correlate a sputum sample.

Any specimen can be regarded as adequate if the material demonstrates a pathological process consistent with the clinical and imaging findings and can be appropriately categorized as "Benign", "Atypical", "Suspicious for malignancy", or "Malignant". However, if nonspecific benign cytopathological material is present on the slides and does not correlate with a suspicious radiological mass or lesion, a malignant process cannot be excluded and the implication is that further biopsy, repeat sampling of the lesion, or other investigation will be required. Cytopathologists can decide to report these cases as "Benign" with a clear description of the material found on the cytopathological preparations, and add a mandatory caveat statement in the report conclusion that "the material may not represent the target lesion on imaging and further biopsy is recommended", or they can report the material as "Non-diagnostic". Each cytopathologist and institution will determine how they report these cases, depending on local historical usage, the availability of imaging to allow for correlation, and billing concerns related to the terms "Insufficient" and "Inadequate", and they should be consistent and clearly communicate the result to their clinicians.

The term "Non-diagnostic" is not recommended for use in cases where there is good benign cytopathological material that does not correlate with a pulmonary nodule or other suspicious imaging, and at the same time, "Insufficient" or "Inadequate" is used to categorize cases where there is a lack of cellular material, poor smearing, poor fixation with artefact, and poor staining, or where there is inflammation or other material obscuring the cytopathological material.

The diversity of cell types and tumour types in the respiratory system and the criteria for specimen adequacy will vary according to the specimen type and sampling technique being used and on the availability of rapid onsite evaluation (ROSE). Currently, there are no universal numerical cellular adequacy criteria. In the case of non-small cell lung cancer diagnosis, the specimen also must be adequate for ancillary testing including ICC and next-generation sequencing for predictive biomarker testing.

The semi-quantitative criteria for sputum and bronchoalveolar lavage (BAL) specimens have remained the same over the past few decades, but adequacy criteria are difficult to define. The presence of respiratory epithelial cells, alveolar macrophages, or inflammatory cells may not provide a useful assessment of adequacy when the cytopathological material is discordant with the imaging findings, such as a distinct, well-defined lung lesion on CXR {675,465}. Therefore, in these settings, a multidisciplinary evaluation of clinical, imaging, and cytopathological features plays a crucial role in assessing sample adequacy.

Box 3.01 Characteristics of an "Insufficient/Inadequate/Non-diagnostic" specimen

- No pathological infectious microorganisms, including bacteria, fungal elements, parasites, parasite ova, or larvae, in the intracellular or extracellular space
- No nuclear or cytoplasmic viral cytopathic effect
- No abundance of inflammatory cells (e.g. lymphocytes, neutrophils, or eosinophils) to suggest an inflammatory or allergic reaction
- No granulomatous inflammation
- No diagnostic matrix or acellular material such as fat, amyloid, clean mucin, proteinaceous fragments, or aspirated foreign material
- Pulmonary macrophages that do not contain haemosiderin pigment, melanin pigment, fatty vacuoles, or other pathological substances suggestive of a pathological condition
- No cytological atypia
- Sputum sample devoid of any pulmonary macrophages, or insufficient material to prepare two smears

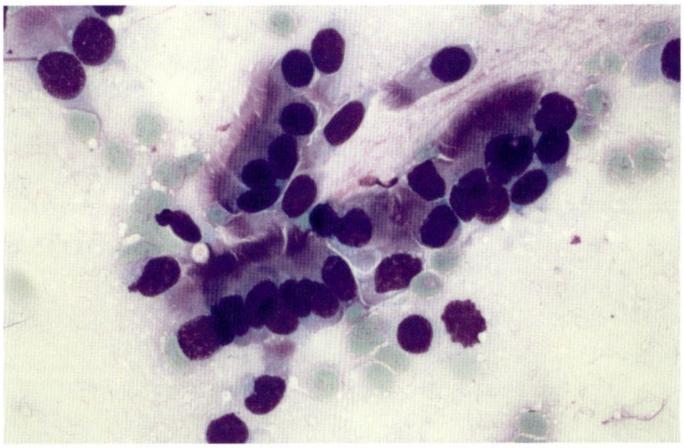

Fig. 3.01 "Insufficient/Inadequate/Non-diagnostic". Benign ciliated respiratory epithelium is present in this endobronchial ultrasound–guided transbronchial FNAB of a patient with a lung mass on CXR in the right middle lobe. This may be reported as "Benign" with a caveat in the conclusion that "this material may not represent the imaging, and repeat study is recommended", or as "Non-diagnostic" (bronchial brushing, Giemsa).

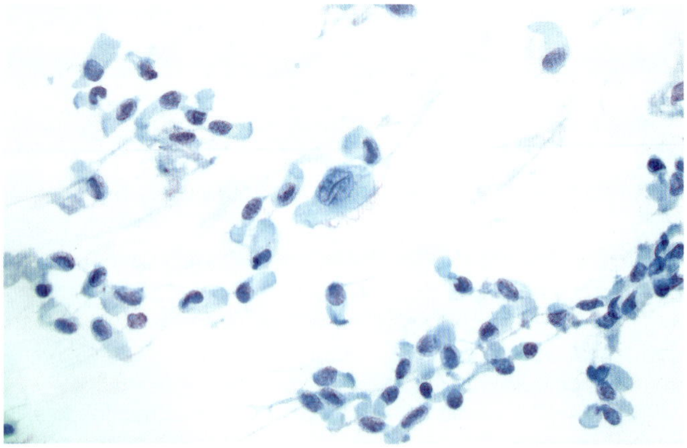

Fig.3.02 "Insufficient/Inadequate/Non-diagnostic". Benign ciliated bronchial epithelium is present in this endobronchial ultrasound–guided transbronchial FNAB of a patient with a lung mass on CXR in the right middle lobe. This may be reported as "Benign" with a caveat in the conclusion that "this material may not represent the imaging, and repeat study is recommended", or as "Non-diagnostic" (Pap).

To recognize and define an "Inadequate" cytopathological specimen, the features of an adequate specimen should be recognized. Specific features to determine adequacy in each of the following specimen types are listed, and it is noted that none require a specific number of cells or cell types.

Sputum

Sputum sample adequacy depends on several factors, including the number of alveolar macrophages, the volume of material processed, the modality of sputum sampling (i.e. whether a spontaneous, induced, or deep-cough specimen is being assessed), and the location and size of the radiologically suspected lesion. An indicator of sputum sample adequacy is a "high number of alveolar macrophages" (although no numerical cut-off point has been defined), along with ciliated columnar bronchial cells {300,149} and a recommended sufficient volume to produce at least two smears {675,465}. Samples should include at least a few alveolar macrophages and ciliated columnar cells on several slides or in a liquid-based cytopathology (LBC) preparation, and if these are absent or obscured the material is categorized as "Inadequate" {465}. A large meta-analysis of classic sputum sample series showed "Insufficient" rates ranging from 0.8% to 29.7%, with an average of 13.8% {71}, but this variability is influenced by the lack of agreement in the definition of an adequate sample. In a recent series, statistically significant differences in adequacy rates were observed between spontaneous and induced sputa, with the latter showing a higher number of adequate samples (91.8%) {624}. In addition, several studies showed a decreased sensitivity of sputum sampling in the detection of diagnostic cells for patients affected by peripherally located lung masses {815}.

Bronchial washing and bronchoalveolar lavage

Bronchial washing (BW) and bronchoalveolar lavage (BAL) have been deemed adequate when they contain > 10 alveolar macrophages per 2 mm^2 using a high-power field diameter of 0.5 mm, which is equivalent to the previously reported value of 20 alveolar macrophages per 10 HPF for most modern microscopes {179}. BB and BAL specimens are considered "Inadequate" when containing numerous bronchial epithelial cells, the number of which should not exceed the number of alveolar macrophages, or when there is obscuring mucopurulent exudate or blood contamination {119,676,729}. BW is preferentially employed for the cytopathological sampling of centrally located lesions, whereas BAL allows sampling of the peripheral lung parenchyma. BAL is usually employed in combination with other cytopathological and histopathological sampling techniques during bronchoscopies, but its diagnostic yield is limited: in a series of 260 bronchoscopies, only 1% of cancer diagnoses would have been missed in the absence of BAL sampling {61}. Recent evidence suggests that routine BW cytopathology may not be justified during bronchoscopy procedures {288}.

Bronchial brushing

Bronchial brushing (BB) specimens, either as direct smears or in LBC preparations, should include abundant bronchial epithelial cells {676}, and macrophages may be present. A lack of bronchial epithelial cells, or poor smearing or fixation of the epithelial component, which is most commonly air-drying artefact of alcohol-fixed Pap-stained smears, is regarded as "Inadequate". BB cytopathology is often performed at the same time as or after a forceps biopsy (with no difference in the diagnostic yield based on the sequence of sampling), or at times after FNAB {938}. Although BB provides the highest diagnostic yield for peripheral lesions beyond the segmental bronchus, the sensitivity of endobronchial FNAB for the sampling of central lesions is reported to be higher than for both BB and BW {815}.

Transthoracic FNAB

A transthoracic FNAB should include some alveolar macrophages, which generally contain carbon with or without haemosiderin, and may include bronchial epithelial cells, reactive type 2 pneumocytes, and tissue fragments of collapsed alveolar septa.

Endobronchial ultrasound–guided transbronchial FNAB

An endobronchial ultrasound-guided transbronchial FNAB (EBUS-TBFNAB) should include reactive bronchial ciliated columnar cells or > 40 lymphocytes in the area of highest cellularity, in greater numbers than a CT-guided transbronchial approach {101,17}. Direct smears or LBC preparations are regarded as "Inadequate" when they are too sparsely cellular and lack alveolar macrophages or bronchial epithelial cells, or

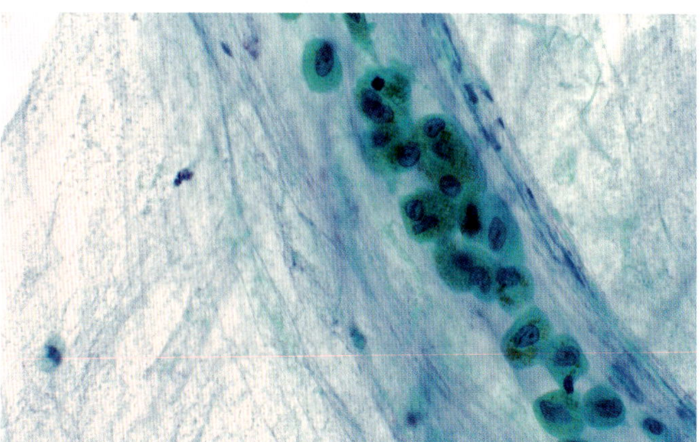

Fig.3.03 Alveolar macrophages. Alveolar macrophages in sputum sample (Pap).

when they are too poorly smeared or fixed to allow cytomorphological assessment.

EBUS-TBFNAB is usually employed for sampling central and endobronchial lung lesions suspicious on imaging and for staging patients with lung cancer through the sampling of mediastinal and hilar lymph nodes. The ultrasound-guided technique has largely substituted the earlier blind procedure originally developed by Wang and colleagues {499}. The "Insufficient" rate depends on different factors, including the presence of a cytopathologist providing ROSE, the cytopathological preparations employed, and the learning curve and expertise of the interventional radiologist or clinician {301}. ROSE is generally recommended at EBUS-TBFNAB to assess specimen adequacy, ensure that the targeted lung lesion is being sampled, and triage the material for ancillary testing, which will minimize the number of repeat procedures required and improve the availability of sufficient material for ancillary testing. ROSE is associated with higher adequate sample rates, with one study showing 7% "Insufficient" FNAB with ROSE versus 25% without ROSE {112}, but when ROSE is not available, multiple (≥ 3) passes are recommended {778}. LBC combined with cell block preparations has been shown by some authors to offer a higher diagnostic yield than conventional smears alone, because it maximizes the yield from needle rinsings, avoids blood contamination that obscures cellular detail, and improves non-small cell lung cancer subtyping by ICC {205,621,797}. However, direct smears (which can be used for directly scraped material for next-generation sequencing) coupled with cell block preparation are preferred by most cytopathologists. It is recommended to use both air-dried Giemsa-stained direct smears, which are commonly used at ROSE, and alcohol-fixed Pap- or H&E-stained smears in all cases, because each stain offers benefits in certain situations. The decision to use direct smears or LBC should be made locally by cytopathologists and their departments, based on historically established local usage and expertise that may favour direct smears, availability of appropriate infrastructure, and cost. If LBC is used for Pap-stained slides, air-dried Giemsa-stained smears will still be required for ROSE, although some cytopathologists use alcohol-fixed rapid Pap or H&E at ROSE. In cases of non-small cell lung cancer diagnosis, for a specimen to be adequate it must provide sufficient material for ancillary testing by ICC {205,621,797}.

In a study of > 13 000 transthoracic FNAB cases, the "Insufficient" rate was low (9%) {1015}. However, a recent meta-analysis of 143 studies showed that the incidence of "Non-diagnostic" results was significantly lower when core needle biopsy was adopted, but it should be noted that "Non-diagnostic" results were more often observed in FNAB from lesions with a final benign diagnosis, indicating a reduction in specificity rather than sensitivity {117,479}. The gauge and the needle type can influence the diagnostic yield of FNAB, with the adoption of a thinner-gauge cutting needle resulting in more samples classed as adequate than aspiration alone {479}. As with the choice of stains and the use of direct smears or LBC, the choice of needle type will be determined by local expertise and experience with the biopsy technique, and the use of ROSE at FNAB (followed by core needle biopsy where required) should be considered to maximize adequate sampling and reduce costs related to repeat procedures. The recent evidence-based guidelines on the collection and handling of thoracic small biopsy and cytopathology specimens strongly recommend ROSE during transthoracic FNAB {778}. In particular, although adequacy rates assessed by cytopathologists, cytopathology biomedical scientists, and cytopathology fellows were comparable, ROSE performed by cytopathologists was more frequently concordant with the final diagnosis {538}.

Risk of malignancy and management recommendations

Canberk S
Bongiovanni M
Raymond WA

Overall, the "Insufficient/Inadequate/Non-diagnostic" category has a risk of malignancy of approximately 40–60%, depending on the mode of cytopathological sampling and the imaging characteristics of the lung lesion {465,318,515}. An "Inadequate" lung cytopathology report should lead to a review of the clinical and imaging findings, preferably in a multidisciplinary setting, and a decision should be made as to whether to repeat the study or proceed to a more invasive test.

Owing to a high risk of malignancy in patients with a mass lesion on imaging, for both exfoliative and FNAB specimens, the number of "Insufficient/Inadequate/Non-diagnostic" samples should be kept to a minimum, and the reason for the use of this "Inadequate" category should be provided in each report. It is recommended that cytopathology services regularly audit their "Inadequate" rates to highlight problems with the procurement of the specimens and the reporting of these cases. The risk of malignancy is reported to be approximately 40% for endobronchial ultrasound–guided transbronchial FNAB (EBUS-TBFNAB), as high as 60% for transthoracic FNAB, and > 60% for exfoliative samples {466,117,105}.

Reporting the reasons for inadequacy in a specimen can contribute to improving the diagnostic yield of a repeat examination {338}. If a sputum sample lacks alveolar macrophages, the report can state this and recommend an adequate deep cough to produce sputum. If a cytopathology specimen is bloody in a patient on anticoagulant therapy, controlled cessation of the treatment can be recommended. In the case of a bronchial brushing (BB) or bronchial washing (BW) of an endobronchial mass that yields only normal bronchial cells owing to the submucosal localization or the fibrotic nature of the tumour, the approach can be changed and an EBUS-TBFNAB performed.

If a sputum sample is "Inadequate", the clinical and imaging findings can be reviewed, and the sputum sampling repeated. This applies both in low- and middle-income countries and in better-resourced countries. If the imaging is suspicious and further biopsy is required, then BW and BB, EBUS-TBFNAB, or transthoracic FNAB or mediastinoscopy can be used to obtain material, depending on the site of the lesion. If these procedures are not available in a low- or middle-income country, then there may be a need to proceed to the biopsy of another site, such as a left supraclavicular lymph node if enlarged, or an open wedge resection of lung.

If a BW and BB are "Inadequate", correlation with clinical and imaging findings is recommended, but in almost all cases repeat BW, BB, EBUS-TBFNAB, or transthoracic FNAB with or without a core needle biopsy will be required. Some clinical teams will have mediastinoscopy available.

If an EBUS-TBFNAB or transthoracic FNAB is "Inadequate" at rapid onsite evaluation (ROSE), as many as four or five repeat passes are recommended {647}. If the specimen is still "Inadequate", or the diagnosis of inadequacy is reported without ROSE at a later date, repeat FNAB with or without core needle biopsy is recommended, and again correlation with the imaging findings is required. Mediastinoscopy may be available. Ancillary testing on the cell block may provide diagnostic material, which can allow the category of the initial cytopathology report to be changed to "Benign", "Atypical", "Suspicious for malignancy", or "Malignant". The multidisciplinary clinical team may decide to progress to lung wedge resection and/or lobectomy, with frozen section providing information to determine the extent of surgery (see Table 1.04, p. 11, and Table 1.05, p. 12, in Chapter 1: *Introduction to the WHO Reporting System for Lung Cytopathology*).

Sample reports: Insufficient/Inadequate/Non-diagnostic

Canberk S
Bellevicine C
Bongiovanni M
Field AS
Maleki Z
Raymond WA
Savic Prince S
Vigliar E

The sample reports provided here are based on the standardized cytopathology report in the *Diagnostic categories and report structure* (p. 8) section of the first chapter. See that section for a discussion on the structure and components.

These are sample reports that include the components required in one possible format; the final report format will depend on local practice and local laboratory information system requirements. For brevity, demographics and information on the macroscopic features and rapid onsite evaluation (ROSE) are not presented here.

For consistency, the term "Insufficient" has been selected for these three sample reports. Cytopathologists and their institutions should decide whether their laboratory will use "Insufficient", "Inadequate", or "Non-diagnostic" for this category and should not use these terms on an ad hoc or interchangeable basis. See the introduction at the beginning of this chapter for a discussion regarding the use of the term "Non-diagnostic".

Each institution should select a term for the main heading of the diagnostic summary, such as "Diagnostic summary" (as used in the examples below), "Diagnosis", or "Final diagnosis", and use it consistently.

Sample report 1

Type of specimen:
Sputum sample (first of three).

Clinical and imaging information:
30 mm solid mass left upper lobe of lung. Presented with haemoptysis. Prior history of colorectal carcinoma. ? metastasis.

Diagnostic summary:
Category: Insufficient
Diagnosis: Insufficient material for diagnostic assessment

Macroscopic description:
3 mL of thick, mucoid, grey frothy material.

Microscopic description:
Only upper aerodigestive tract components are present, with no bronchial macrophages. The material is insufficient for diagnostic assessment.
Comment: Repeat study or consideration of bronchial wash/brush or FNAB is recommended.

Sample report 2

Type of specimen:
Bronchial wash and brush left upper lobe bronchus.

Clinical and imaging information:
30 mm solid mass left upper lobe of lung. Presented with haemoptysis. Prior history of colorectal carcinoma. ? metastasis.

Diagnostic summary:

Specimen 1:
Bronchial wash
Category: Benign
Diagnosis: Benign bronchial material. However, there is a mass lesion on imaging and this sample may not represent the target lesion.

Specimen 2:
Bronchial brush
Category: Insufficient
Diagnosis: Severe air-drying artefact prevents diagnostic assessment.

Macroscopic description:
Specimen 1: Bronchial wash left upper lobe bronchus: 4 mL pink frothy saline rinse.
Specimen 2: Bronchial brush left upper lobe bronchus: 2 alcohol-fixed direct smears.

Microscopic description:

Specimen 1: These highly cellular smears show bronchial epithelium in tissue fragments and as single dissociated cells, with a small number of macrophages and lymphocytes.
Comment: There is benign material. However, there is a mass lesion on imaging and this sample may not represent the target lesion. Repeat study or FNAB should be considered if clinically indicated.

Specimen 2: There is a small amount of material showing severe air-drying artefact, preventing cytopathological assessment.
Comment: There is insufficient material for diagnostic purposes. Repeat study or FNAB should be considered if clinically indicated.

Sample report 3

Type of specimen:
FNAB of left upper lobe lung. Endobronchial ultrasound.

Clinical and imaging information:
30 mm solid mass left upper lobe of lung. Presented with haemoptysis. Prior history of colorectal carcinoma. ? metastasis.

Diagnostic summary:
Category: Insufficient
Diagnosis: Insufficient material for diagnostic assessment

Macroscopic description:
3 air-dried slides, 3 alcohol-fixed slides
3 mL pink normal saline needle rinsings

Microscopic description:
Blood only is present on the smears. There is no diagnostic material in the cell block.
Comment: There is insufficient material for diagnostic assessment. Repeat study should be considered if clinically indicated.

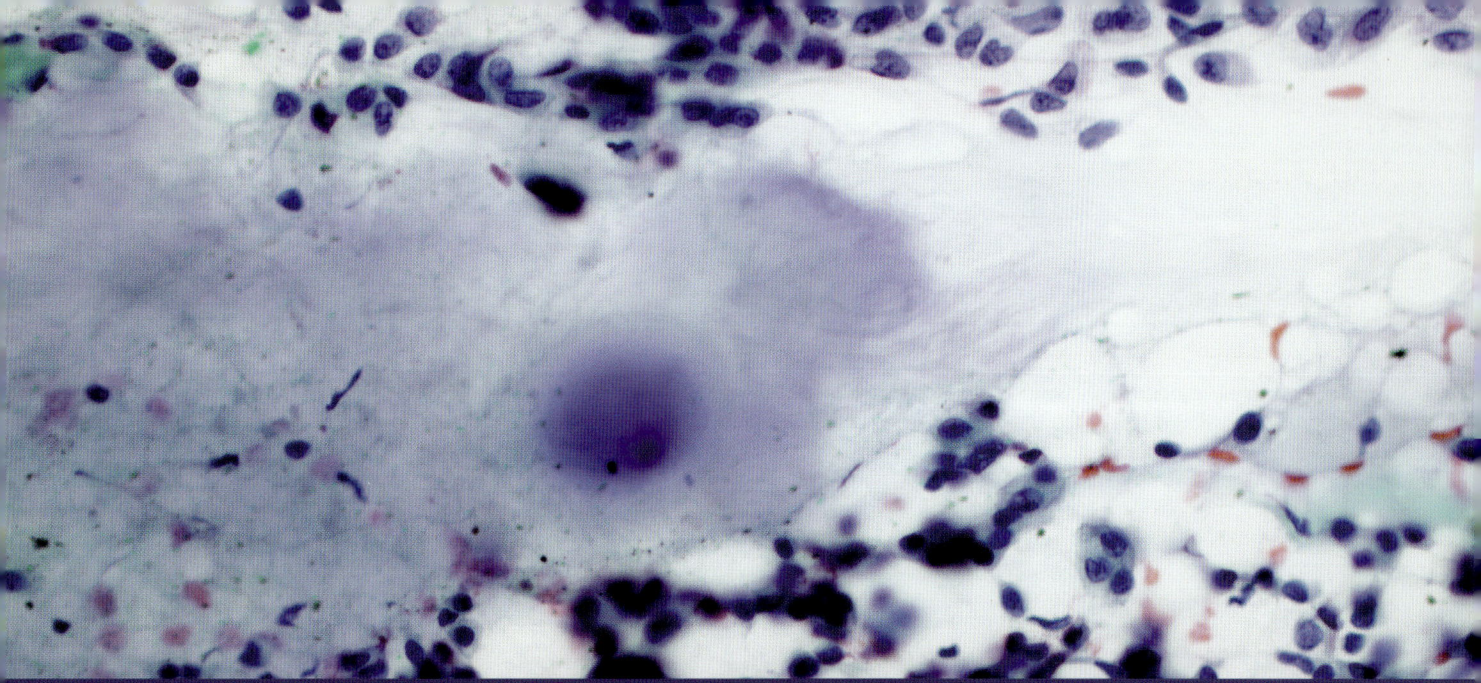

4

Diagnostic category: Benign

Edited by: Chandra A, Field AS, Layfield LJ, Mehrotra R, Osamura RY, Schmitt F, VanderLaan PA

Introduction

Engels M
Michael CW

Sputum samples, bronchial washings, bronchial brushings, and bronchoalveolar lavage (BAL) are used to investigate suspected infections and to rule out malignancy. Sputum sampling has a pooled sensitivity and specificity of 60% and 90% respectively, and the diagnostic yield approaches 95% when combined with bronchial samples {201,424}. Currently, bronchial washing / BAL is the specimen of choice for the evaluation of suspected infectious and interstitial lung disease; these specimens are used for cytopathological assessment including cell counts, identifying lipid- or haemosiderin-laden macrophages, and testing for amiodarone toxicity, as well as to provide material for microbiological testing {569}. The bronchial washing procedure is routinely performed at the same time as bronchial brushing. A fresh sample is required for cultures. However, liquid-based fixatives are suitable for molecular testing, as is scraped material from direct smears {799}.

A "Benign" categorization can be issued in adequate exfoliative specimens that lack malignant cells, and there may be no diagnosis of a specific benign process or lesion. If an FNAB of a nodule yields benign lung components or an inflammatory process and imaging shows a lesion that suggests a benign neoplasm, a "Benign" report can be issued with routine follow-up. If an FNAB of a nodule that on imaging is regarded as suspicious for malignancy yields benign lung components, the case can be categorized as "Benign" and the report should describe the material present and then in the diagnostic summary or conclusion clearly state a caveat that "the material may not represent the lesion seen on imaging". Some cytopathologists may categorize such cases as "Non-diagnostic". The final diagnosis should be established in the context of the triple test, with correlation of the cytopathology findings with the clinical and imaging findings {80}. This is especially important in benign neoplasms such as hamartoma, where the material may resemble normal lung elements. If a diagnosis is not established by FNAB in a case where clinical or imaging findings are suspicious for malignancy, further evaluation such as repeat FNAB, core needle biopsy, or limited resection should be performed.

Definition

Engels M
Michael CW

A specimen categorized as "Benign" demonstrates unequivocal benign cytopathological features, which may or may not be diagnostic of a specific process or benign neoplasm.

Discussion and background

Engels M
Michael CW

The "Benign" category includes inflammatory processes and benign neoplasms found in all types of respiratory cytopathology specimens. The category includes those cases where the material is diagnostic of a specific process (such as acute or granulomatous inflammation) or a specific tumour (such as a pulmonary hamartoma), as well as those cases where the normal components of lung tissue (including bronchial cells, alveolar macrophages, alveolar septa and type 2 pneumocytes) are found. Correlation with imaging is required wherever available. The "Benign" categorization should be followed by as specific a diagnosis as possible. If the cytopathological findings are benign but do not correlate with the imaging when it is indeterminate or suspicious, then the case can be categorized as "Benign", the cytopathological findings should be described, and in the conclusion a caveat should be stated that "the cytopathological material may not represent the lesion seen on imaging". Recommendations for further diagnostic workup should be given {80,196,65}.

Inflammatory lesions that are categorized as "Benign" are presented in this chapter, using a pattern-based approach, in three sections, covering acute inflammation/suppuration, histiocytic/lymphocytic/eosinophilic inflammation, and granulomatous disorders. If possible, the specific type of inflammation should be diagnosed, including wherever possible a specific infectious agent (e.g. *Aspergillus* spp., *Pneumocystis jirovecii*, or CMV), or another specific inflammatory process should be diagnosed or suggested (e.g. lipid pneumonia or pneumonia caused by foreign body aspiration). This routinely involves special stains for organisms, such as the Ziehl–Neelsen or related stain for mycobacterial infection, Gram stain for bacteria, Grocott methenamine silver for fungi, and ICC as appropriate. Wherever possible, correlation with microbiological studies is required. If an exact diagnosis is not possible, description and assignment to one of the morphological patterns is helpful for the differential diagnosis of the lesion. A recommendation for further diagnostic workup is appropriate {408,645,15,290}.

The presentation of benign neoplastic tumours follows the presentation in the fifth-edition WHO classification of thoracic tumours and includes pulmonary hamartoma, sclerosing pneumocytoma, bronchial papillomas, salivary gland tumours, pulmonary chondroma, paraganglioma, perivascular epithelioid cell tumour (PEComa), schwannoma, meningioma, and granular cell tumour. Not every entity described in histopathology has also been described in cytopathology, so not every entity listed in the WHO classification is presented in this volume {979,828}.

Risk of malignancy and management recommendations

Engels M
Michael CW
Navani N
Satoh Y

The published risk of malignancy (ROM) for pulmonary cytopathology cases categorized as "Benign" is highly variable. In most studies, the ROM is between 24% and 42%, and it does not vary to any great extent between the different types of cytopathology specimens {574,465,65,105}. A study with stringent criteria for the adequacy of transbronchial FNAB specimens reported a very low ROM of 3% for "Adequate" specimens with a categorization of "Negative", but the term "Negative" as used in this study differs from the "Benign" category of the WHO Reporting System in that it excludes cases with adequate benign material where the cytopathological finding did not correlate with the imaging findings; it also has to be balanced against a higher "Insufficient" rate in this study {405}. In defining adequacy criteria for each type of cytopathological specimen there should be a balance between minimizing the number of "Insufficient" specimens and the risk of a false negative diagnosis {405}. Further studies will be valuable for the clarification of the ROM of cases in the "Benign" category.

The "Benign" cytopathology report should be correlated with the clinical and imaging features. The aims of the cytopathology study are to exclude malignancy and to diagnose infections, various inflammatory processes, and benign neoplasms. If the cytopathology report correlates with the clinical and imaging findings, and confirms an inflammatory process or a benign neoplasm, then recommended routine follow-up may be to review the patient in 3–6 months after treatment of any infection, or to get an immediate surgical assessment if the patient has symptoms related to the neoplasm, such as respiratory obstruction.

If a sputum sample "Benign" categorization does not correlate with the clinical and/or imaging findings, then bronchial wash (BW), bronchial brush (BB), and FNAB should be considered for further defining the lesion. Spontaneous or induced sputum sampling can be a first-line test in patients with central nodules or haemoptysis and offers a pooled sensitivity of 66%. Three consecutive samples are recommended, and as many as five samples are suggested, to rule out cancer. Sputum sampling has a relatively high false negative rate because it fails to sample a lesion, which is frequently beneath the bronchial mucosa. If a sputum sample "Benign" report does not correlate with the clinical and/or imaging findings, the patient should be referred to bronchoscopy, where BW and BB can be obtained, especially for central visible lesions. These techniques have a combined sensitivity of 88% {569,858}.

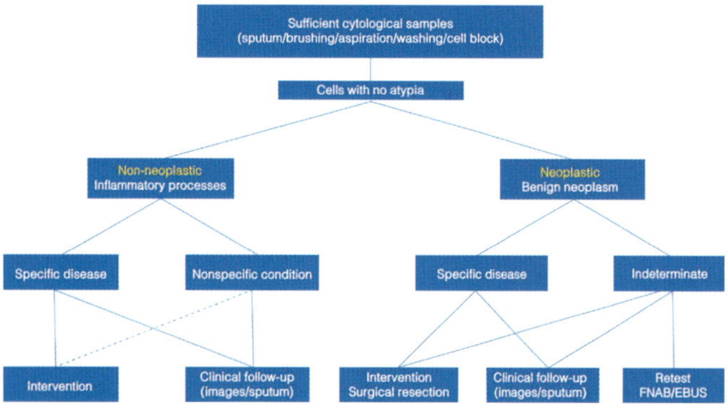

Fig. 4.01 Algorithm for diagnostic workup in benign lung conditions

The hallmark of granulomatous entities, which can be infectious or non-infectious in etiology, is the presence of necrotizing and non-necrotizing granulomas, with or without necrosis in the background. In the presence of these findings, the cytopathologist or cytotechnologist at rapid onsite evaluation (ROSE) or in the laboratory should determine how to triage the sample for further workup, including special stains, cultures, PCR molecular testing, and sensitivity analysis {290}. BW and BB have a low diagnostic yield for detecting granulomatous disease, but BW when combined with sputum sampling has a sensitivity of 88% for detecting acid-fast bacilli. Postbronchoscopy sputum samples can also be collected, with a sensitivity of 35%. Unless the samples are transferred immediately, they should be kept at 0–4 °C.

Bronchoalveolar lavage (BAL) is the method of choice for the diagnosis of a wide range of interstitial lung diseases, with a sensitivity of 85% (94% when combined with biopsy) {162}. If a BW, BB, or BAL "Benign" report does not correlate with the clinical and/or imaging findings, then endobronchial ultrasound or transthoracic FNAB should be considered.

In general, endobronchial ultrasound–guided transbronchial FNAB is best for central submucosal lesions, and transthoracic FNAB is best for peripheral lesions {569,568}. CT-directed sampling can be performed for well-defined nodules or non-infectious tumour-like lesions. Benign lesions account for 30% of transthoracic FNAB specimens {465}. If an FNAB does not correlate with the clinical and/or imaging findings, transbronchial core needle biopsy should be considered immediately if ROSE has been performed, or at a later procedure. If transbronchial core needle biopsy is not available, consideration should be given for open surgery.

Treatment of benign neoplasms depends on whether the tumour is symptomatic or not, and on the type of tumour. The optimal treatment for endobronchial or symptomatic lesions is limited surgical resection, such as wedge resection, particularly for lesions with reported aggressive potential {79}. Otherwise these tumours tend to be slow-growing, with an excellent prognosis, and can be clinically followed up {170}.

Acute inflammation and suppuration

Engels M
Lokuhetty D
Pantanowitz L

Definition

Acute inflammation is an inflammatory pattern dominated by neutrophils, with or without necrosis. It may result in suppuration (the formation of pus).

Clinical features and imaging

Patients with acute pulmonary inflammation usually present with an acute febrile illness with cough and dyspnoea, purulent expectoration, and sometimes haemoptysis, and on imaging there are diffuse or lobular infiltrations {745,358}.

Histopathology

The lung tissue is infiltrated predominantly by neutrophils, whereas macrophages predominate in the resolution phase. With added suppuration, the tissue architecture is lost owing to necrosis, and the area is filled with intact and degenerating neutrophils as well as necrotic detritus, forming an abscess. Granulation tissue develops around the abscess {445}.

Key diagnostic cytopathological features

- Neutrophils showing varying stages of degeneration predominate in a fibrinous, proteinaceous background with or without degenerative changes
- Acutely inflamed tissue fragments of bronchial epithelial cells and fragments of inflamed alveolar septa (in FNAB smears)
- Variable numbers of macrophages, eosinophils, lymphocytes, and plasma cells, which increase during resolution
- Detritus and cellular debris in the background
- Bacteria (which can be of a single type or mixed types) or fungal elements are commonly seen in Pap-stained and Giemsa-stained specimens
- Aspiration pneumonia has pus and foreign-body (often birefringent) vegetable material and non-birefringent muscle fragments, as well as multinucleated giant cells with squamous metaplasia in the epithelial component in later specimens
- Pulmonary infarct presents with hyperplastic bronchial cells showing nuclear atypia, haemosiderophages, and a variable neutrophilic and macrophagic component
- Lipoid pneumonia shows lipid-laden macrophages and a variable number of neutrophils

Discussion and differential diagnosis

An acute inflammatory reaction may occur in a variety of clinical conditions, including acute pneumonia caused by bacterial, fungal, or mycobacterial infection; pulmonary infarction; lung abscess; and aspiration of foreign material. Some infectious agents that induce a granulomatous reaction in immunocompetent patients may result in a suppurative inflammation in immunocompromised patients. This holds true especially for mycobacterial and fungal infections. In aspiration pneumonia, fragments of birefringent plant cells and muscle fibres derived from food may be observed. Acute inflammation can also be seen in various vasculitides. Acute inflammation is uncommon in malignancies unless there is an associated pneumonia related to bronchial obstruction. An acute inflammatory reaction should induce a thorough search for the causative agent. Many bacteria and fungi are visible in routine stains (see Table 4.03, p. 59, in *Granulomatous disorders*).

In pulmonary infarction and in other severe acute inflammatory changes, hyperplasia and atypia of bronchial epithelium may occur and present with marked nuclear and cytoplasmic changes. The affected epithelium shows enlarged nuclei, often with prominent nucleoli, and nucleomegaly can occur. Cytoplasmic changes include clear vacuoles and loss of cilia or the terminal bar. Squamous metaplasia is frequently present, often with nuclear atypia. The differential diagnosis of these changes

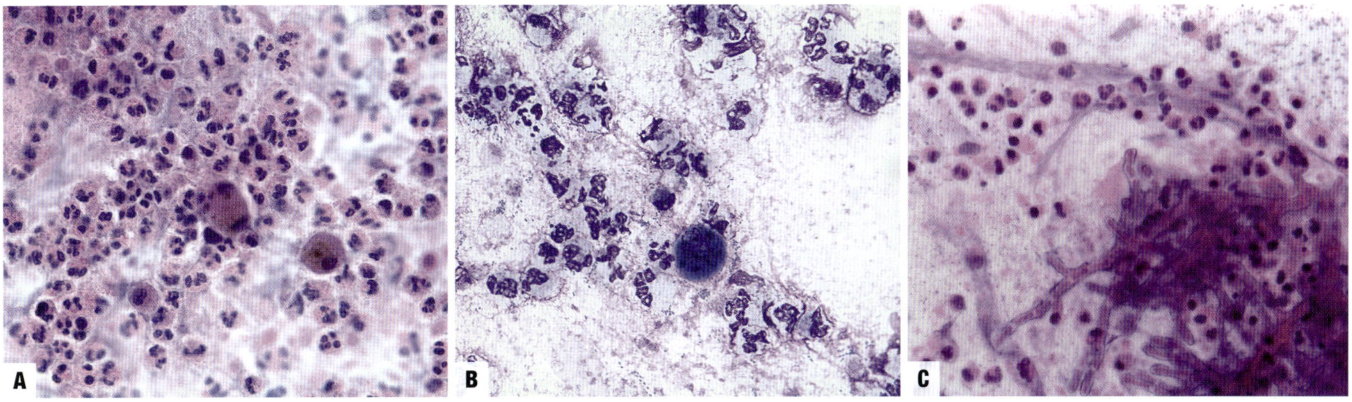

Fig. 4.02 A Acute pneumonia. Abundance of neutrophils and two alveolar macrophages (bronchial washing, H&E). **B** Acute pneumonia. Plentiful neutrophils, one alveolar macrophage, and bacteria in the background (bronchial washing, Giemsa). **C** *Aspergillus* infection. Acutely branching septate hyphae in a background of abundant neutrophils (bronchial washing, H&E).

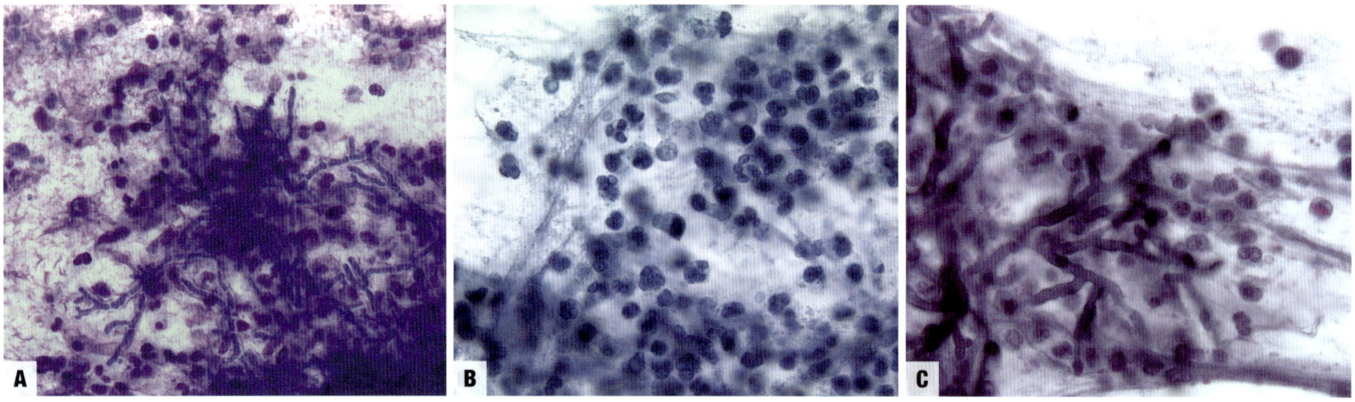

Fig. 4.03 **A** *Aspergillus* infection. *Aspergillus* infection with acutely branching hyphae in a background of debris and neutrophils (bronchial washing, Giemsa). **B** Acute pneumonia. Acute pneumonia with abundant neutrophils, some showing degrees of degeneration (bronchial washing, Pap). **C** *Aspergillus* infection. Acutely branching septate hyphae in a background of abundant neutrophils (bronchial washing, Pap).

includes adenocarcinoma and squamous cell carcinoma. The most important distinguishing feature is the cytomorphological continuum: from normal epithelium, to slight changes, to more severe changes, and finally to reactive atypia in severe inflammation. If cilia are found, this strongly supports a benign inflammatory process. Often, suspicious nuclear findings can also be seen in neighbouring ciliated cells.

Ancillary testing

Many bacteria and fungi can be seen in routine Giemsa and Pap staining, but PASD, Gram, acid-fast stains, and the Grocott methenamine silver stain applied to direct smears, cytospins, and cell blocks are all required to adequately assess suppurative material {258}. ICC on cell block material can be used, particularly for viral infections. Cultures for bacteria and fungi, and PCR for viral infections, mycobacteria, *Pneumocystis jirovecii*, and other fungi, are all indicated {15,290,258}.

Histiocytic, lymphocytic, and eosinophilic inflammatory patterns

Engels M
Lokuhetty D

Definition

A histiocytic inflammatory pattern is an inflammatory reaction with a predominance of histiocytes, whereas lymphocytic and eosinophilic inflammatory patterns are inflammatory reactions with numerous lymphocytes and eosinophils, respectively.

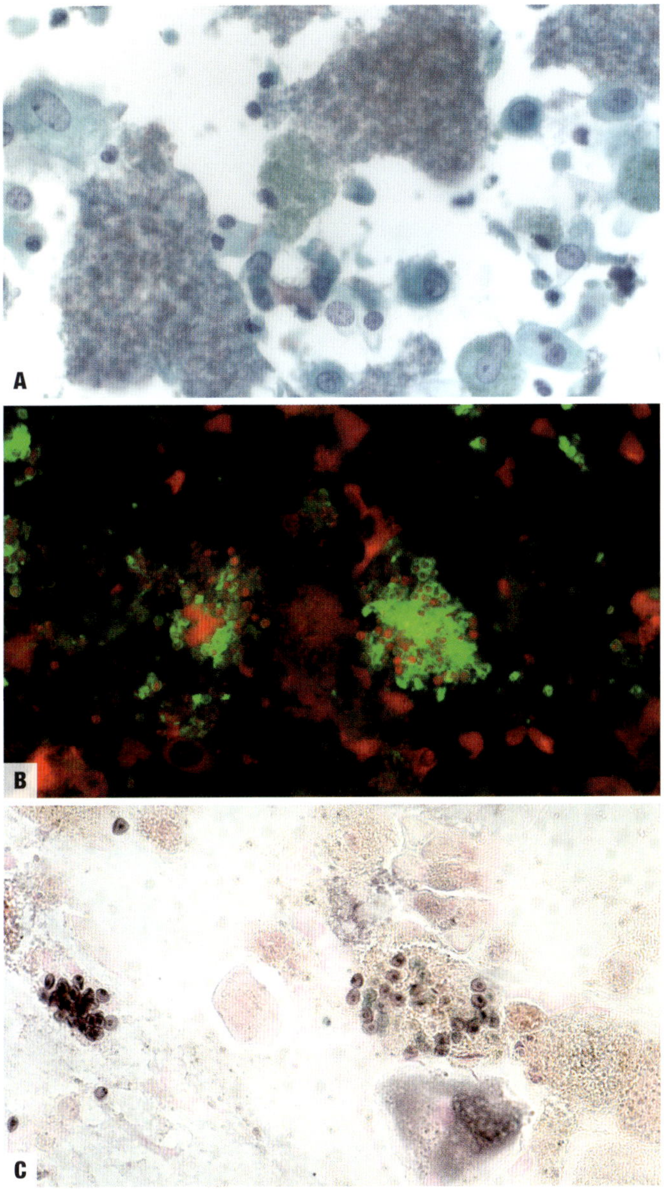

Fig. 4.04 *Pneumocystis jirovecii.* **A** *P. jirovecii* showing the classic foamy exudate with vague outlines of cysts (bronchoalveolar lavage [BAL], Pap). **B** *P. jirovecii* shown by green immunofluorescence (BAL, immunofluorescence). **C** *P. jirovecii* showing typical dot-like intracystic density (BAL, methenamine silver).

Clinical features and imaging

Clinical presentations vary widely depending on the etiology: patients with acute pneumonia present with fever and dyspnoea, and those with chronic inflammatory processes present with slowly increasing dyspnoea, whereas many disease processes have an indolent course with minimal symptomatology (see Table 4.01, p. 56) {452,53}.

Imaging findings also vary and include local or bilateral pulmonary infiltrates and nodular or reticular-nodular patterns with or without enlarged hilar lymph nodes.

Histopathology

A number of diseases give rise to these three cytopathological patterns, each with a predominant cell type. The histopathology varies with the predominant cell present and includes lipid-laden macrophages with a chronic foreign body reaction in lipoid pneumonia {414}; a lymphoid infiltrate of variable cytopathological appearance expanding the marginal zones of reactive lymphoid follicles and lymphoepithelial lesions

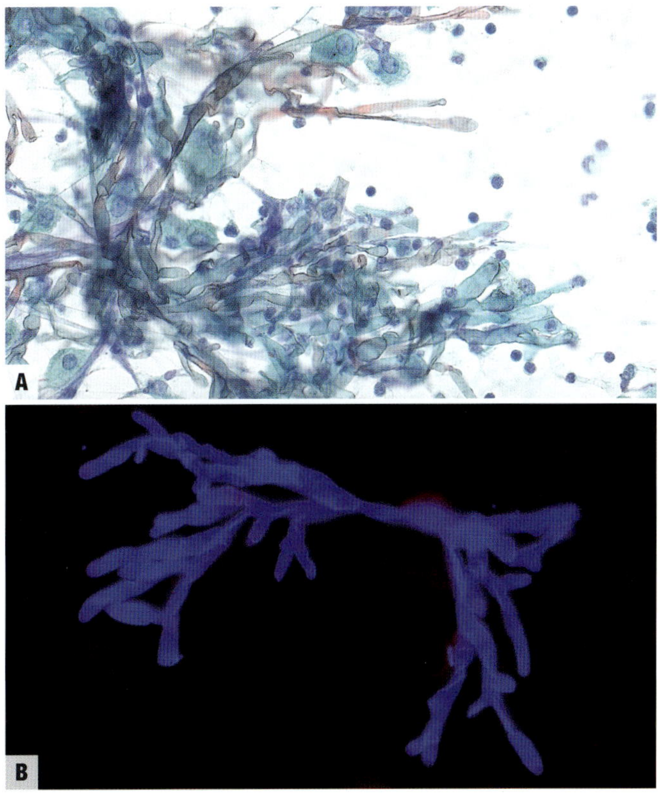

Fig. 4.05 Mucormycosis in a patient with COVID-19. **A** COVID-19 pneumonia in a 69-year-old patient 6 weeks after commencing treatment with corticosteroids: thick non-septate hyphae consistent with mucormycosis, confirmed by microbiology studies (bronchoalveolar lavage [BAL], Pap). **B** Mucormycosis with thick branching hyphae highlighted by immunofluorescent staining.

in MALT lymphomas {82}; eosinophilic infiltrates in alveolar spaces and interstitium with eosinophilic abscesses in acute eosinophilic pneumonia {199}; allergic granulomas and eosinophilic vasculitis in eosinophilic granulomatosis with polyangiitis (formerly Churg–Strauss syndrome) {912}; bronchocentric granulomas, mucoid impaction of bronchi, tissue eosinophilia, and fungal elements in allergic bronchopulmonary aspergillosis {84}; acute eosinophilic alveolitis and histiocytic infiltration depending on the stage of the disease in tropical pulmonary eosinophilia {595}; and collections of Langerhans cells and other inflammatory cells in small airways, resulting in nodular inflammatory lesions in pulmonary Langerhans cell histiocytosis {881}.

Key diagnostic cytopathological features

Histiocytic pattern

- Numerous histiocytes of variable cytomorphology, including multinucleated giant cells
- Macrophages may contain lipid, haemosiderin, surfactant protein, dust particles, and mineral fibres

Lymphocytic pattern

- Numerous lymphocytes and various lymphoid cells of varying size and morphology
- Admixtures of plasma cells, histiocytes, and eosinophils

Eosinophilic pattern

- Numerous eosinophils
- Occasionally Charcot–Leyden crystals

Discussion and differential diagnosis

The commonest proliferation of macrophages is seen with carbon-laden macrophages in cigarette smokers and people living in smoke-polluted settings, whereas in pneumoconiosis the macrophages contain dust particles, which most commonly are carbon and may include birefringent silica and other pollutants (see Table 4.02, p. 57, for the differential diagnosis). Histiocytes predominate in samples of organizing pneumonia and in atypical mycobacterial infections. In lipoid pneumonia, lipid-laden macrophages can be seen and contain Oil Red O–positive exogenous lipid vacuoles, and foamy histiocytes contain endogenous lipids derived from cholesterol in cell membranes in fine vacuoles that may also be positive for Oil Red O. Foamy histiocytes are also found in e-cigarette or vaping product use–associated lung injury (EVALI), which is becoming more important. In amiodarone-induced lung toxicity, macrophages with very fine, clear, Oil Red O–negative vacuoles are seen. In pulmonary alveolar proteinosis, macrophages are filled with flocculent surfactant protein, and in diffuse alveolar haemorrhage, with haemosiderin. Mineral asbestos fibres may be visible as ferruginous bodies within macrophages {53,771,880,857,196, 390}.

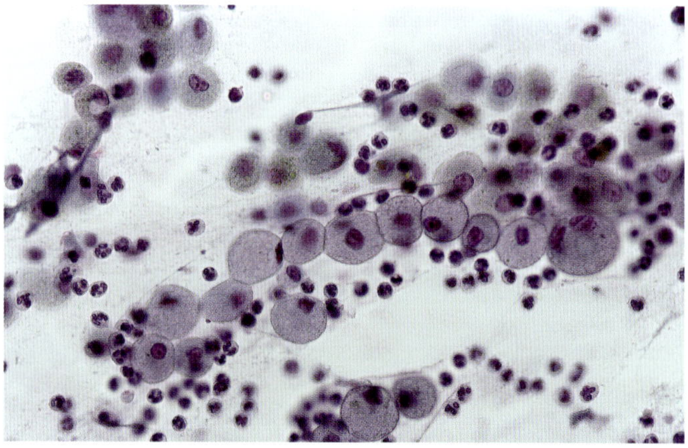

Fig. 4.07 Amiodarone-induced lung toxicity. Foamy histiocytes with abundant cytoplasm filled with small vacuoles, with neutrophils in the background (bronchial washing, Pap).

Benign lymphoid follicles in the bronchial mucosa may be sampled by FNAB or bronchial brush and show predominantly small lymphocytes with a variable number of larger lymphoid cells. Elevated lymphocyte counts in bronchoalveolar lavage (BAL) and an altered distribution of subtypes are seen in interstitial lung diseases, sarcoidosis, Behçet disease, and hypersensitivity pneumonitis. Malignant lymphoma with a low proliferation rate may mimic inflammatory reactions {142,481, 823,434}.

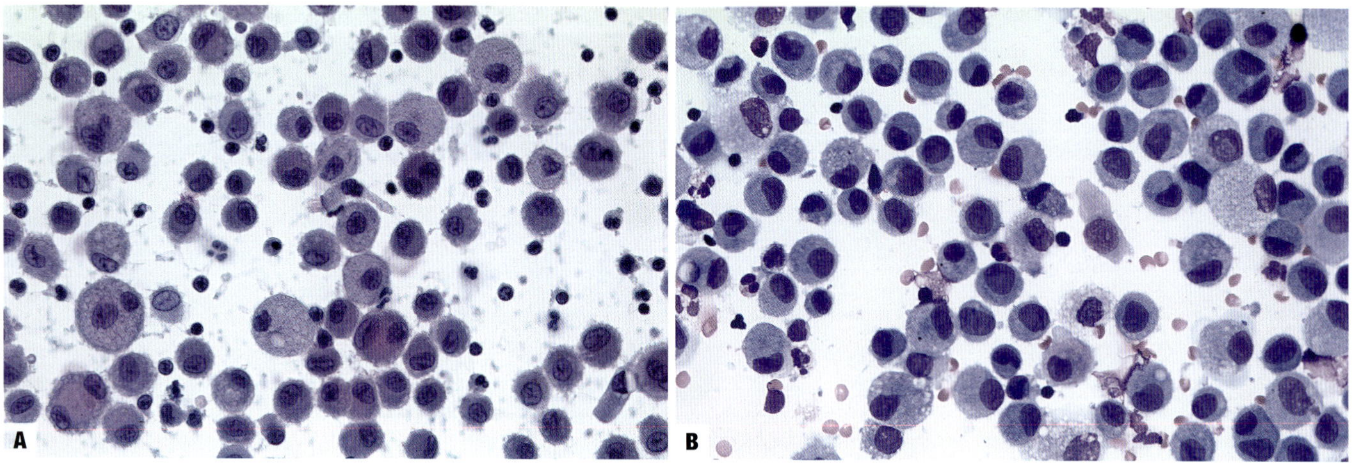

Fig. 4.06 Lipoid pneumonia. **A** Alveolar macrophages, some with abundant cytoplasm filled with fine vacuoles (bronchial washing, Pap). **B** From the same case: alveolar macrophages, many of which have abundant cytoplasm filled with fine vacuoles (bronchial washing, Giemsa). This case is also shown in Fig. 4.09B.

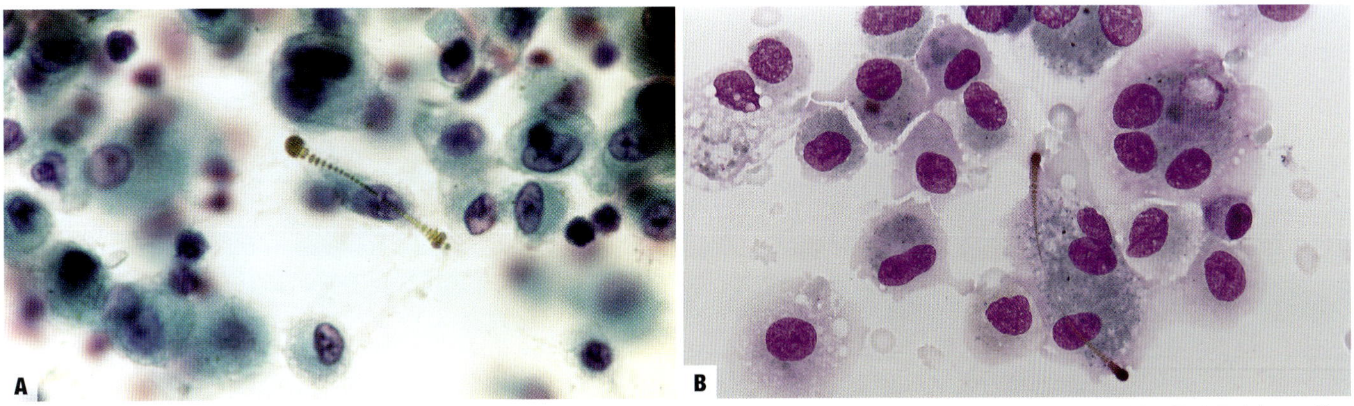

Fig. 4.08 Asbestos fibre. **A** Ferruginous body, possibly in an alveolar macrophage, with other macrophages in the background (bronchial washing, Pap). **B** Asbestos fibre phagocytosed by a large alveolar macrophage, with other macrophages containing carbon in the background (bronchoalveolar lavage [BAL], Giemsa).

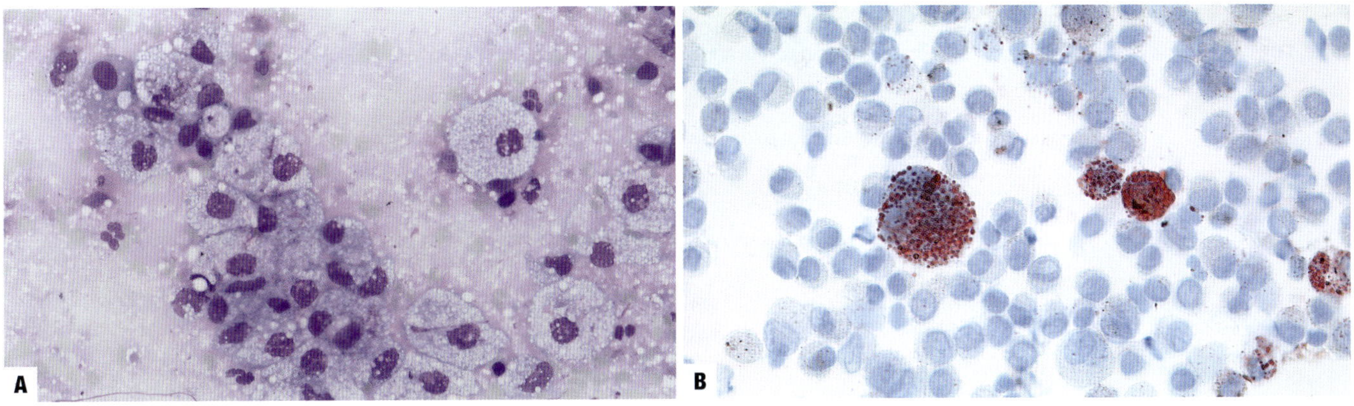

Fig. 4.09 Histiocytic reaction. **A** Foamy histiocytes (bronchoalveolar lavage [BAL], Giemsa). **B** Foamy lipid-laden macrophages positive with the Oil Red O stain (BAL, Oil Red O).

Eosinophilia may occur in acute and chronic eosinophilic pneumonia, vasculitis, asthmatic inflammatory material, allergic bronchopulmonary aspergillosis, eosinophilic granulomatosis with polyangiitis (formerly Churg–Strauss syndrome), and parasitic or fungal infections {199,925,629,965}.

In patients infected with COVID-19, BAL is reserved for those with an atypical clinical presentation, to exclude an alternative diagnosis and to detect coinfections. Hospitalized patients with COVID-19 pneumonia are particularly at risk of developing secondary fungal infections, as are immunocompromised patients who can have a prolonged course of COVID-19 pneumonia.

Ancillary testing

Special stains include the Oil Red O stain for neutral fats, the PASD stain for surfactant protein, and the Prussian blue or Perls stain for iron, and these are routinely performed at the same time with the auramine or Ziehl–Neelsen or related stain for mycobacterial infection and the methenamine stain for fungi, to exclude infectious causes. Many bacteria and fungi are visible in routine Giemsa and Pap staining {258}. ICC may be used when assessing lymphoid material, but the standard practice is to use flow cytometry on lymphoid samples to exclude a B-cell monoclonality and assist with other lymphoid marker analyses.

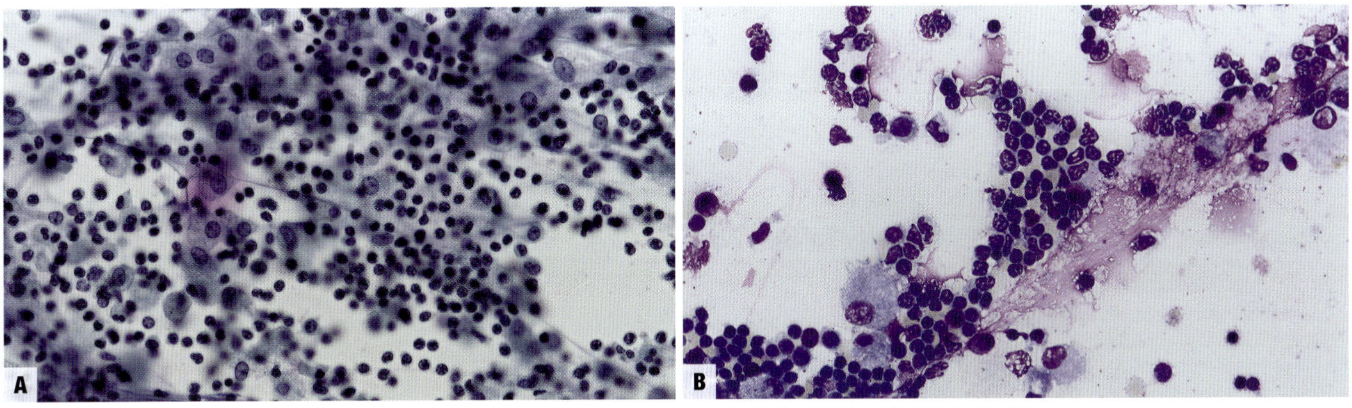

Fig. 4.10 Lymphocytic reaction. **A** Large numbers of small lymphocytes with scattered macrophages (bronchial washing, Pap). **B** In the same case: numerous small lymphocytes and some alveolar macrophages, with mucin in the background (bronchial washing, Giemsa).

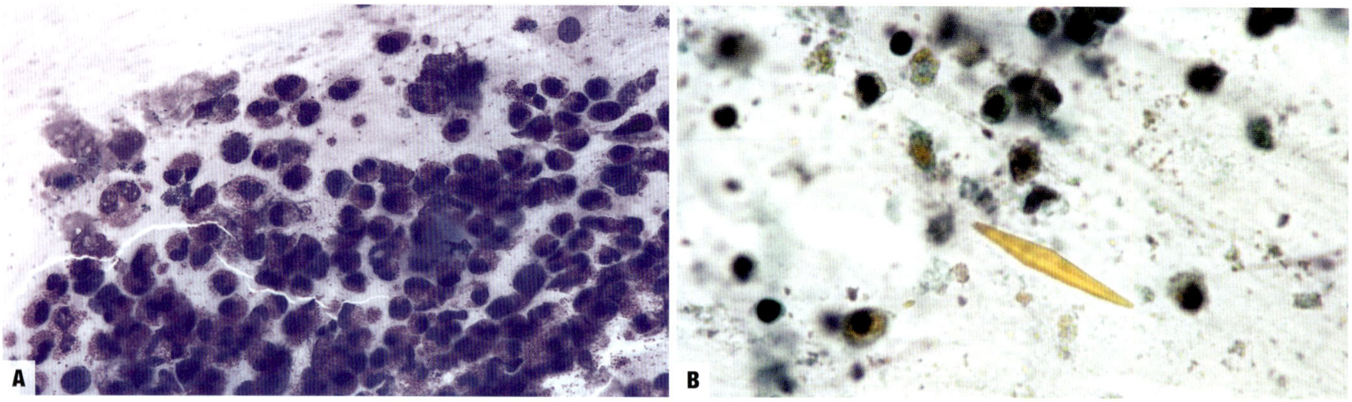

Fig. 4.11 Eosinophilic pneumonia. **A** Eosinophilic pneumonia with large numbers of eosinophils (bronchial washing, Giemsa). Charcot–Leyden crystals were also present. **B** A Charcot–Leyden crystal, with eosinophils in the background (bronchial washing, Pap).

Table 4.01 Diseases with histiocytic, lymphocytic, and eosinophilic patterns: clinical presentation and imaging {452,53,565,252}

Specific disease	Clinical presentation	Imaging (high-resolution CT)
Silicosis	Cough and dyspnoea with gradual onset; exposure history	Dense, well-circumscribed nodules
Organizing pneumonia	Cough, dyspnoea	Ground-glass opacities, consolidation, reticulation, parenchymal distortion
Atypical mycobacterial infection	Cough, sputum, haemoptysis, fatigue, malaise and weight loss	Bronchiectasis, small and large nodules, consolidation, centrilobular nodules, and cavitary lesions
Lipoid pneumonia	Cough, dyspnoea, haemoptysis; history of use of mineral, vegetable, or animal oil	Extensive ground-glass opacities or consolidation
EVALI	Shortness of breath, cough, haemoptysis; use of e-cigarettes or vaping products	Bilateral, diffuse, ground-glass infiltrates
Amiodarone-induced lung toxicity	Variable insidious or acute presentation; various inflammatory reactions including eosinophilic pneumonia, chronic obstructive pulmonary disease, NSIP-like ARDS; history of medication with amiodarone (antiarrhythmic drug)	New chest infiltrates
Pulmonary alveolar proteinosis	Dyspnoea with subacute onset	Alveolar-filling pattern
Diffuse alveolar haemorrhage	Acute dyspnoea, hypoxaemia; history of collagen vascular disease, especially systemic lupus erythematosus	Patchy or diffuse areas of ground-glass attenuation
Lymphocytic interstitial pneumonia	Cough, fever, dyspnoea; often associated with underlying immunological disease	Bilateral ground-glass attenuation, scattered cysts
Hypersensitivity pneumonitis	Acute or chronic presentation; exposure history to specific compounds	Acute: bilateral ground-glass opacities and poorly defined nodules Chronic: reticular fibrotic pattern, honeycomb change, traction bronchiectasis, ground-glass opacities
Sarcoidosis	Bilateral hilar lymphadenopathy; uveitis or erythema nodosum often present	Hilar/mediastinal lymphadenopathy, nodules along bronchovascular bundles
Behçet disease	Haemoptysis, history of uveitis, ulcers in mouth and genitals	Poorly defined areas of increased opacity, thrombosis of pulmonary vessels, focal atelectasis
Malignant lymphoma, low-grade	Cough, dyspnoea	Lymphadenopathy, ground-glass opacities
Eosinophilic pneumonia	Cough, fever, dyspnoea; acute or chronic presentation; rapid response to corticosteroids	Bilateral peripheral subpleural airspace consolidation
Bronchial asthma	Periodic wheezing and dyspnoea	No specific changes
Allergic bronchopulmonary aspergillosis	Episodic asthmatic attacks, expectoration of mucus plugs	Transient infiltrates
Eosinophilic granulomatosis with polyangiitis (Churg–Strauss disease)	Asthma, rash, peripheral neuropathy	Bilateral areas of ground-glass opacity, or consolidation with a bilateral symmetrical distribution
Parasitic and fungal infections	Fever, cough, dyspnoea	Variable, depending on infectious agent and immune status of host

ARDS, acute respiratory distress syndrome; EVALI, e-cigarette or vaping product use–associated lung injury; NSIP, nonspecific interstitial pneumonia.

Table 4.02 Diseases with histiocytic, lymphocytic, and eosinophilic patterns: cytopathological features, differential cytopathology in bronchoalveolar lavage (BAL), and ancillary testing {452,53,565,252,314,443,434}

Specific disease	Cytopathological features	Differential cytopathology in BAL	Ancillary testing
Silicosis	Silica-laden macrophages		
Organizing pneumonia	Increase of lymphocytes, foamy macrophages	Lymphocytes > 25%	
Atypical mycobacterial infection	Macrophages filled with acid-fast rods		Ziehl–Neelsen and auramine stains; PCR; culture
Lipoid pneumonia	Lipid-laden macrophages, Oil Red O+		Oil Red O
EVALI	Lipid-laden macrophages, Oil Red O+		Oil Red O
Amiodarone-induced lung toxicity	Macrophages with fine clear vacuoles		Oil Red O
Pulmonary alveolar proteinosis	Macrophages filled with PASD-positive material; cholesterol crystals		PASD
Diffuse alveolar haemorrhage	Haemosiderin-laden macrophages, intact red blood cells		Iron stain
Lymphocytic interstitial pneumonia	Increase of lymphocytes	Lymphocytes > 15%	
Hypersensitivity pneumonitis	Increase of lymphocytes, foamy macrophages, mast cells, plasma cells	Lymphocytes > 50%	
Sarcoidosis	Increase of lymphocytes	Lymphocytes > 15%	Elevated CD4:CD8 ratio
Behçet disease	Slight increase of lymphocytes		Elevated CD4:CD8 ratio
Malignant lymphoma, low-grade	Lymphocytosis, mostly small lymphoid cells, increase of plasma cells, some multinucleated histiocytes	Lymphocytes > 15%	Flow cytometry; ICC may assist in some cases
Eosinophilic pneumonia	Marked eosinophilia	Eosinophils > 25%	
Bronchial asthma	Slight eosinophilia	Eosinophils > 1%	
Allergic bronchopulmonary aspergillosis	Slight eosinophilia, fungal structures	Eosinophils > 1%	
Eosinophilic granulomatosis with polyangiitis (Churg–Strauss disease)	Slight eosinophilia, histiocytes, granuloma, blood	Eosinophils > 1%	
Parasitic and fungal infections	Fungal structures or fragments of parasites	Eosinophils > 1%	Methenamine silver and PASD stains; ICC; PCR

EVALI, e-cigarette or vaping product use–associated lung injury.

Granulomatous disorders

Engels M
Lokuhetty D
Pantanowitz L

Definition

Granulomatous disorders are entities or lesions containing characteristic granulomas consisting of epithelioid cells and histiocytic multinucleated giant cells with a variable admixture of lymphocytes, neutrophils, and eosinophils. Necrosis may or may not be present.

Clinical features and imaging

Presenting symptoms vary depending on the primary disorder and are often mild and vague, with low-level fevers, but progress to weight loss and debilitation compounded by cough, haemoptysis, and deteriorating lung function. Imaging also varies with the cause, but commonly CXR and CT show enlarged lymph nodes and variable pulmonary infiltrates, raising the differential diagnosis of the primary tuberculosis primary complex and sarcoidosis. Postprimary tuberculosis shows variable hilar and mediastinal lymphadenopathy, pulmonary infiltrates, and cavities, with or without progressive fibrosis. Sarcoidosis presents in most cases with bilateral hilar lymphadenopathy with or without bilateral perihilar or other pulmonary infiltrates {63,641}.

Histopathology

A granuloma is a focal aggregation of epithelioid histiocytes, lymphocytes, and histiocytic giant cells. Their size may vary. Depending on the underlying entity or disease, the granulomas may be discrete or coalescing, have a peripheral lymphoid cuff and/or a peripheral fibrotic zone, have central necrosis, be either caseous or non-caseous in type, and be associated with suppuration. Histiocytic giant cells may also vary in morphology, depending on the arrangement of nuclei within the cell. At times, etiological agents may be identified on routine/special stained sections within or outside the histiocytic giant cells and granulomas {645}.

Key diagnostic cytopathological features

- Epithelioid histiocytes form distinct granulomatous tissue fragments with a variable number of histiocytic multinucleated giant cells that show grouped uniform nuclei, usually in abundant cytoplasm, and lymphocytes
- Epithelioid histiocytes have elongated, often indented (so-called barefoot) nuclei; fine chromatin; and inconspicuous nucleoli
- Cytoplasm is vaguely demarcated and often syncytial in the granulomas
- If necrosis is present it may be granular and caseous or non-caseous and is usually central
- There is a variable amount of hyaline sclerosis around the granulomas
- A variable number of small lymphocytes are present – they may be predominant, whereas eosinophils or neutrophils may be predominant in other cases

Reference(s): {123,258}

Discussion and differential diagnosis

Granulomas occur in a variety of diseases. Infectious agents are an important cause of granulomatous disorders, especially *Mycobacterium tuberculosis*, atypical mycobacteria, and other bacteria including *Francisella tularensis*; and fungal infections including *Aspergillus* spp., *Blastomyces*, *Coccidioides immitis*, *Cryptococcus*, histoplasmosis, mucormycosis, and *Pneumocystis jirovecii*. Several bacteria and fungi can be identified in routine stains, but the assessment of granulomatous cytopathology material requires appropriate special stains (see Table 4.03) {15,290,258,570,123,276}. Correlation with microbiological studies, including cultures and PCR studies, is mandatory where available.

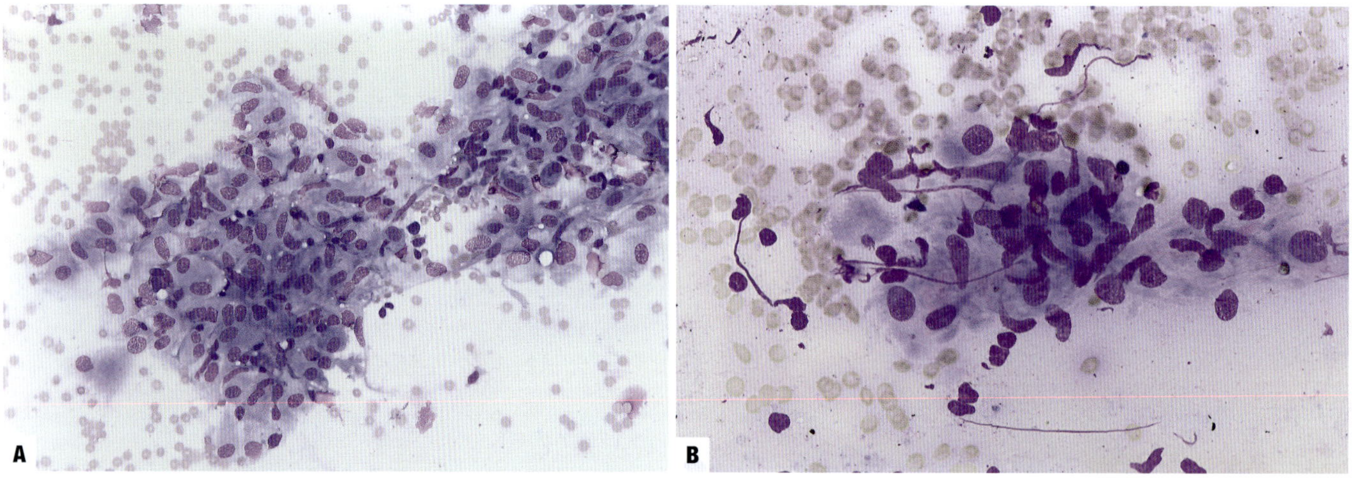

Fig. 4.12 Sarcoidosis. **A** Large granuloma made up of epithelioid histiocytes, with no necrosis (Giemsa). **B** Small, non-necrotizing granuloma of epithelioid histiocytes (Giemsa).

Table 4.03 Granulomatous inflammation: bacteria and fungi in cytopathological specimens {459}

Infectious agent	Morphology in cytological specimens	Stains, ancillary testing	Reference(s)
Actinomyces	Masses consisting of numerous thin, filamentous, beaded, branched bacteria; diameter: 1.0–1.5 μm	GMS, Gram	{552}
Aspergillus	Uniform, septate hyphae (diameter: 3–6 μm) with acute 45° branching; occasionally fruiting bodies or oxalate crystals	GMS	{263,710}
Blastomyces	Yeast-like spherical cells with broad-based budding; diameter: 5–15 μm	GMS	{710}
Candida	Slender pseudohyphae (diameter: 3–5 μm), budding yeast forms	GMS	{710}
Coccidioides immitis	Large spherules (diameter: 10–80 μm) filled with endospores (diameter: 2–5 μm); necrotizing granulomatous inflammation	GMS	{132}
Cryptococcus	Narrow-based budding yeast with variable diameter (5–20 μm); non-staining distinct capsule	GMS, mucicarmine	{853}
Histoplasma	Small yeast forms (diameter: 2–4 μm), seen as negative images in the foamy or vacuolated cytoplasm of macrophages	GMS	{277}
Mycobacterium tuberculosis	Slender, acid-fast rods (diameter: 0.2–0.6 μm), extracellular; caseous necrosis in the background	Acid-fast stains, PCR, culture	{123}
Nocardia	Thin, long, filamentous, beaded bacteria with 90° branching; diameter: 0.5–1.0 μm	PCR	{15,552,97}
Pneumocystis jirovecii	Foamy alveolar casts consisting of multiple rounded, crescentic, or cup-shaped cysts; diameter: 2–5 μm	GMS, PCR	{15}
Zygomycetes	Wide (diameter: 6–15 μm), ribbon-like, pauciseptate hyphae with 90° branching	PASD, GMS	{710}

GMS, Grocott methenamine silver stain.

If no infectious cause is found, further workup in correlation with the medical history and imaging is required. Important non-infectious causes include autoimmune diseases, such as granulomatosis with polyangiitis (previously known as

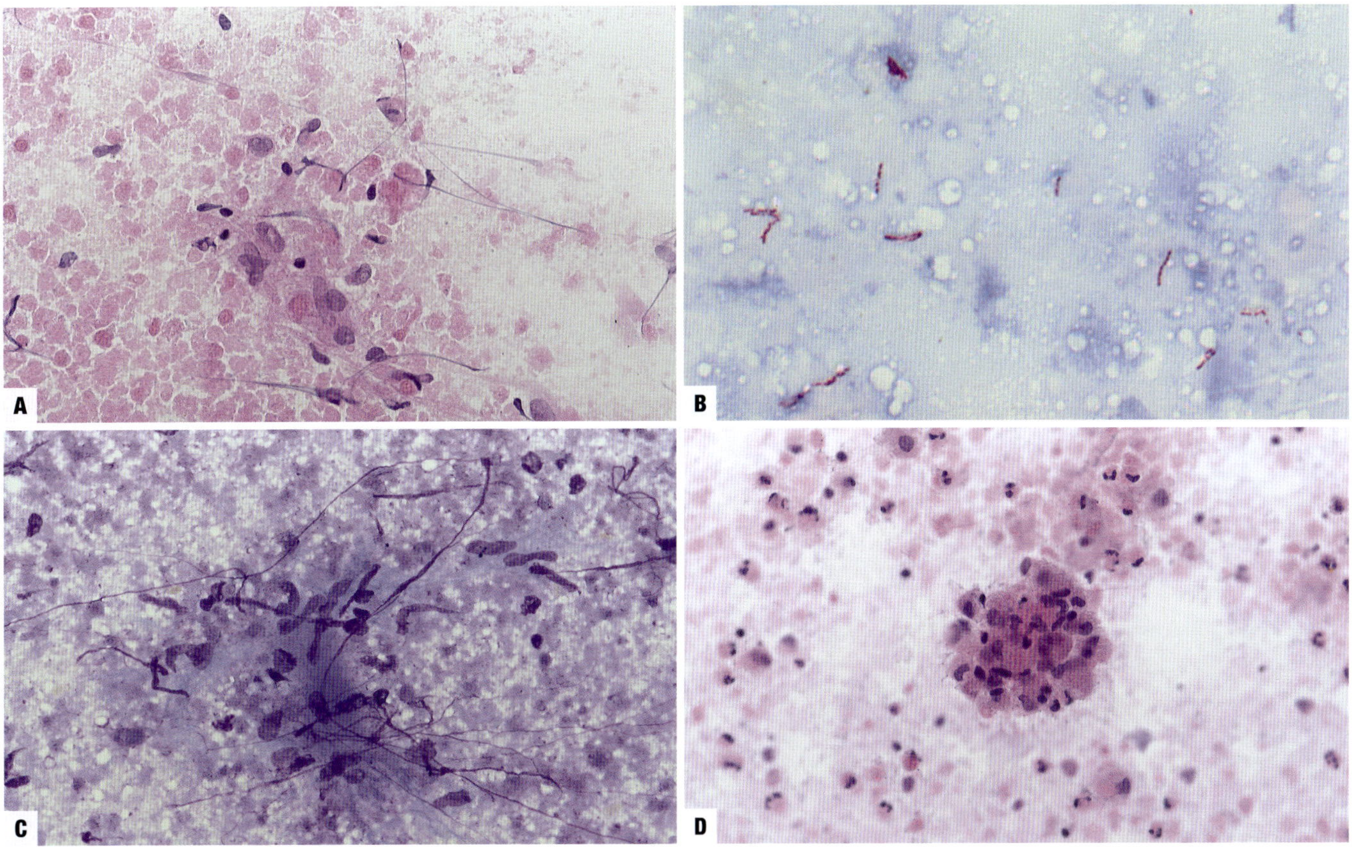

Fig. 4.13 Tuberculosis. **A** Minute, poorly formed granuloma of epithelioid histiocytes surrounded by caseous necrosis (H&E); same case as in Panel C. **B** Endobronchial ultrasound–guided mediastinal lymph node FNAB shows many curved and beaded acid-fast bacilli of *Mycobacterium tuberculosis* in a background of necrosis (Ziehl–Neelsen). **C** Small epithelioid granuloma in a background of caseous necrosis (Giemsa). **D** Small granuloma consisting of histiocytes with more foamy cytoplasm in a background of suppurative necrosis (H&E).

Wegener granulomatosis) and eosinophilic granulomatosis with polyangiitis (previously known as Churg–Strauss syndrome), foreign body reactions, hypersensitivity pneumonitis, and drug-related reactions. A common differential diagnosis in respiratory cytopathology is sarcoidosis, in which clearly demarcated epithelioid granulomas show no necrosis and few multinucleated giant cells. Granulomas with suppuration are seen in granulomatosis with polyangiitis {645,32,629,823,151,198}.

Ancillary testing

For infectious agents, see Table 4.03 (p. 59).

Inflammatory and reactive changes in glandular cells and squamous cells

Engels M

Chapter 4

Definition

Inflammatory and reactive changes in glandular or squamous cells are benign alterations of cytomorphology that may mimic neoplastic lesions and occur in inflammatory conditions of various etiologies.

Clinical features and imaging

Inflammatory, reactive, and regenerative changes may be very marked in a variety of clinical settings, including pneumonia, pulmonary fibrosis, bronchiectasis, pulmonary infarction, and cavitation related to abscesses and granulomatous infections, as well as after instrumentation and tracheal intubation, after radiation therapy and chemotherapy, and in cases related to fungal and viral infections {615,360,785,901,852}.

Histopathology

The histopathology varies with the etiology. Papillary hyperplasia shows folding of mucosa to form papillary projections of the bronchial epithelial surface consisting of normal ciliated and goblet cells, with smaller intermediate cells in the deeper layers. Reactive bronchial epithelium may show enlarged nuclei within an obviously benign tissue fragment {615}. Basal cell hyperplasia is an abnormal multiplication of basal cells forming several layers, and it frequently coexists with squamous metaplasia. Type 2 pneumocyte hyperplasia shows large cells with cuboidal cytoplasm and large nuclei, each with a prominent macronucleolus, lining the lumina of alveoli, and it may mimic atypical alveolar hyperplasia. Squamous metaplasia can replace respiratory mucosa with non-keratinizing squamous epithelium, while some scattered residual respiratory cells or cells with partial

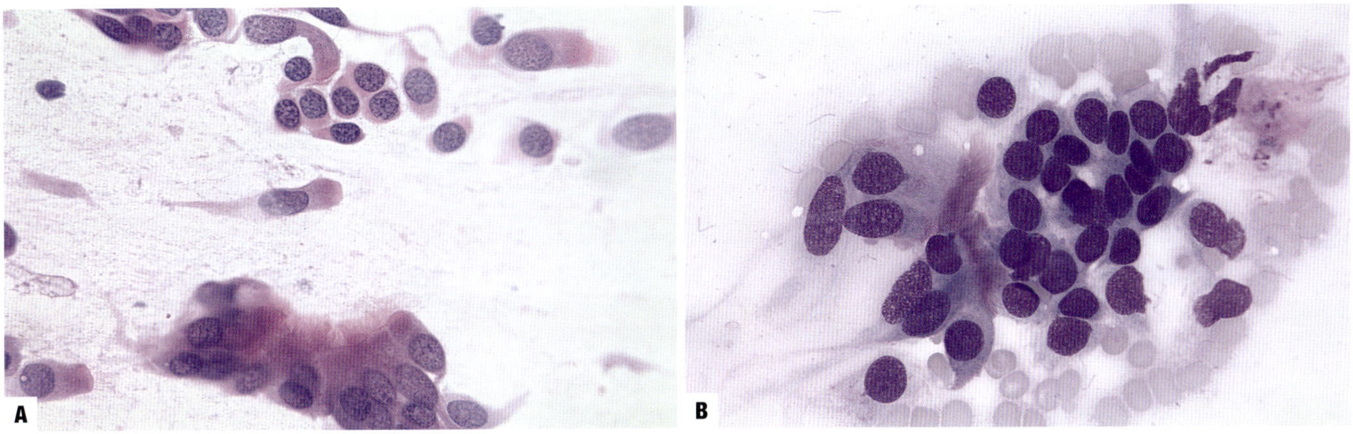

Fig. 4.14 Basal cell hyperplasia. **A** Small flat sheet of bland basal cells in the upper half of the photo; in the lower half, normal ciliated bronchial epithelium (bronchial brushing, H&E). **B** From the same case: small flat sheet of bland basal cells at the right; at the left, normal ciliated epithelium (bronchial brushing, Giemsa).

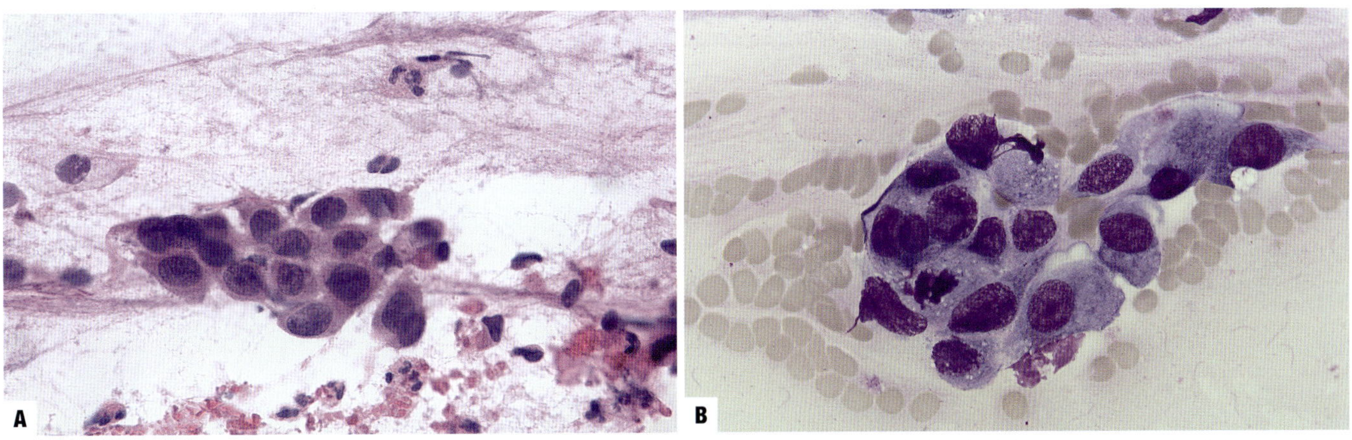

Fig. 4.15 Repair after instrumentation. **A** Small flat sheet of reactive bronchial epithelium with large nuclei, macronucleoli, a bland chromatin pattern, and well-demarcated cytoplasm (bronchial brushing, H&E). **B** From the same case: small flat sheet of reactive bronchial epithelium with large nuclei and regular nuclear membrane, some macronucleoli, a bland chromatin pattern, and one mitotic figure (bronchial washing, Giemsa).

differentiation are present; the metaplastic cells are seen amid columnar cells without cilia or a terminal bar and with intracytoplasmic mucin. Squamous metaplasia frequently coexists with basal cell hyperplasia.

Key diagnostic cytopathological features

Bronchial cell hyperplasia

- Large papillary tissue fragments of columnar cells
- Palisading of peripheral cells
- Terminal bars and/or cilia present
- Nuclei are oval and may contain single nucleoli but are relatively uniform within any tissue fragment

Basal cell hyperplasia

- Cohesive sheets
- Small uniform cells, scant cytoplasm, and a high N:C ratio
- Round to oval nuclei, even chromatin, inconspicuous or absent nucleoli
- Occasional cells show maturation towards columnar cells
- Clean background

Reactive bronchial epithelium, repair and regeneration

- Papillary tissue fragments that may be 3D or cohesive sheets
- Large polygonal cells with abundant cytoplasm
- Cilia and terminal bars may be lost
- Nuclei are enlarged and oval, with a regular smooth nuclear membrane and a central macronucleolus
- Cells with abnormal nuclei can occur within a benign tissue fragment with cilia

Type 2 pneumocyte hyperplasia

- Large cells
- Single cells or small round complexes with knobbly borders
- Some large nuclei with large nucleoli
- Cytoplasm may be vacuolated

Squamous metaplasia

- Sheets and single cells
- Round to slightly irregular nuclei
- Variable to high N:C ratio
- Variable chromatin, occasional nucleoli
- Dense eosinophilic cytoplasm with some keratinization

Cytopathic changes in viral infection

- CMV: large cells with large round to oval nuclei showing a single large intranuclear viral inclusion with chromatinic rimming, giving an owl-eye appearance; some cells will show multiple small basal cytoplasmic inclusions

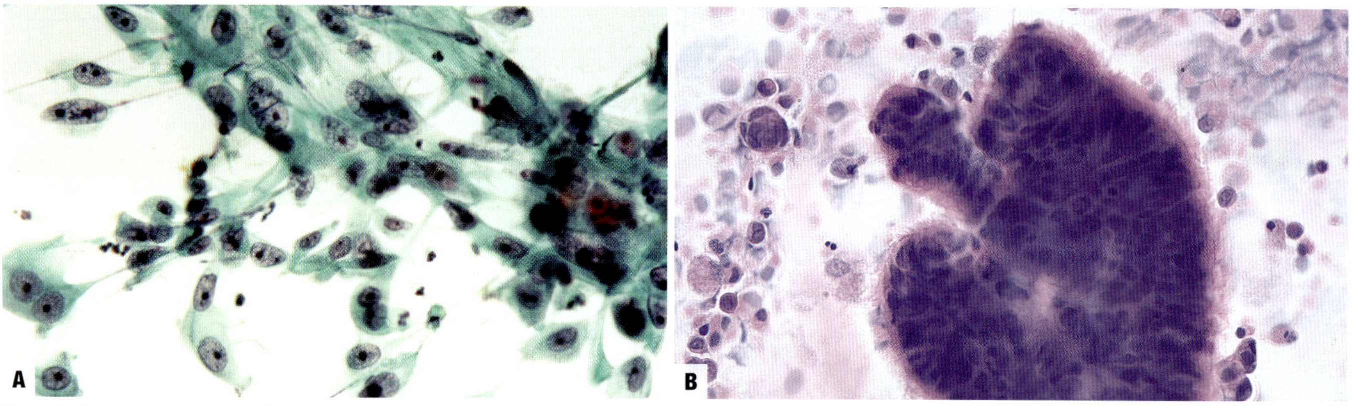

Fig. 4.16 A Reactive bronchial epithelium. Loosely cohesive tissue fragment of large bronchial epithelial cells with mild anisonucleosis, enlarged nuclei, regular nuclear membranes, prominent macronucleoli, and a fine chromatin pattern. The cells are pulled out with long cytoplasmic interconnections between the cells. Some cells are binucleated (bronchial washing, Pap). **B** Bronchial cell hyperplasia. Bronchial cell hyperplasia with crowded tissue fragment of oriented columnar cells with nuclear multilayering and cilia (bronchial washing, H&E).

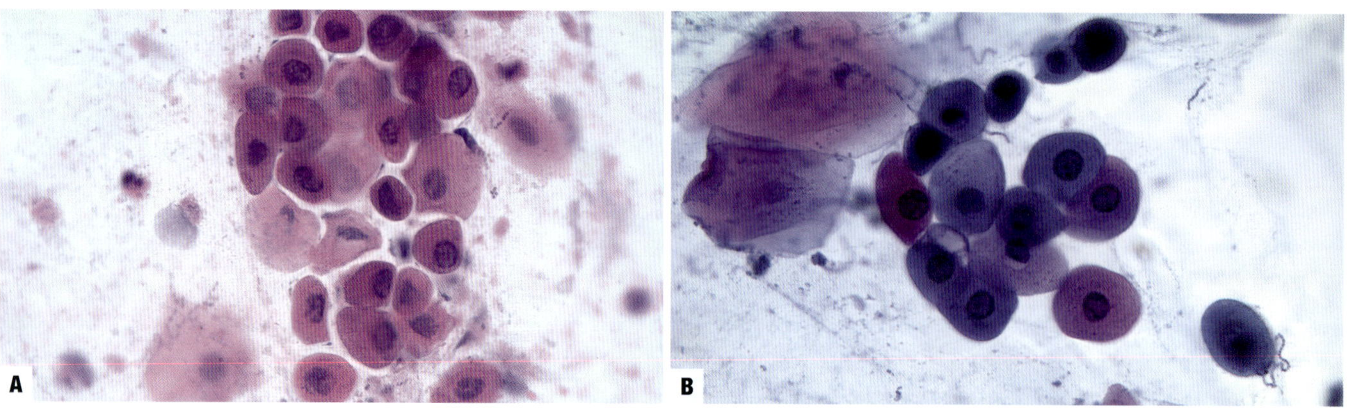

Fig. 4.17 Squamous metaplasia. **A** Metaplastic squamous cells of medium size, with round to oval mildly pleomorphic nuclei that have bland chromatin, and with dense, opaque cytoplasm (bronchial washing, H&E). **B** From the same case: metaplastic squamous cells of medium size, with low N:C ratio, round to oval hyperchromatic nuclei, and dense and opaque but not keratinized cytoplasm. At the upper left are two large squamous cells of the upper respiratory tract (bronchial washing, Pap).

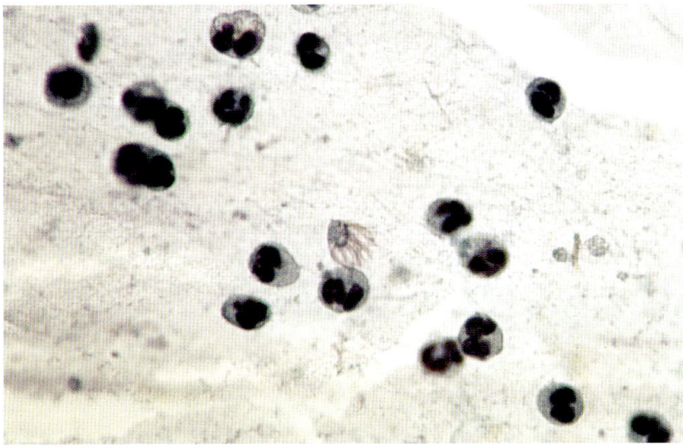

Fig. 4.18 Ciliocytophthoria in viral infection. Detached ciliary tuft with some attached cytoplasm of a bronchial cell with neutrophils in a bronchial washing (bronchial washing, Pap).

- Herpes simplex virus: virion forms a nuclear inclusion filling the entire nucleus with a frayed nuclear envelope, dark degenerative nuclear inclusion bodies, and often multinucleated giant cells
- Adenovirus: smudge cells, with mild cellular enlargement and smudged nonpunctate chromatin, often associated with detached ciliary tufts (ciliocytophthoria), which is a helpful finding but not pathognomonic

Chemotherapy- and radiotherapy-related changes

- Both squamous epithelium and respiratory epithelium are affected
- Enlarged cells with vacuolated cytoplasm, which may be relatively dense
- One or several enlarged nuclei, smudged chromatin
- Large nucleoli occur frequently
- Squamous metaplasia
- Enlargement of type 2 pneumocytes
- Chemotherapy-related changes: appear within a few weeks, resolve within a month or two after finishing the chemotherapy
- Radiation-induced changes: acute changes appear within 6 months; chronic changes may persist for years or for life

Reference(s): {615,360,785,16,176,457,712,539}

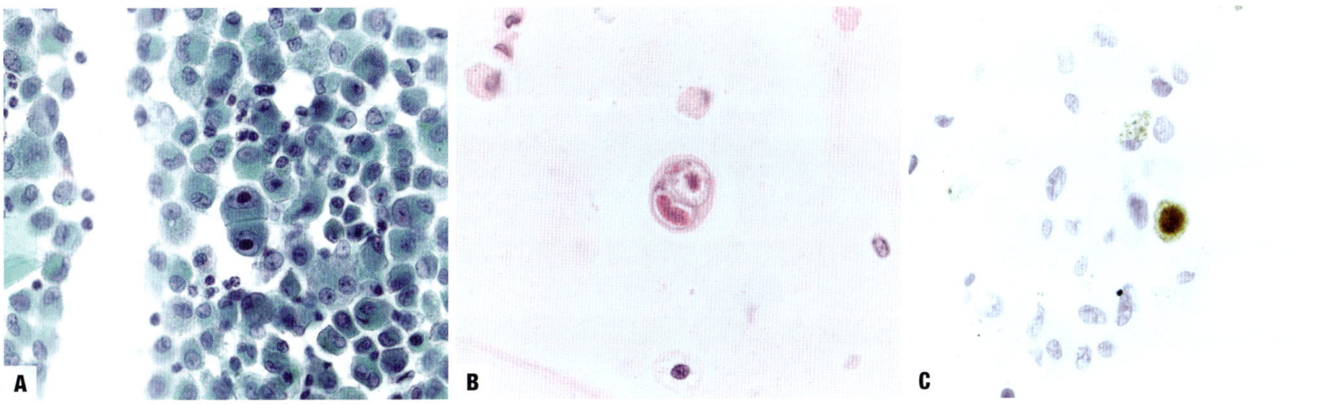

Fig. 4.19 CMV. **A** In the centre are two infected cells, each with a large, opaque viral inclusion surrounded by clearing (the characteristic owl-eye appearance), in a background of plentiful macrophages (bronchoalveolar lavage [BAL], Pap). **B** Binucleated pneumocyte with characteristic large eosinophilic nuclear inclusion with surrounding clearing (BAL, H&E). **C** Pneumocyte with positive CMV nuclear ICC staining (bronchial washing).

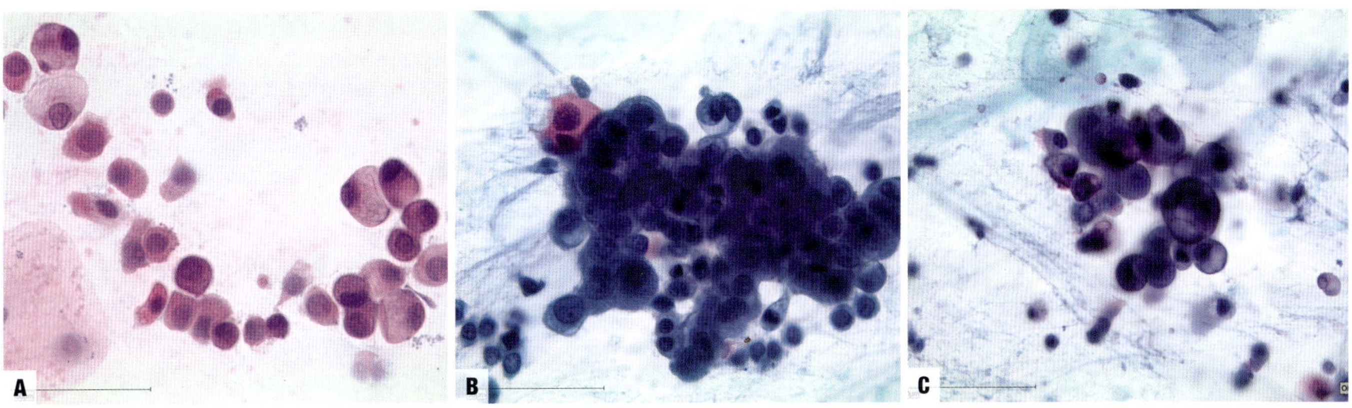

Fig. 4.20 Chemotherapy-related changes. **A** Imaging showed pulmonary infiltrates during chemotherapy for malignant lymphoma (R-CHOP 14). Bronchial epithelium with reactive changes including enlarged nuclei with smudged chromatin, fine cytoplasmic vacuoles, and loss of cilia (bronchial washing, H&E). **B** Pulmonary infiltrates during chemotherapy for malignant lymphoma (R-CHOP 14). Bronchial epithelium with reactive changes including large, crowded tissue fragments of cells with enlarged nuclei, some macronucleoli, and focal loss of cilia (bronchial washing, Pap). **C** Pulmonary infiltrates during chemotherapy for malignant lymphoma (R-CHOP 14). Bronchial epithelium with severe reactive changes, including cytomegaly, some cells with enlarged hyperchromatic nuclei that have blurred chromatin, large cytoplasmic vacuoles, and focal loss of cilia (bronchial washing, Pap).

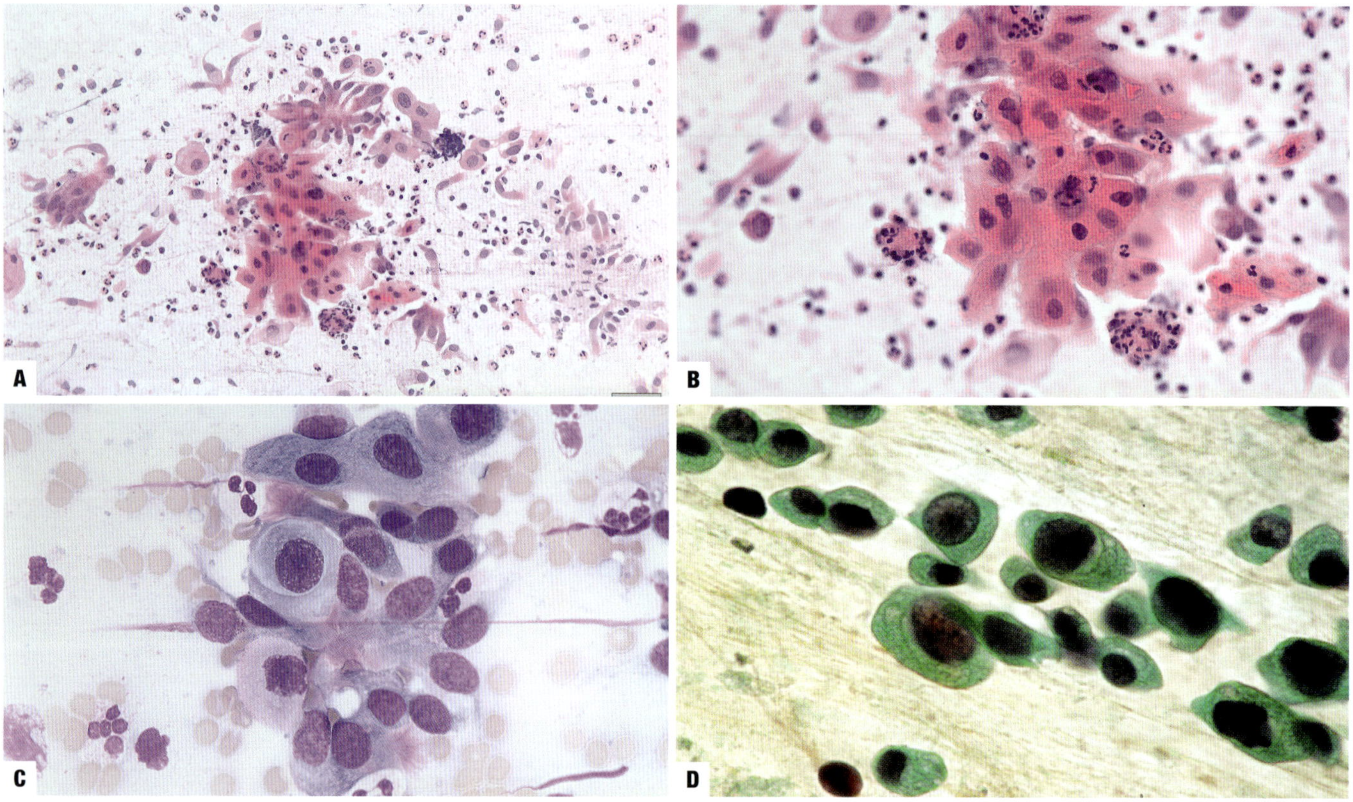

Fig. 4.21 Chemotherapy-related changes. **A–C** Pulmonary mass lesion and history of high-dose chemotherapy, autologous and allogenous stem cell transplantation for malignant lymphoma 5 years previously. **A** Squamous metaplasia with nuclear atypia in a background of ciliated bronchial cells and numerous neutrophils (bronchial brushing, H&E). **B** Squamous metaplasia with nuclear atypia, low N:C ratio, and abundant dense eosinophilic cytoplasm in a background of ciliated bronchial cells and numerous neutrophils (bronchial brushing, H&E). **C** Several cells show squamous metaplasia with nuclear atypia and denser concentric cytoplasm, in a background of ciliated bronchial cells neutrophils (bronchial brushing, Giemsa). **D** Imaging showed pulmonary infiltrates after high-dose chemotherapy for acute myeloid leukaemia. Bronchial epithelium with reactive changes including enlarged nuclei with smudged chromatin, dense cytoplasm, and loss of cilia (sputum sample, Pap).

Discussion and differential diagnosis

Reactive changes in the respiratory tract may sometimes exhibit features that make it difficult to exclude malignancy. A spectrum of reactive changes, from mild to marked, favours a benign diagnosis. Bronchial cell hyperplasia and repair may mimic adenocarcinoma. The presence of cilia and/or a terminal bar strongly suggests that inflammatory atypia is present.

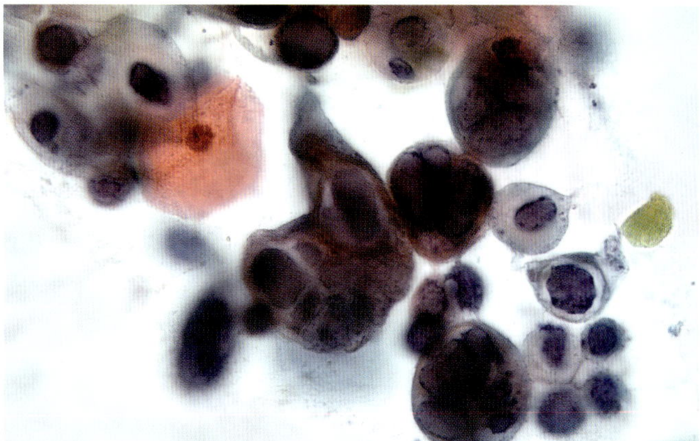

Fig. 4.22 Herpes simplex virus infection. Multinucleated bronchial cells with typical nuclei showing irregular rim of chromatin and central blurred inclusion of herpes simplex virus (tracheal washing, Pap).

Basal cell hyperplasia may mimic small cell carcinoma. The regular shape of the nuclei in basal cell hyperplasia and the even chromatin pattern are similar to those of the ciliated cells in the neighbourhood, whereas cells of a small cell carcinoma often show irregular nuclear contours and a punctate dark and light chromatin with nuclear moulding and chromatinic smearing, with apoptotic debris in the background. Basal cells usually are arranged in flat sheets with a regular pattern.

Reactive bronchial epithelium may mimic adenocarcinoma or non-keratinizing squamous cell carcinoma. The nuclear changes can be severe in reactive bronchial epithelium and may be misleading. Sometimes cells with severe nuclear changes are found within an intact tissue fragment of ciliated cells, and the changes can be assumed to be reactive and not malignant. A spectrum of changes from normal to atypical, instead of two distinct populations of normal cells and malignant cells, is an important feature in inflammatory changes.

Type 2 pneumocyte hyperplasia may also mimic adenocarcinoma, and a certain diagnosis is not possible in every case. In the context of longstanding inflammation, oxygen therapy, or regeneration after lung injury, type 2 pneumocyte hyperplasia is more probable than malignancy. Usually the number of atypical type 2 pneumocytes will decline over time if the cause of the inflammation is removed. In the case of atypia, repeat studies should be recommended.

Squamous metaplasia may be difficult to distinguish from squamous cell carcinoma. In inflammation, especially in fungal infection and in cavitary lesions, squamous metaplasia including keratinization may show marked nuclear atypia. In squamous cell carcinoma of the lung, keratinized and non-keratinizing tumour cells are usually found. These non-keratinizing tumour cells, which are often arranged in crowded 3D tissue fragments, are rare in squamous metaplasia.

In chemotherapy- and radiotherapy-related changes, the therapy-induced changes can be severe and mimic residual or recurrent carcinoma. Correlation with the history and bronchoscopy findings is important to avoid a false positive diagnosis.

Reference(s): {615,614,852,704,785,360}

Ancillary testing

In selected cases, ICC may be helpful, and it may be diagnostic of CMV, herpes simplex virus, and adenovirus on cell blocks of suspected viral infection cases.

Pulmonary hamartoma

Chen L
Geisinger KR
McLean E
Pijuan L

Definition

Pulmonary hamartoma is a benign neoplasm that consists of at least two mesenchymal elements, combined with entrapped respiratory epithelium.

Clinical features and imaging

Pulmonary hamartoma is the most common benign neoplasm of the lung, accounting for approximately 8% of solitary lung nodules, and is more common in men than in women {915,937}. Pulmonary hamartomas are often peripherally located, although rarely they are endobronchial {173}.

On imaging, pulmonary hamartomas are solitary, well circumscribed, and heterogeneous. CT scans are in general more sensitive than CXR for identifying adipose tissue and calcifications. However, there is significant overlap between hamartomas and other benign and malignant neoplasms on imaging {293}.

Histopathology

Pulmonary hamartomas are composed of a disorganized proliferation of mesenchymal tissues (typically cartilage) and may also include adipose tissue, fibrous tissue, or smooth muscle. There are often entrapped adjacent airways lined by cuboidal to low columnar respiratory epithelium. Occasionally, metaplasia, hyperplasia, and reactive atypia can be observed in the epithelium {979}.

Key diagnostic cytopathological features

- Cellularity varies from low to high
- A typical biphasic pattern of tissue fragments of fibromyxoid stroma and epithelium is seen at low power
- The fibromyxoid stroma is typically wispy with irregular feathered outlines, basophilic (Pap), and intensely metachromatic magenta (Giemsa), and it contains bland fusiform and stellate stromal cells with small nuclei

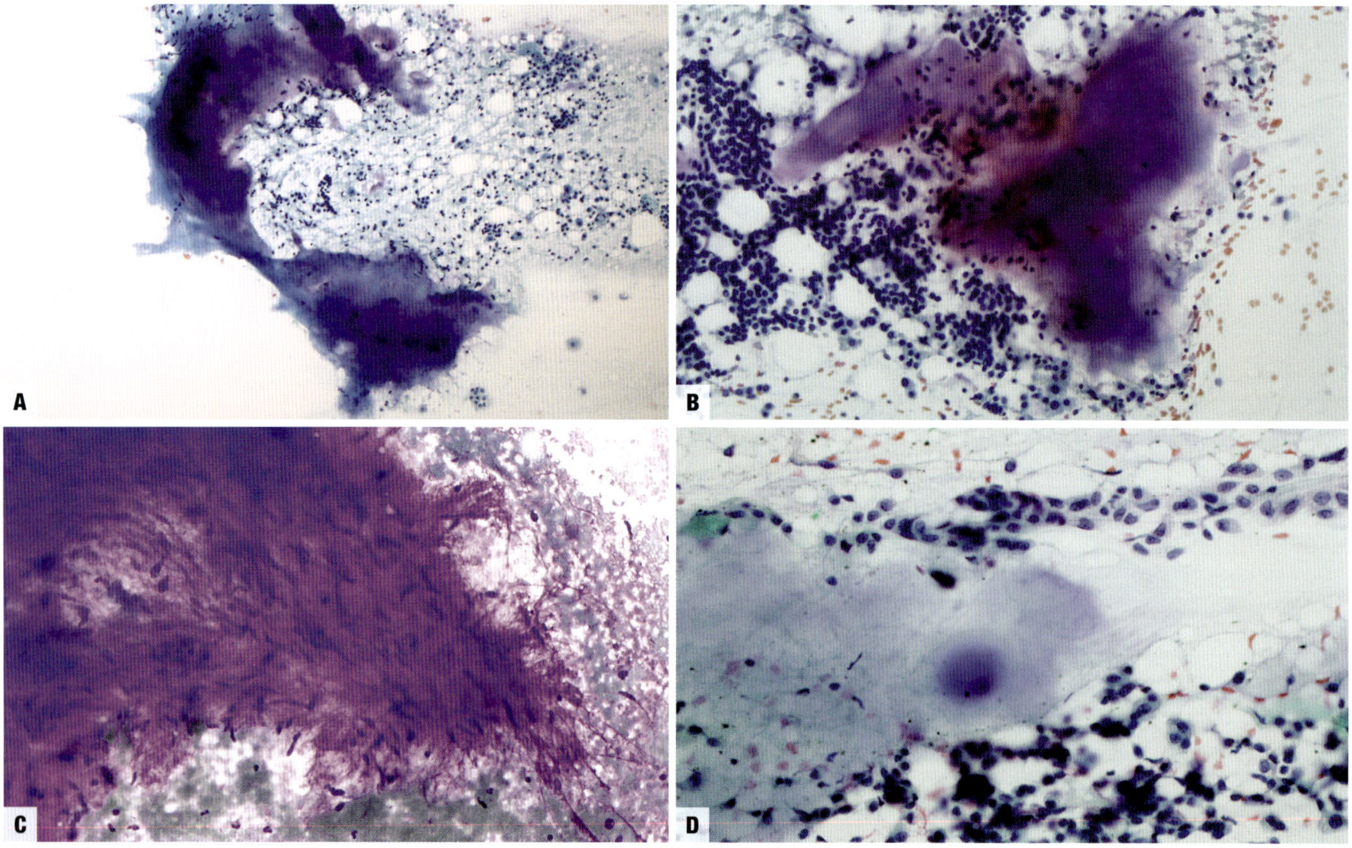

Fig. 4.23 Pulmonary hamartoma. **A** Low-power appearance of FNAB showing a biphasic pattern of fibromyxoid stroma and epithelial components (Pap). **B** On higher-power magnification, the fibrillar fibromyxoid stroma contains scattered fusiform spindled cells. Also present are numerous type 2 pneumocytes (Pap). **C** On high-power magnification, FNAB shows the typical metachromatic fibrillar stroma with embedded bland spindle to stellate cells with inconspicuous nuclei (Giemsa). **D** High-power magnification of FNAB showing mature cartilage with rare lacunar chondrocyte surrounded by abundant bronchial cells and type 2 pneumocytes (Pap).

- The epithelial component can sometimes be prominent, with bronchial cells in sheets or metaplastic cells, and it can show reactive atypia
- Mature cartilage tissue fragments are usually sparse and stain dark blue (Pap) and bright magenta (Giemsa); the lacunar chondrocytes can show slight nuclear variability but lack significant cytopathological atypia
- Other mesenchymal elements, such as adipose tissue, bone, and muscle, can be present

Reference(s): {933,232,978,984,798}

Discussion and differential diagnosis

FNAB has a high diagnostic accuracy for pulmonary hamartoma when the typical cytopathological features are displayed. One study demonstrated that FNAB has 100% accuracy {798}. However, the College of American Pathologists (CAP) Interlaboratory Comparison Program has shown that pulmonary hamartoma is a common source of false positive results {350}, when it is mistaken for carcinoid tumour, pulmonary adenocarcinoma, and small cell carcinoma. Correctly recognizing the mesenchymal component of the FNAB smears is key. An uncommon variant, mucinous adenomyomatous pulmonary hamartoma, can mimic primary mucinous neoplasms of the lung (e.g. mucinous adenocarcinoma), owing to its irregular monotonous growth of non-ciliated mucinous cells in a smooth mucin-rich smear {387,770}.

The differential diagnosis of pulmonary hamartoma also includes biphasic neoplasms, such as pulmonary salivary gland–type tumours, including pleomorphic adenoma (which is usually centrally rather than peripherally located, as is pulmonary hamartoma) and adenoid cystic carcinoma. Although both pulmonary hamartoma and pleomorphic adenoma can have fibromyxoid stroma, pleomorphic adenoma usually lacks other mesenchymal components {21}. The FNAB of pulmonary adenoid cystic carcinoma usually shows cohesive tissue fragments of basaloid cells with a high N:C ratio, and homogeneous hyaline globules of metachromatic basement membrane–like material, which contrasts with the fibrillary stroma and chondroid elements of pulmonary hamartoma {822,718}.

Pulmonary chondroma is a rare tumour that often arises in the setting of Carney triad and is morphologically similar to pulmonary hamartoma but generally lacks adipocytes, muscle, and entrapped respiratory epithelium {758}. Loss of the SDHB subunit of succinate dehydrogenase has been shown to be specific to pulmonary chondroma, whereas pulmonary hamartoma usually retains expression {125}.

Ancillary testing

The fibromyxoid stroma of pulmonary hamartoma can express S100. The epithelial component of entrapped bronchial and alveolar cells can be positive for CK7 and thyroid transcription factor 1 (TTF1) {978}. It has been demonstrated that clonal translocation at chromosome 6p21 occurs in the mesenchymal cells of pulmonary hamartoma, but the value of molecular tests for confirming the diagnosis is limited {266}.

Sclerosing pneumocytoma

VanderLaan PA
Baloch ZW
Maleki Z
Pitman MB

Definition
Sclerosing pneumocytoma, previously termed "sclerosing haemangioma", is a rare indolent pulmonary tumour originating from primitive pneumocytes, composed of a dual population of cuboidal surface cells and round stromal cells with bland cytomorphology.

Clinical features and imaging
Sclerosing pneumocytoma occurs predominantly in middle-aged, non-smoking women of eastern-Asian descent and is often incidentally detected on chest imaging. Most patients are either asymptomatic or present with cough, haemoptysis, or chest pain {501}. Tumours range from 10 to 50 mm, averaging 20 mm, and calcification and cystic change is uncommon. They are typically characterized by a solitary solid, well-circumscribed, round to oval peripheral parenchymal nodule showing strong contrast enhancement on CT, and they tend to be non–FDG-avid on PET-CT {842}. Rarely, multiple tumours may occur {664,592}. These tumours almost always act in a benign fashion, although rare reports of lymph node metastasis have been reported {210}.

Histopathology
Sclerosing pneumocytoma is composed of two main cell types: cuboidal/surface cells and round/stromal cells. There are four main histopathological growth patterns – solid, haemorrhagic/angiomatous, papillary, and sclerotic – and most tumours show a mixture of architectural patterns {664,75}.

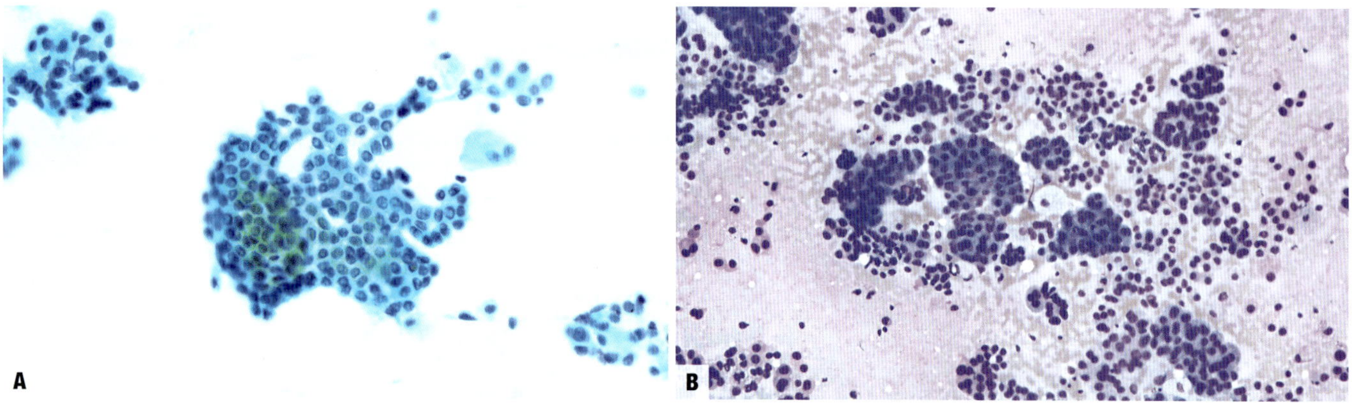

Fig. 4.24 Sclerosing pneumocytoma. **A** Cohesive tissue fragment with 3D and flat sheet regions made up of cuboidal to polygonal cells with a high N:C ratio, and mildly pleomorphic small nuclei with occasional grooves and pseudoinclusions and small nucleoli (Pap). **B** Cellular smear showing cohesive, balled-up papillary tissue fragments and small sheets sometimes showing an acinar architecture, along with a small number of dispersed cells (Giemsa).

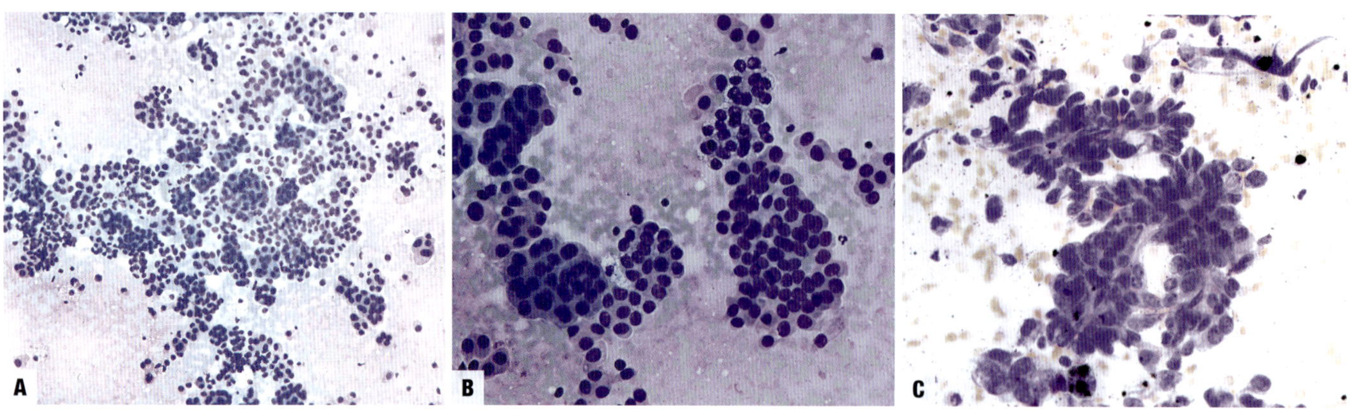

Fig. 4.25 Sclerosing pneumocytoma. **A** Highly cellular smear showing cohesive, balled-up papillary tissue fragments and small sheets sometimes showing an acinar architecture, along with a small number of dispersed cells (Giemsa). **B** Cohesive, balled-up papillary tissue fragments and small sheets sometimes showing an acinar architecture, with few dispersed polygonal cells, showing round to minimally pleomorphic nuclei and scant inclusions. One small sheet at 12 o'clock shows fine vacuolation of the cytoplasm, perhaps a degenerative change (Giemsa). **C** A papillary fragment with a delicate central blood vessel and covered by columnar cells with overlapping elongated and somewhat hyperchromatic nuclei. Scattered spindle cells are also seen, with round to oval nuclei and elongated cytoplasm, present in a background of red blood cells and haemosiderin-laden macrophages (Giemsa).

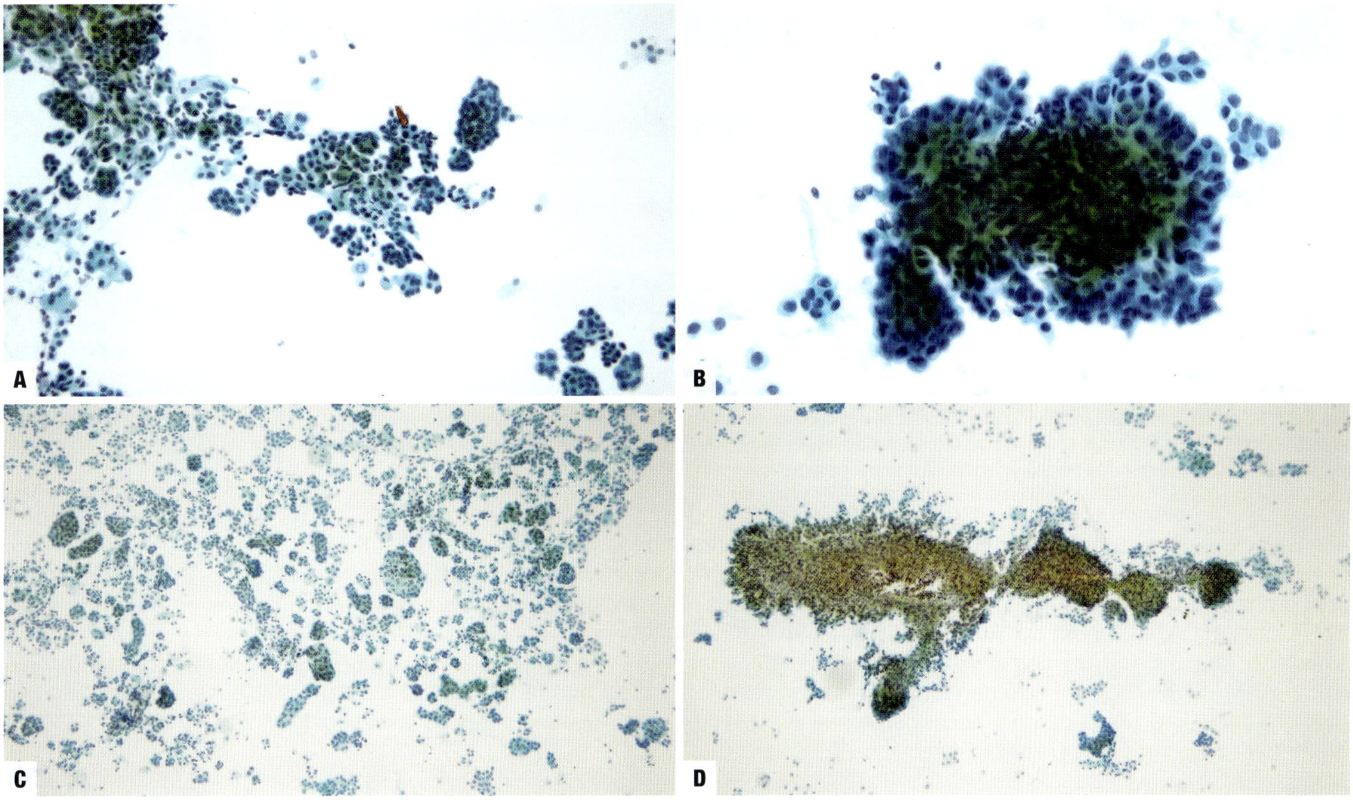

Fig. 4.26 Sclerosing pneumocytoma. **A** Small papillary tissue fragments and cohesive acinar tissue fragments of small cells (Pap). **B** Dense fibrovascular papillary tissue fragment covered in cuboidal epithelium, with small, round to oval nuclei and a high N:C ratio (Pap). **C** Highly cellular smear showing small papillary and acinar tissue fragments with some dispersal of single cells (Pap). **D** Larger papillary tissue fragment with smaller papillary protrusions covered in a bland epithelium (Pap).

Key diagnostic cytopathological features

- Variably cellular smears with cohesive tissue fragments or dispersed epithelioid cells
- Papillary tissue fragments with stromal cores covered by cuboidal epithelial cells with prominent nucleoli; sheets and acini with hyalinized stromal fragments are also seen
- Dual cell population: (1) surface cells: polygonal to cuboidal cells with moderate amounts of vacuolated cytoplasm; (2) stromal cells: round to spindle cells with more dense cytoplasm
- Nuclei show varying degrees of atypia and usually mild anisonucleosis, and they may contain intranuclear pseudoinclusions, nuclear grooves, and indistinct nucleoli
- Mitotic figures are rare and cholesterol crystals/clefts may be seen, but necrosis and overtly malignant features should be absent
- Bloody background with foamy macrophages (many of which contain haemosiderin) and multinucleated giant cells

Reference(s): {524,339,209,1017,210}

Discussion and differential diagnosis

Sclerosing pneumocytoma has usually been regarded as a pulmonary adenoma, along with the less common alveolar adenoma, papillary adenoma, mucinous cystadenoma, and mucous gland adenoma, for many of which there is insufficient information in the cytopathology literature.

Establishing a definitive diagnosis of sclerosing pneumocytoma on cytopathology alone can be difficult, if not impossible, in the absence of clinical and imaging findings. Identification of a two-cell population (i.e. the surface and round cells) with a papillary architecture in a bloody background with haemosiderin-laden macrophages in conjunction with the ICC profile described below can establish a diagnosis of sclerosing pneumocytoma in the proper clinical and imaging context. Overall, the bland appearance of the cells largely recapitulates pneumocyte morphology and immunoprofile. Cell blocks can be helpful in highlighting the distinctive histopathological growth patterns.

The differential diagnosis of sclerosing pneumocytoma includes non-neoplastic entities such as reparative and inflammatory changes, as well as neoplasms such as alveolar adenoma, haemangioma, well-differentiated non-mucinous lung adenocarcinoma with or without lepidic or papillary growth pattern, pulmonary hamartoma, and carcinoid tumour {339, 209,524,664}. Carcinoid tumours tend to show a more uniform pattern of bland round or spindle cells with nuclei showing a fine granular chromatin. Identification of benign cartilaginous and adipose tissue elements admixed with bland epithelial cells can point towards a pulmonary hamartoma, although care should be taken to ensure they are not bronchial contaminants.

Ancillary testing

ICC can be helpful in highlighting the two-cell populations seen in most sclerosing pneumocytomas. The surface cells are positive for cytokeratins (including CK7 and pancytokeratin), EMA, thyroid transcription factor 1 (TTF1), and napsin A, similarly to pulmonary pneumocytes and well-differentiated

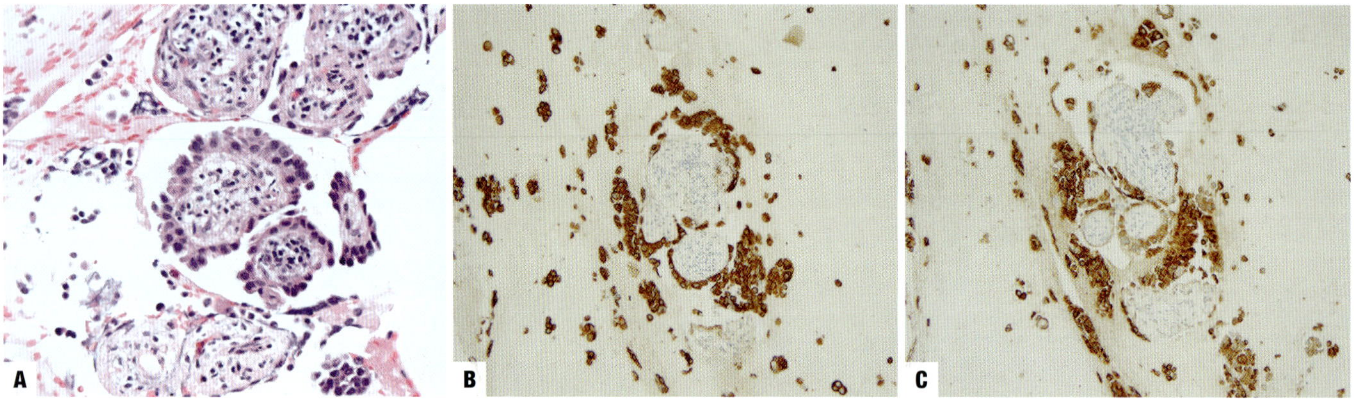

Fig. 4.27 Sclerosing pneumocytoma. **A** Papillary architecture with cuboidal cells with round to oval nuclei surrounding the fibrovascular cores (cell block, H&E). **B** Thyroid transcription factor 1 (TTF1) ICC shows strong staining of the superficial cells surrounding the tissue fragments (cell block). **C** Epithelial membrane antigen ICC shows strong staining of the superficial cells surrounding the tissue fragments. A similar pattern is seen with TTF1 (cell block).

non-mucinous lung adenocarcinomas. The round cells tend to be positive for TTF1 and EMA, and sometimes for SMA and progesterone receptor (PR), but they tend to be negative for napsin A and most cytokeratins {664}. Both surface cells and round cells are negative for S100, HMB45, and melan-A (MART1). They are also negative for neuroendocrine markers (including chromogranin and synaptophysin), which are helpful in ruling out a carcinoid tumour {524}. Sclerosing pneumocytomas are negative for other metastatic papillary carcinoma markers such as PAX8, GATA3, and CDX2.

Molecular analysis has shown mutations in the mTOR pathway–related genes, including *AKT1*, *PIK3R1*, and *PTEN* {75}. *BRAF* p.V600E mutations have also been reported {380}. Currently, ancillary molecular testing has little role in either diagnostic or treatment-related issues for this indolent tumour.

Solitary tracheobronchial papilloma

Baloch ZW

Definition

Pulmonary papillomas are divided into three types: (1) multiple papillomatosis, usually found in children, affecting the larynx and (rarely) the lower respiratory tract; (2) inflammatory endobronchial polyps, originating in the setting of chronic respiratory infection; and (3) solitary tracheobronchial papilloma (STBP), which is subclassified into squamous, glandular, and mixed squamous and glandular subtypes. This section focuses on STBP.

Clinical features and imaging

Patients with STBP can present with either wheezing or pneumonia due to airway obstruction or haemoptysis, although in some cases, STBP can be found incidentally on imaging, either as an endobronchial mass in the segmental bronchi or as a plaque-like mucosal lesion near the carina {267,322,454,420, 828,550}. Squamous cell STBP has been shown to be related to HPV infection and is commonly encountered in middle-aged smokers, with a male predominance, whereas the mixed squamous and glandular type is usually seen in non-smoker older men {327}. Squamous cell STBPs are usually exophytic masses, although inverted types have been reported. These tumours can spread to multiple sites within the tracheobronchial tree, recur, and progress to squamous cell carcinoma {368,665}.

Histopathology

STBPs are subclassified as squamous, glandular, and mixed squamous and glandular types {486,514,454}. Squamous STBP can show a polypoid mass with a central core, covered by multilayered squamous epithelium that may show HPV koilocytic atypia and varying degrees of squamous dysplasia and transformation to squamous cell carcinoma. Glandular STBP can occur also as a polypoid mass, covered by tall columnar respiratory epithelium with prominent microvilli and usually lacking cellular atypia.

Key diagnostic cytopathological features

Squamous STBP

- Loosely cohesive tissue fragments and scattered keratinizing and non-keratinizing squamous cells, some with anucleate squamous cells
- Background of inflammatory and keratinous debris, but no cellular debris or tumour necrosis
- Squamous cells with koilocytic atypia and (rarely) dysplastic changes
- Most cases lack mitotic figures

Glandular STBP

- Tissue fragments and singly scattered enlarged or hyperplastic columnar cells with retained cilia
- Rare reports of mixed squamous and glandular STBP showing features of both squamous and glandular STBP

Reference(s): {454,760,90,392}

Discussion and differential diagnosis

STBPs are rare neoplasms; cases have been reported on the basis of bronchial brushings and FNAB specimens, but they are difficult to diagnose solely from cytomorphology {454,760,90,392}. Correlating imaging appearances with cytomorphology is essential, and core needle biopsy at rapid onsite evaluation (ROSE) should be recommended. The differential diagnosis of STBP includes squamous metaplasia, well-differentiated squamous cell carcinoma, well-differentiated adenocarcinoma, and low-grade mucoepidermoid carcinoma for glandular or mixed subtypes {454}.

Ancillary testing

HPV has been linked to the pathogenesis of STBP, most commonly HPV types 6 and 11 along with types 16 and 18 and other high-risk subtypes, which can be associated with transformation to higher-grade lesion {1016,708,454,885,410,884}.

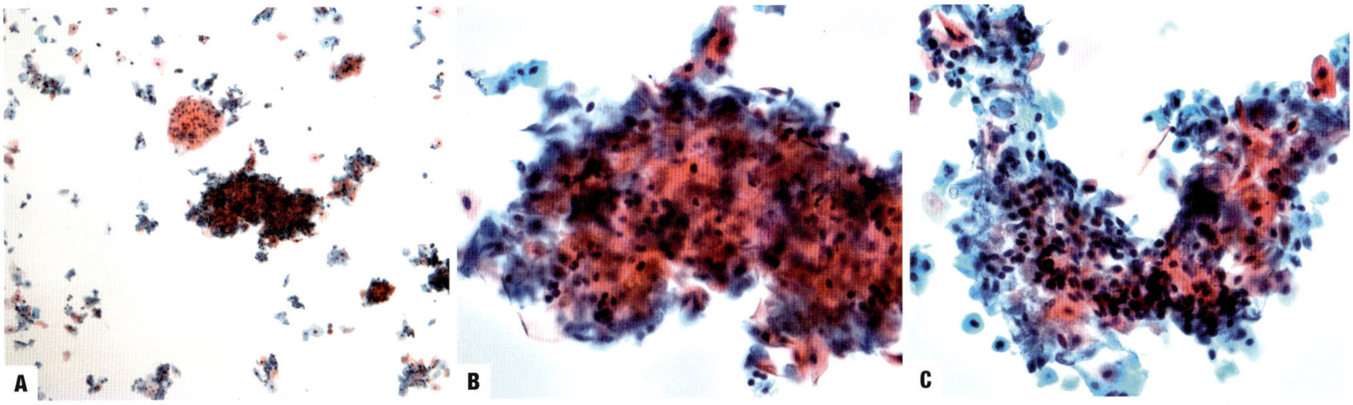

Fig. 4.28 Bronchial papilloma. **A** Loosely cohesive tissue fragments and singly scattered nucleated and anucleated keratinized squamous cells (bronchoalveolar lavage [BAL], liquid-based cytopathology, Pap). **B,C** Tissue fragment of keratinized squamous epithelium showing mild to moderate nuclear atypia, without associated tumour necrosis (BAL, liquid-based cytopathology, Pap).

Salivary gland neoplasms

Maleki Z

Definition

Benign salivary gland neoplasms of the respiratory tract include pleomorphic adenoma, myoepithelioma, and oncocytoma and closely resemble their salivary gland counterparts.

Clinical features and imaging

Clinical symptoms are related to the location and size of the tumours and include cough, wheeze, haemoptysis, and postobstructive changes such as pneumonia. On CXR and CT, the tumour typically appears as a central well-circumscribed polypoid mass arising within the bronchus.

Histopathology

Pleomorphic adenoma is a biphasic tumour consisting of nests, tubules, glands, and branching ducts, with a variable amount of fibromyxoid or chondromyxoid stroma. The epithelial cells are cuboidal, and the myoepithelial cells are large with clear cytoplasm, forming the outer layer of the ducts or tubules, and present in the stroma as spindle cells. Myoepithelioma shows solid, canalicular, or mixed patterns of myoepithelial cells, with no duct formation, and the cells can be epithelioid, plasmacytoid, spindle, clear, or hyaline. The matrix can be hyaline or myxoid. Oncocytoma is composed of large cells with abundant eosinophilic cytoplasm, large vesicular nuclei, and prominent nucleoli. The neoplasm may show papillary configurations, focal necrosis, cystic change, and haemorrhage with cholesterol clefts {96}.

Key diagnostic cytopathological features

Pleomorphic adenoma

- Epithelial cells are small, cuboidal with a high N:C ratio, occasionally basaloid, and seen singly and in tissue fragments forming stellate-shapes, strands, and tubules
- Myoepithelial cells are plasmacytoid, spindle, or clear cells, and they are dispersed singly, in small tissue fragments or embedded in the matrix
- Chondromyxoid or fibrillary matrix that is magenta (Giemsa) or pale green (Pap)
- Low mitotic activity and no necrosis

Myoepithelioma

- Myoepithelial cells with clear, spindle, epithelioid, or plasmacytoid features seen singly or in loose tissue fragments
- Uniform round to oval nuclei and eosinophilic or clear cytoplasm
- Nuclear inclusions can be seen in plasmacytoid cells
- Variable amount of fibrillary or myxoid matrix

Oncocytoma

- Loosely cohesive tissue fragments of large epithelioid cells in a clean background
- Large cells with abundant granular cytoplasm; round nuclei; and small, prominent nucleoli

Reference(s): {223}

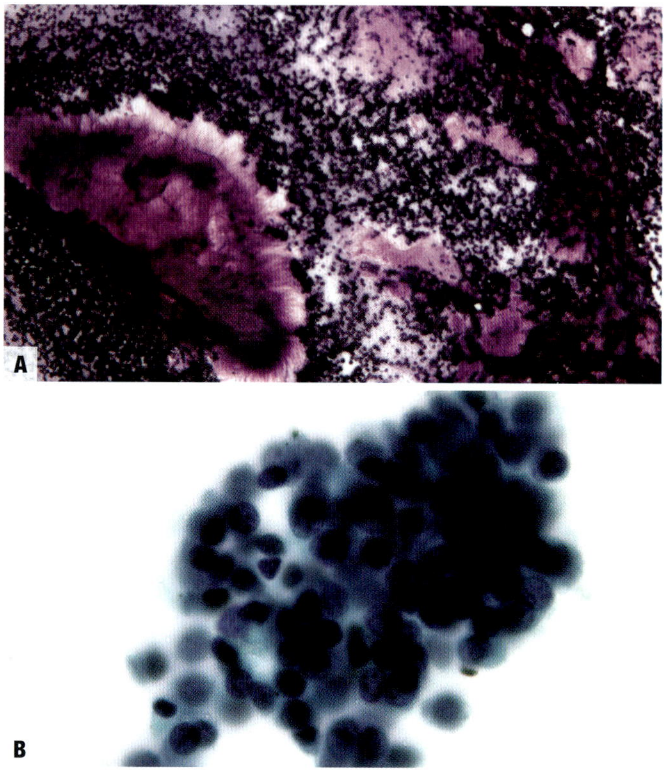

Fig. 4.29 Pleomorphic adenoma. **A** Transbronchial FNAB showing a tissue fragment of magenta stroma with a fibrillary quality, most pronounced at the edge – the so-called troll hair appearance. Notice small tissue fragments of bronchial cells in the background (Giemsa). **B** Transbronchial FNAB showing a tissue fragment of the myoepithelial cells, some with a plasmacytoid appearance (liquid-based cytopathology, Pap).

Discussion and differential diagnosis

The clinical behaviour of respiratory tract pleomorphic adenoma varies from benign to more aggressive. The differential diagnosis includes pulmonary hamartoma, myoepithelioma, epithelial-myoepithelial carcinoma, adenoid cystic carcinoma, pulmonary blastoma, and carcinosarcoma. Tumours with a stromal component are in the differential diagnosis with myoepithelioma, including adenoid cystic carcinoma, pleomorphic adenoma, and epithelial-myoepithelial carcinoma. Carcinoid tumour, metastatic oncocytic carcinoma of the thyroid, and metastatic oncocytic carcinoma of the kidney are in the differential diagnosis with oncocytoma. Overall, the prognosis of these tumours is favourable.

Ancillary testing

The epithelial cells in pleomorphic adenoma are positive for CK7, CAM5.2, AE1/AE3, and S100, and the myoepithelial cells are positive for p63, p40, S100, SMA, and GFAP in pleomorphic adenoma and in myoepithelioma {789}. Oncocytoma is positive for CAM5.2 and negative for chromogranin, PAX8, and S100. Surgical resection is the recommended treatment.

PEComa

Michael CW

Definition

Pulmonary perivascular epithelioid cell tumour (PEComa) is a benign neoplasm of lung that arises from epithelioid perivascular cells.

Clinical features and imaging

PEComas, which have been known as "clear cell tumour of lung", are more common in elderly patients. They have a slight female predominance and occasionally are associated with tuberous sclerosis and lymphangioleiomyomatosis {268,836}. They occur anywhere in the lungs, but most commonly in the lower lobes as a solitary peripheral lung nodule {268}. Peripheral nodules are asymptomatic, whereas central lesions may present with shortness of breath, high fever, cough, haemoptysis, or thrombocytosis {796,826}.

PEComas are often incidentally discovered by CXR as peripheral coin-shaped, well-demarcated nodules, with no cavitation or calcifications {120}. The reported size ranges from 1 mm to 120 mm {409}. CT shows intense postcontrast enhancement due to the rich vascular stroma {268,423}. PET shows mild FDG uptake {947}.

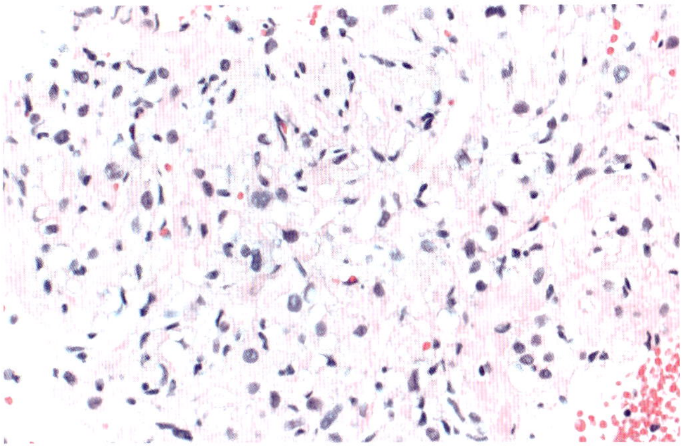

Fig. 4.31 PEComa. Cell block containing a syncytial fragment of epithelioid cells traversed by thin-walled blood vessels. The cells are round to spindle, with poorly defined eosinophilic granular cytoplasm and round to oval nuclei with significant size variation (H&E).

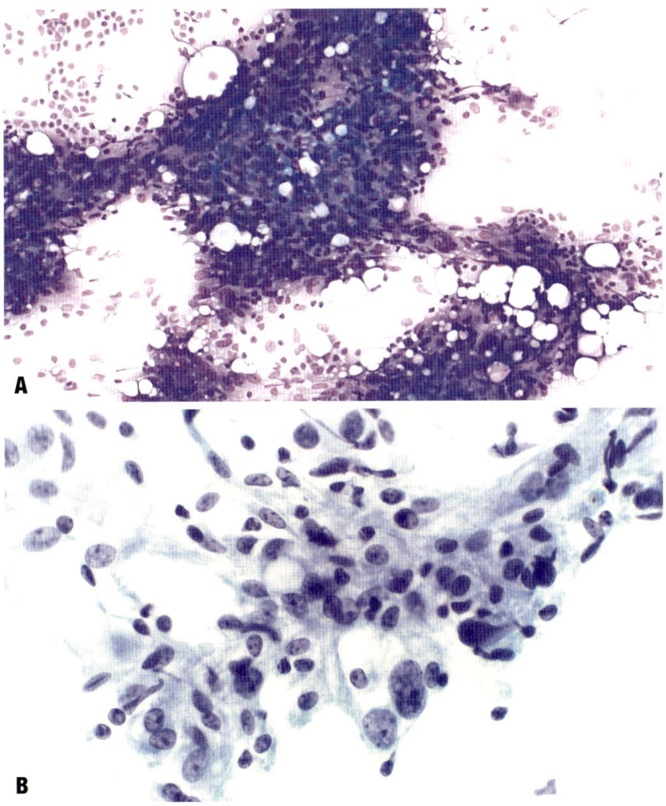

Fig. 4.30 PEComa. **A** Cellular smear comprising syncytial tissue fragments of epithelioid cells with round to oval nuclei and delicate blood vessels in a background of numerous bare nuclei (Giemsa). **B** A syncytial tissue fragment of spindle to round cells with poorly defined cytoplasm and anisonucleosis. The nuclei are round to oval, with finely dispersed chromatin and inconspicuous nucleoli (Pap).

Histopathology

PEComa presents as a well-circumscribed, unencapsulated nodule with a red-tan cut surface. Microscopically it presents as sheets or vague nests of cells surrounded by thin blood vessels. The cells are round to oval and occasionally spindle, with abundant clear or slightly eosinophilic cytoplasm and well-defined cell borders. The nuclei are not mitotically active, and they vary in size and shape but are usually oval with finely granular chromatin and occasional small nucleoli {274}. Electron microscopy reveals that the cytoplasm is rich in free and membrane-bound glycogen and premelanosomes {273}.

Key diagnostic cytopathological features

- Moderately cellular smears
- Small to large cohesive tissue fragments traversed by thin capillaries, and scattered spindle cells
- Bland cells with round to oval nuclei with mild anisonucleosis, indistinct nucleoli, and no atypia or mitoses make up the tissue fragments
- Abundant clear or finely vacuolated cytoplasm and distinct cell borders
- Rare intranuclear pseudoinclusions
- Background of blood, lymphocytes, macrophages, and numerous single round to oval bare nuclei

Reference(s): {703,922}

Discussion and differential diagnosis

The differential diagnosis includes other primary or metastatic clear cell carcinomas, including primary lung adenocarcinoma and acinic cell carcinoma and metastatic renal cell carcinoma. Less frequently, it includes adrenal cortical carcinoma; glycogen-rich clear cell breast carcinoma; clear cell hepatocellular carcinoma; clear cell tumours from the ovary, uterus, and cervix; and melanoma {703,922,963, 863,10,34,967,349}.

Ancillary testing

PEComas give a positive PAS reaction, reflecting the abundant glycogen content. ICC is positive for HMB45, S100, melan-A (MART1), vimentin, MYOD1, desmin (focally), SMA, α1-antitrypsin, factor XIIIa, NSE, synaptophysin, cathepsin B, and CD57 (LEU7). One report showed a strong reaction for CD1a, but this was not reproduced in other studies {100,275,273,2,669,255}. The cells are negative for pancytokeratin AE1/AE3, CK7, CK20, and EMA {922,703}.

Spindle cell tumours

Hiroshima K

Definition

Benign spindle cell tumours and related spindle cell tumours that may have a low risk of recurrence or metastasis include a broad range of tumours in which bland spindle cells predominate or are the sole cell type.

Clinical features and imaging

Most spindle cell tumours arising in the lung do not have distinctive clinical or imaging features. In the thoracic cavity, most schwannomas arise in the posterior mediastinum in the paravertebral region. Schwannomas can also occur in other mediastinal compartments and the pleura {74}. Schwannomas typically occur as slow-growing solitary tumours. Most are asymptomatic and are detected on imaging or at autopsy.

Histopathology

Conventional schwannomas are spindle cell neoplasms showing alternating areas of the compact Antoni A pattern and the hypocellular, more open Antoni B pattern. Areas of nuclear palisading, also known as Verocay bodies, may be seen. The spindle cells have pale eosinophilic cytoplasm and ovoid or buckled nuclei with tapered ends. Some tumours may show cytoplasmic nuclear pseudoinclusions, mild pleomorphism, and mitotic activity. Ancient schwannomas feature scattered atypical or bizarre nuclei with dark, smudgy chromatin, considered a degenerative change.

Pulmonary hamartomas have fibromyxoid stroma along with chondroid stroma and entrapped bronchial epithelium.

Fibromatoses, also known as desmoid tumours, have long, sweeping fascicles of bland fibroblasts and myofibroblasts without cytopathological atypia.

Leiomyomas consist of cells closely resembling normal smooth muscle cells, with eosinophilic cytoplasm and uniform blunt-ended, cigar-shaped nuclei, arranged in orderly intersecting fascicles.

Solitary fibrous tumours consist of haphazardly arranged spindle to ovoid cells with pale eosinophilic, indistinct cytoplasm, within a variably collagenous stroma that may be myxoid, admixed with branching and hyalinizing staghorn-shaped or haemangiopericytomatous blood vessels, and in some cases they may have a high mitotic count, with or without increased cellularity, atypia, necrosis, and an infiltrative growth pattern.

Inflammatory fibroblastic tumours have variable amounts of three patterns: a myxoid pattern of plump or spindle myofibroblasts in an oedematous background with plasma cells, lymphocytes, and eosinophils, mimicking granulation tissue; a hypercellular pattern with a fascicular spindle cell proliferation; and a collagenized stromal hypocellular pattern.

Key diagnostic cytopathological features

Benign spindle cell tumours usually show low cellularity, with spindle cells predominantly in small tissue fragments that may show a fascicular architecture or myxoid change or a variable amount of collagenous material separating the spindle cells, which contain bland elongated nuclei. Dispersed single spindle cells are less prominent. In FNAB cytopathology, most of these cases will not have sufficiently distinctive features for a specific diagnosis; they will be reported as "benign spindle cell tumour", and ICC on cell blocks may allow a more specific diagnosis. Mitoses and necrosis are not seen, except in rare cases of solitary fibrous tumour, and their presence should suggest that the tumour may be a related malignant spindle cell tumour, including spindle cell variants of lung carcinoma and mesothelioma, or a metastasis.

Discussion and differential diagnosis

Spindle cell lesions encountered in lung FNAB include a broad spectrum of inflammatory lesions, benign neoplasms, and neoplasms that can recur or rarely metastasize, and they have to be distinguished (if possible) from high-grade spindle cell tumours, which are most commonly metastases of soft tissue neoplasms. The differential diagnosis of spindle cell neoplasms is assisted by correlation with imaging and negative microbiological studies and by finding few or no inflammatory cells.

Some lesions and neoplasms may be specifically diagnosed, particularly with the assistance of ancillary testing, whereas others will simply have inflammatory or spindle cell material that correlates with the imaging and clinical findings and is regarded as benign. In other cases, the FNAB material may show significant atypical cytopathological features, such as high spindle cell cellularity, nuclear atypia, necrosis, and mitoses, and be categorized as "Atypical". If a spindle cell tumour that can occasionally recur or rarely metastasize (e.g. solitary fibrous tumour) is specifically diagnosed, this is best categorized as "Atypical" or "Suspicious for malignancy", but the specific diagnosis guides management.

Inflammatory and reactive processes that produce spindle cells include a wide range of infections and organizing fibrotic lesions, and the number of associated acute or chronic inflammatory cells (including plasma cells, eosinophils, and multinucleated giant cells) correlated with the clinical history, imaging, special stains (for specific bacterial, fungal, or mycobacterial infections), and microbiological findings can be diagnostic {953,352}. Granulation tissue and fragments of often partially crushed alveolar septa may appear to consist mainly of spindle cells. Fibrosing mediastinitis may also be considered, depending on the FNAB site {856}.

Schwannomas show cohesive tissue fragments, with fibrillary, fibrotic, and/or myxoid stroma sometimes forming rough meshworks of intersecting stroma in a clean background, with focal palisading of the spindle, wavy, or fish-hook–like nuclei with pointed ends, fine chromatin, smooth and regular nuclear membranes, and inconspicuous nucleoli and no mitoses, and bipolar spindle cytoplasm. Ancient schwannomas may show

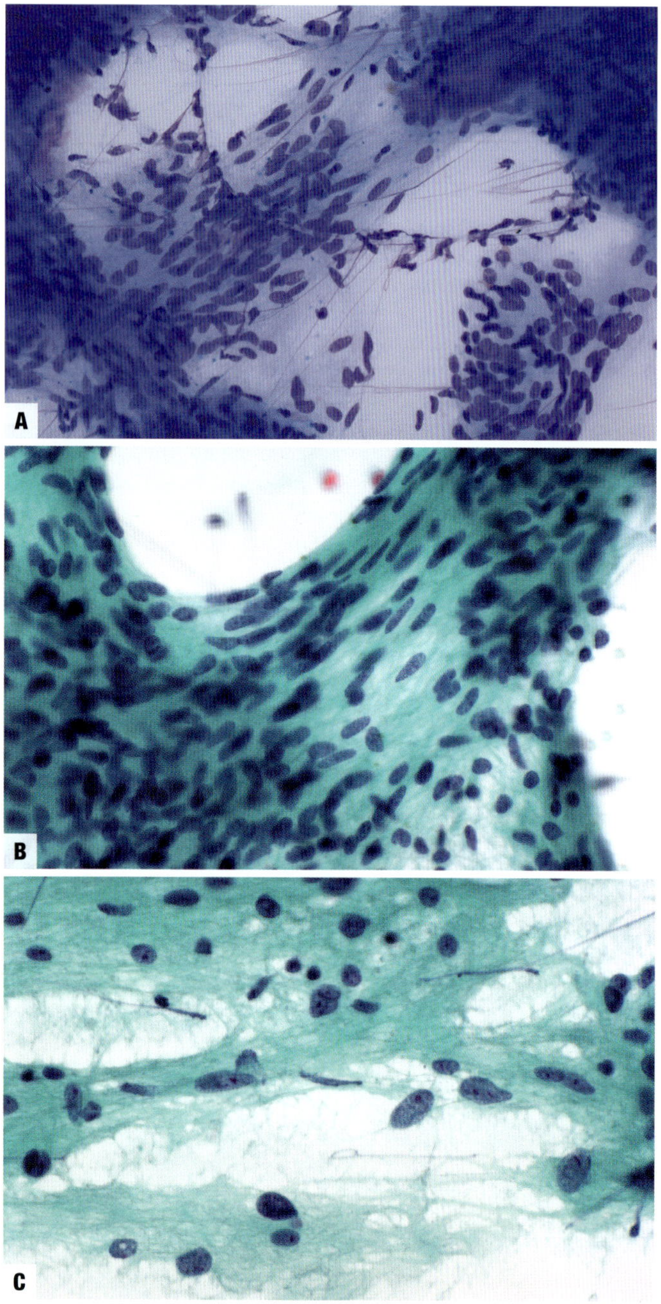

Fig. 4.32 Schwannoma. **A** Round to oval nuclei are arranged in a palisading pattern embedded in a fibrillary matrix (Giemsa). **B** Tissue fragments appear highly cellular and the cytoarchitectural arrangement of the cells is fascicular, corresponding to histopathological areas of Antoni A. Spindle cells with oval to pointed nuclei are embedded in a fibrillary matrix. Nuclear membranes are smooth and regular, and the chromatin texture is fine (Pap). **C** Loosely cohesive tissue fragment of spindle cells with round to oval nuclei, some with pointed tips, embedded in a fibrillary matrix. Some anisonucleosis and an intranuclear cytoplasmic pseudoinclusion are identified (Pap).

scattered hyperchromatic pleomorphic nuclei {217,128,583, 189,308,326}. Schwannomas may be difficult to distinguish from other spindle cell processes and neoplasms on cytopathological smears alone, and correlation with the clinical history, imaging, and site is required; the use of ICC on cell block and core needle biopsies is a useful adjunct {6,856}.

Pulmonary hamartomas may have a spindle cell component along with the fibromyxoid stroma and chondroid stroma and usually bronchial epithelial tissue fragments.

Fibromatoses (also known as desmoid tumours) show low but variable cellularity, spindle cells separated by magenta stroma (Giemsa) arranged in cohesive long fascicular fragments, a small number of single bland spindle fibroblasts/myofibroblasts with tapering elongated cytoplasm, oval to elongated nuclei with evenly dispersed fine chromatin, and rare inflammatory cells {721,658}. Mitoses may occasionally be seen, but no atypical mitoses are present.

Leiomyomas in FNAB smears show variable cellularity, irregularly contoured cohesive tissue fragments of variable cellularity, and often a parallel arrangement of spindle cells with moderate amounts of relatively dense cytoplasm with distinct boundaries. The bland ovoid nuclei have blunt ends (cigar-shaped nuclei); fine, even chromatin distribution; and in some cases, occasional mitoses and focal nuclear atypia with enlargement and pleomorphism {953,51}. Necrosis or increased mitotic activity are not present {949}. Differentiating a leiomyoma from normal muscular tissue may be difficult on cytopathological material, because many leiomyomas are not hypercellular and have low mitotic activity {949}.

Solitary fibrous tumour FNAB yields low to moderate cellularity, reflecting the histopathological spectrum of hyalinized to more cellular, classic haemangiopericytoma tumours. The relatively discohesive cellular tissue fragments have irregular fascicles consisting of bland spindle cells with often pale indistinct cytoplasm and a fusiform nucleus, finely dispersed chromatin, and an inconspicuous nucleolus {357}. Collagenous stroma is prominent in some tissue fragments. These tumours have been reported to recur or metastasize on rare occasions, and the pathology is not predictive of behaviour {893,68}.

Inflammatory myofibroblastic tumour shows scant cellularity varying to hypercellularity, reflecting the histopathological spectrum, from myxoid or hyaline stroma containing loosely arranged spindle or stellate cells with variable inflammatory cells, through to a compact proliferation of spindle cells arranged in a storiform architecture, and then hypocellular sclerotic fibrotic tumours with scattered spindle and inflammatory cells. The cells vary from bland fibroblast-like cells, to spindle cells, to epithelioid cells with prominent nuclear atypia and prominent nucleoli, and the tumours can be rich in plasma cells and lymphocytes. Necrosis or marked mitotic activity are not present {287,829, 872}. Very occasionally these tumours have been reported to recur or metastasize {78}.

Ancillary testing

All schwannomas show diffuse nuclear and cytoplasmic staining for S100, particularly in Antoni A areas. SOX10 nuclear staining is usually extensive {638,403}. GFAP and CD34 staining is variable. Mediastinal schwannomas can show staining for cytokeratin AE1/AE3, often extensively {250}.

Leiomyomas are positive for SMA and desmin and negative for S100, KIT (CD117), DOG1, BCL2, β-catenin, and ALK.

Desmoid fibromatoses usually show patchy SMA expression and rarely are reactive for desmin, whereas nuclear β-catenin expression is usually seen secondary to *CTNNB1* or *APC* mutations in as many as 75% of cases, particularly most sporadic cases {113,473,219,59,309}. CD34, DOG1, S100, and KIT (CD117) are negative.

Solitary fibrous tumours are typically positive for CD34, CD99, BCL2, EMA, SMA, and nuclear STAT6 immunoreactivity {145, 756,893}, which may be lost in dedifferentiated tumours. S100, DOG1, and KIT (CD117) are negative.

Inflammatory myofibroblastic tumours show variable positivity for SMA, calponin, and desmin; positivity for pankeratin in less than one third of cases; and negativity for CD34, S100, and DOG1. Cytoplasmic immunoreactivity for ALK is distinctive and detectable in 50–60% of cases, and it correlates well with the presence of *ALK* gene rearrangement {291,169,89,24}. ALK-negative inflammatory myofibroblastic tumours occur in adult patients and have greater nuclear pleomorphism, atypia, and atypical mitoses {163}. Microbiological studies and special stains are negative.

Meningiomas

Satoh Y
Pitman MB

Definition

Pulmonary meningiomas are meningothelial (arachnoid cell) neoplasms identical to those that arise from the dura mater of the CNS, but in patients without a demonstrable CNS lesion.

Clinical features and imaging

Most pulmonary meningiomas produce no symptoms and are discovered incidentally on CXR, whereas some patients present with respiratory symptoms including cough and haemoptysis {934,367,585}. Imaging shows a single or (rarely) multiple slow-growing, round, well-circumscribed nodule(s) with lobulated margins on CT, and soft tissue attenuation and high metabolic activity on FDG PET {926,367}. Most lesions are peripheral and localized to the lung, with no predilection for any lobe {585,801}.

Histopathology

Most tumours are low-grade, well circumscribed, solid proliferations of bland tumour cells growing in whorls and lobular nests in the meningothelial tumour, or showing spindle architecture in the fibroblastic tumour. Rare examples of high-grade meningiomas with anaplastic (grade 3) {966,711} and chordoid (grade 2) features have been reported {692,775}. CNS surgical pathology criteria can be used for grading from grade 1 to grade 3.

Key diagnostic cytopathological features

- Hypercellular
- Cohesive small sheets and tissue fragments sometimes showing a whorled pattern
- Spindle or epithelioid cells with elongated or fusiform nuclei, and when seen singly the cytoplasm may be wispy
- Fine nuclear chromatin and small, inconspicuous nucleoli with scattered intranuclear pseudoinclusions; degenerative changes can produce nuclear hyperchromasia, enlargement, and atypia
- Psammoma bodies may be present
- Mitotic figures and necrosis are absent but may be present in high-grade tumours

Reference(s): {926,644,934,585}

Discussion and differential diagnosis

The primary differential diagnosis is metastatic meningioma, which should be excluded clinically. Other tumours in the differential diagnosis include spindle cell thymoma, solitary fibrous tumour, and monophasic synovial sarcoma. Meningothelioid nodules are only distinguished on resection by their poorly defined borders and interstitial and frequently perivenular pattern of growth. The presence of intranuclear pseudoinclusions and psammoma bodies can create confusion with metastatic thyroid carcinoma {644}.

Ancillary testing

Meningiomas label strongly for vimentin and variably for EMA, progesterone receptor (PR), SSTR2A, CD56, and S100 {644}. Pancytokeratin, melanoma markers (HMB45 and melan-A [MART1]), neuroendocrine markers (synaptophysin and chromogranin), GFAP, and OCT4 are negative {972,87}. Most meningiomas in the CNS show allelic loss on chromosome 22 and *NF2* mutations {972}.

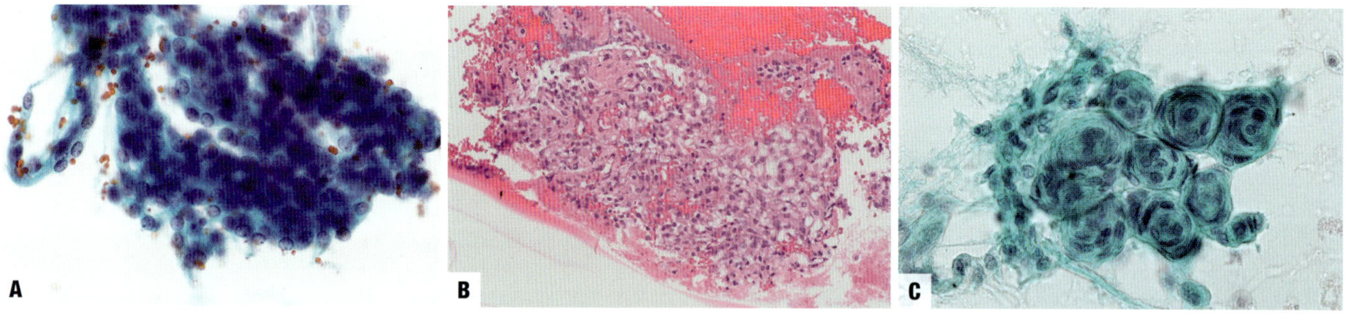

Fig. 4.33 Meningioma. **A** Low-grade pulmonary meningioma. Cohesive tissue fragment consisting of spindle or epithelioid tumour cells. Nuclei are elongated or fusiform with fine nuclear chromatin and small, inconspicuous nucleoli (Pap). **B** Bland epithelioid or spindle tumour cells growing in whorls and lobular nests (cell block, H&E). **C** Pulmonary meningioma. Meningothelial meningioma with whorl formation in a tissue fragment (liquid-based cytopathology, Pap).

Granular cell tumour

Pitman MB
VanderLaan PA

Definition

Granular cell tumour is a tumour showing neuroectodermal differentiation and is believed to be of Schwann cell origin.

Clinical features and imaging

Granular cell tumours are typically small (< 50 mm). They present mainly within the 30- to 60-year-old age group but can arise at any age, and they show a slight female predominance {182,127}. Although they most commonly arise in the tongue, hypopharynx, oesophagus, colon, skin, and breast {247,251}, granular cell tumours can arise anywhere in the body, including the lung. Pulmonary granular cell tumours are usually associated with the airways at bifurcation sites, with an endobronchial component in approximately 90% of cases, although rare peripherally located parenchymal tumours have also been described {204,183}. Granular cell tumours are almost always benign neoplasms, but malignant granular cell tumours can occur, representing only 1–2% of all granular cell tumours {137, 381}.

Granular cell tumours are often incidentally detected by CXR or CT, but larger tumours can cause bronchial obstruction and symptoms such as wheezing, cough, dyspnoea, haemoptysis, chest pain, or pneumonia. Imaging may show a postobstructive opacity that may have irregular borders or enhancement on MRI, thus yielding a differential diagnosis of atelectasis, infection, or neoplasia {247}. PET is negative for metabolic activity.

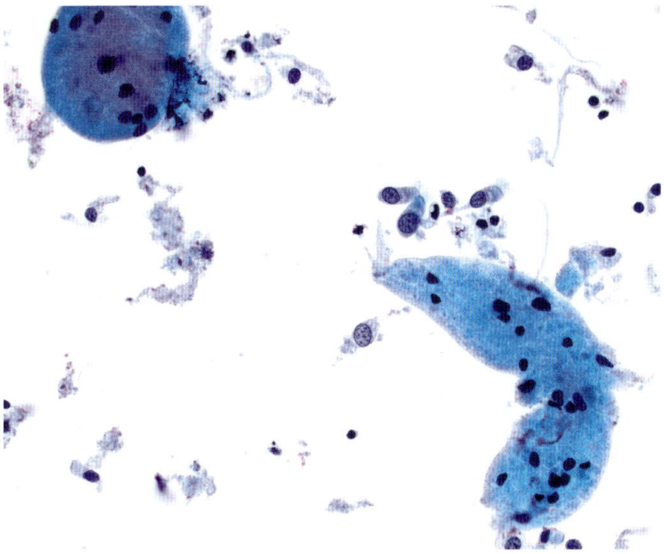

Fig. 4.34 Granular cell tumour. The dense granularity of the tumour cells is readily apparent in liquid-based cytology preparations (liquid-based cytopathology, Pap).

Histopathology

The histopathology of granular cell tumours is the same regardless of the site of origin. Tumours are composed of sheets, nests, cords, or trabeculae of distinctive polygonal tumour cells with round central nuclei and abundant granular cytoplasm.

Key diagnostic cytopathological features

- Moderately cellular
- Loosely cohesive sheets and some single cells
- Medium-sized to large, monomorphic round to oval polygonal cells
- Characteristic abundant eccentric eosinophilic granular cytoplasm, which is fragile, leading to spilled granules in the background
- Granules are seen better on H&E- or Pap-stained smears than on Giemsa-stained smears
- Liquid-based cytopathology demonstrates more cohesive, smooth-margined, small tissue fragments with indistinct individual cell borders
- Nuclei are round and are small to medium in size, with occasional small nucleoli

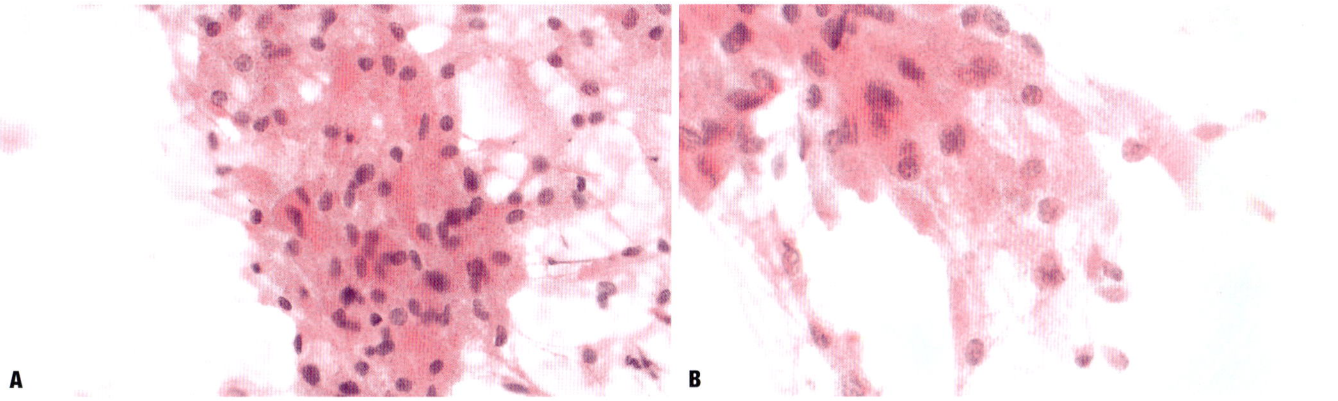

Fig. 4.35 Granular cell tumour. **A** Densely granular cytoplasm of bland polygonal cells is the key diagnostic feature of granular cell tumours (H&E). **B** The key diagnostic feature of granular cell tumour is the intensely eosinophilic, coarsely granular cytoplasm (H&E).

- Mitotic activity and necrosis are absent, and if necrosis is present the rare malignant granular cell tumour should be considered

Reference(s): {204,190,262}

Discussion and differential diagnosis

The differential diagnosis of granular cell tumours in the lung is different to that at other sites and includes carcinoid tumours with oncocytic morphology and pulmonary macrophages, which show more vacuolated cytoplasm, often containing carbon pigment, and do not demonstrate the distinct cytoplasmic coarse granularity that is so characteristic of granular cell tumours. Metastases to the lung of tumours with granular cytoplasm, such as acinic cell carcinoma of the salivary gland or acinar cell carcinoma of the pancreas, warrant consideration {305,133}.

Ancillary testing

Granular cell tumours are positive for PAS with and without diastase, and positive by ICC for S100, myelin basic protein (MBP), calretinin, α-inhibin, and CD68. Granular cell tumours are negative for all cytokeratins, desmin, thyroid transcription factor 1 (TTF1), and the endocrine markers chromogranin and synaptophysin. Pulmonary carcinoid tumours are positive for pancytokeratin, endocrine markers, and TTF1. Acinic cell carcinomas also stain with PAS and PASD and may show focal staining for endocrine markers, but they are distinguished by showing complete membranous staining for SOX10 and DOG1. Pancreatic acinar cell carcinomas are positive for pancytokeratin, trypsin, and BCL10. Macrophages stain for CD68 {474,118}.

Ectopic thyroid and parathyroid tissues

Baloch ZW

Definition

Ectopic thyroid and parathyroid are developmental abnormalities due to abnormal migration of the thyroid anlage or parathyroid tissue during embryogenesis.

Clinical features and imaging

Ectopic thyroid has a reported incidence in the general population of 1 case per 100 000–300 000 person-years {42}. In the great majority (~90%) of cases, ectopic thyroid is seen along its migration pathway; however, in as many as 10% of cases it can be seen in other locations, such as the mediastinum, lung, oesophagus, aorta, heart, adrenal gland, and gallbladder {42, 363,768,900,213}. Only rare cases of intrapulmonary ectopic thyroid tissue have been reported {214,139,138}.

On imaging, ectopic thyroid in either mediastinum or lung can mimic primary or metastatic tumours at these sites {214,139,138}.

Ectopic parathyroid is more commonly related to the inferior parathyroid gland than to the superior parathyroid gland {818, 284,92,436,213}. The ectopic locations for superior parathyroid glands include the tracheoesophageal groove, posteromedial to the thyroid, the carotid sheath, within the thyroid, and the mediastinum. The common ectopic locations for the inferior glands are the intrathymic and perithymic soft tissues, the thyrothymic ligament, the carotid sheath, within the thyroid, and the anterior mediastinum. Rare cases of intratracheal parathyroid tissue have been reported {818,436,284,92}. The majority of ectopic parathyroid glands are clinically silent; however, parathyroid neoplasms (usually adenomas) can develop, causing hyperparathyroidism {344,960}.

Ultrasound usually fails to localize parathyroid neoplasms arising in ectopic locations, whereas technetium-99m sestamibi CT and PET-CT have shown high sensitivity and specificity for localizing these lesions {960,639,70}.

Histopathology

The histopathological features of ectopic thyroid and parathyroid tissue and their associated neoplasms are similar to those occurring in the thyroid and parathyroid in their usual anatomical location.

Key diagnostic cytopathological features

Ectopic thyroid

- Substernal goitre or a parasitic goitrous nodule on FNAB shows cytomorphological features of thyroid tissue: abundant thin colloid, macrophages, and monolayer sheets of follicular cells without nuclear atypia
- Follicular nodular disease nodules will show follicular sheets, tissue fragments of follicles of varying size including macrofollicles, and usually abundant thin colloid; cystic change with siderophages may also be present
- Follicular adenoma arising in ectopic locations will show predominant microfollicles, thick luminal colloid, and a lack of nuclear features of papillary thyroid carcinoma, and will be diagnosed as follicular neoplasm
- Rare cases of papillary carcinoma arising in ectopic thyroid tissue will show the diagnostic nuclear features of elongation, fine dusty chromatin (Pap), grooves, and pseudoinclusions, with or without papillary tissue fragments

Reference(s): {959,62,861,868,1020,662,512}

Ectopic parathyroid

- Parathyroid neoplasms, which are usually adenomas arising in ectopic locations, are usually hypercellular and consist of epithelial cells with round nuclei and clear to slightly dense cytoplasm arranged in monolayer sheets and acini
- Fine blood vessels may traverse the tissue fragments, and papillary architecture may be seen

Reference(s): {868,935,691}

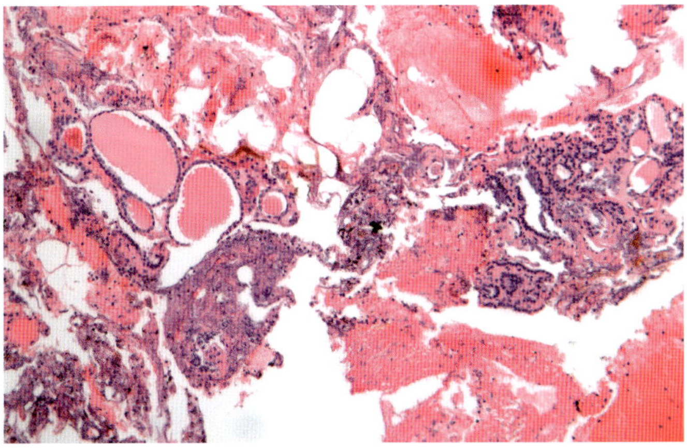

Fig. 4.36 Ectopic thyroid. Cell block of FNAB of an anterior mediastinal mass showing benign thyroid tissue (H&E).

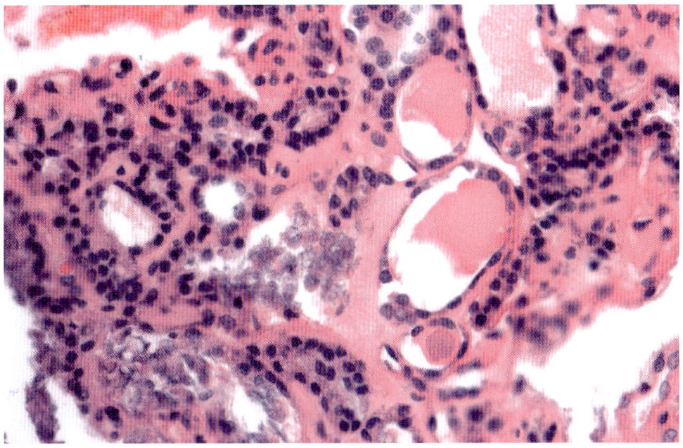

Fig. 4.37 Ectopic thyroid tissue. High magnification of cell block showing benign thyroid follicles (H&E).

Discussion and differential diagnosis

Ectopic thyroid tissue or its associated neoplasms arising in the mediastinum and lung can mimic primary and metastatic neoplasms at these locations. This diagnosis can only be rendered after excluding metastasis from a thyroid primary {1020}. Parathyroid tissue in an ectopic location can mimic low-grade neuroendocrine neoplasms and thyroid tumours {802,639}.

Ancillary testing

The cytomorphological diagnosis of thyroid tissue can be confirmed by positive ICC for thyroid transcription factor 1 (TTF1), thyroglobulin, and PAX8. In some cases, an aliquot of the FNAB rinse can be submitted for thyroglobulin assessment {37,500, 747}. Parathyroid origin can be confirmed by demonstrating high PTH concentration in the FNAB rinse or by ICC positivity for PTH, GATA3, and chromogranin {244,114,188}.

Sample reports: Benign

Field AS

The sample reports provided here are based on the standardized cytopathology report in the *Diagnostic categories and report structure* (p. 8) section of the first chapter. See that section for a discussion on the structure and components.

These are sample reports that include the components required in one possible format; the final report format will depend on local practice and local laboratory information system requirements. For brevity, demographics and information on the macroscopic features and rapid onsite evaluation (ROSE) are not presented here.

Each institution should select a term for the main heading of the diagnostic summary, such as "Diagnostic summary" (as used in the examples below), "Diagnosis", or "Final diagnosis", and use it consistently.

Sample report 1

Type of specimen:
Sputum sample (first of three).

Clinical and imaging information:
Bilateral lung infiltrates with hilar lymphadenopathy. Fever. Haemoptysis.

Diagnostic summary:
Category: Benign
Diagnosis: Mycobacterial infection

Macroscopic description:
6 mL of thick, mucoid, grey frothy material.

Microscopic description:
Scattered multinucleated giant cells and small epithelioid granulomas are present in a background of granular necrosis, with macrophages, lymphocytes, and debris. Curved beaded bacilli are seen in the Ziehl–Neelsen stain for mycobacteria.
Comment: Mycobacterial infection is present. Correlation with microbiological studies is required.

Sample report 2

Type of specimen:
Bronchial wash and brush right lower lobe.

Clinical and imaging information:
Irregular 50 mm solid mass right lower lobe. Presented with right lower lobe pneumonia. Immunocompromised patient.

Diagnostic summary:

Specimen 1:
Bronchial wash right lower lobe bronchus
Category: Benign
Diagnosis: Acute inflammation

Specimen 2:
Bronchial brush right lower lobe bronchus
Category: Benign
Diagnosis: Acute inflammation with fungi. See report below.

Macroscopic description:
Specimen 1: Bronchial wash right lower lobe bronchus: 5 mL grey viscous fluid
Specimen 2: Bronchial brush right lower lobe bronchus: 2 alcohol-fixed direct smears

Microscopic description:

Specimen 1: Pus is present with plentiful neutrophils, macrophages, and debris, as well as a small number of bronchial cells. Ziehl–Neelsen stain for mycobacteria is negative, and PASD for fungi is negative.
Comment: Acute inflammation is present. Correlation with microbiological studies is required.

Specimen 2: Tissue fragments of bronchial cells, macrophages, and neutrophils are present, with necrotic debris. The Giemsa and PASD show aggregates of fungi with acutely branching hyphae, confirmed in the Grocott methenamine silver stain, which shows septa, suggestive of *Aspergillus* spp.
Comment: Correlation with microbiological studies and imaging is required.

Editorial note:
There is a mass lesion in the lung. The bronchial washing and bronchial brushing show acute inflammatory changes, and some cytopathologists may prefer to use the category "Non-diagnostic" for this, despite the presence of the fungal elements suggesting a possible aspergilloma. Correlation with clinical and imaging findings is required.

Sample report 3

Type of specimen:
Endobronchial ultrasound–guided FNAB of left upper lobe lung.

Clinical and imaging information:
20 mm solid rounded mass left lower lobe of lung. Presented with wheeze and history of previous pneumonia.

Diagnostic summary:
Endobronchial ultrasound–guided FNAB of left upper lobe lung
Category: Benign
Diagnosis: Suggestive of pulmonary hamartoma

Macroscopic description:
3 air-dried slides, 3 alcohol-fixed slides
3 mL pink normal saline needle rinsings

Microscopic description:
These mildly cellular smears show fragments of myxoid stroma and chondroid material with occasional bronchial epithelial tissue fragments in a bloody background. There is no diagnostic material in the cell block.
Comment: The features are suggestive of a pulmonary hamartoma.

Editorial note:
In this report the exact site of the FNAB specimen from the request form has been included in the diagnostic summary, which is presented as an option in the structured report.

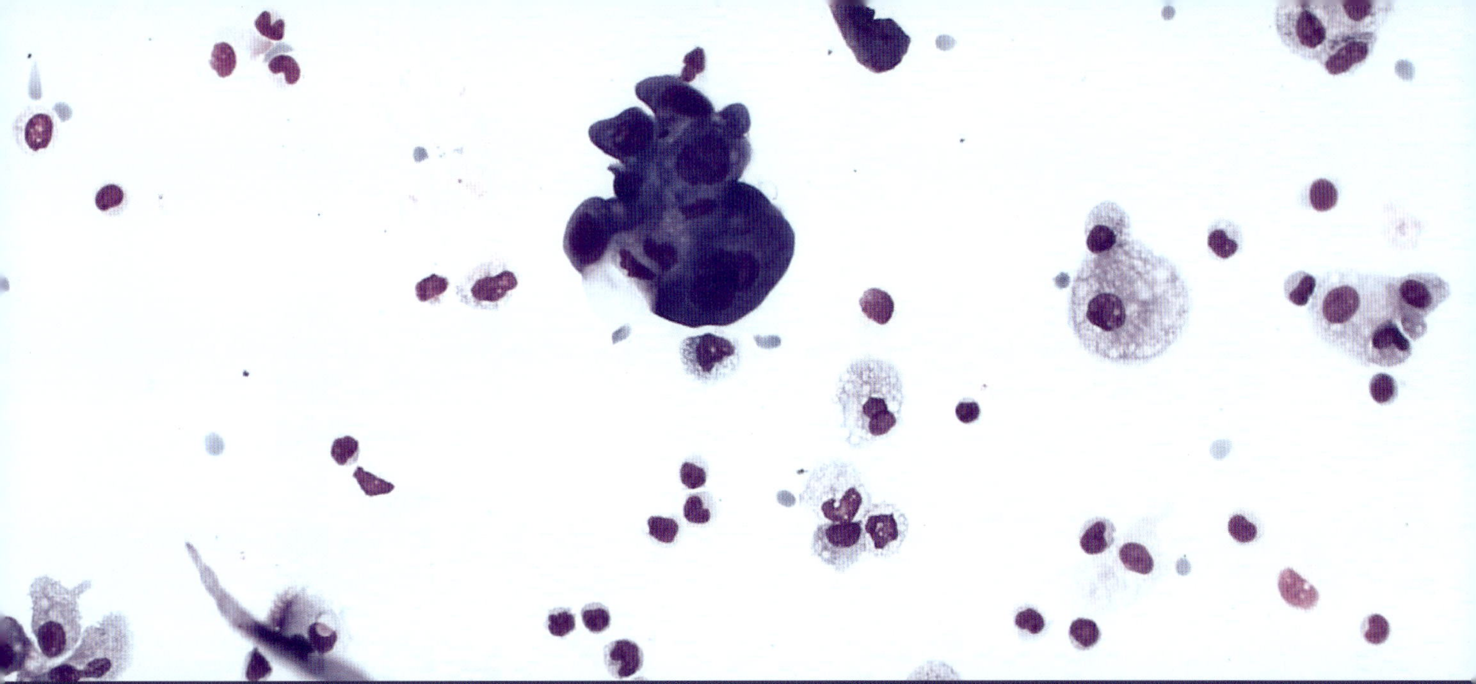

5

Diagnostic category: Atypical

Edited by: Chandra A, VanderLaan PA

Introduction

Baloch ZW
Kawahara K
Sheaff MT

In respiratory cytopathology specimens the use of the "Atypical" category is based on an assessment of the following: the pattern of dispersal of tissue fragments and individual cells, the architectural features of the tissue fragments, the nuclear features of the epithelial or lymphoid cells present, and background features. The majority of these features may appear benign or reactive, but some findings may suggest malignancy {360,465,742,468, 464}. The atypical features should be specified, the differential diagnosis discussed, and the most likely diagnosis suggested in a report categorized as "Atypical" {43,463,105,338}.

All cellular elements of the respiratory tract, including the oropharyngeal squamous cells, metaplastic squamous cells, respiratory bronchial epithelial cells, terminal bronchiolar or alveolar lining cells, and pulmonary macrophages, may demonstrate architectural and/or cellular atypia {615}. The majority of cytopathological cases categorized as "Atypical" will have histopathological correlates, which are benign lesions demonstrating reactive and reparative changes, including infectious etiologies, squamous metaplasia, and nuclear atypia secondary to iatrogenic effects, in particular radiation therapy and chemotherapy {463,465,360}.

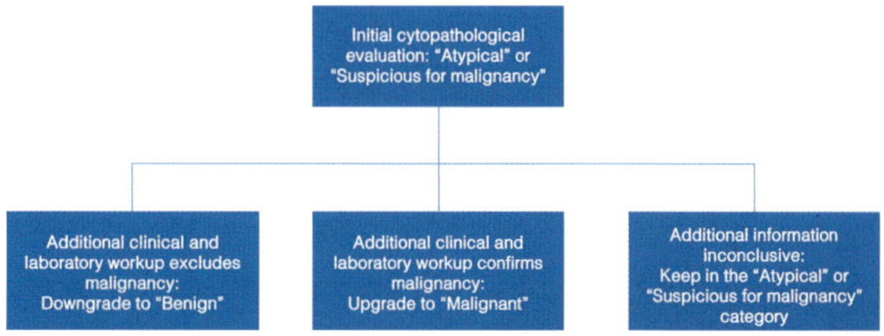

Fig. 5.01 Workflow for lung lesions categorized as "Atypical". The use of "Atypical" and "Suspicious for malignancy" categories as holding categories while awaiting additional workup.

It is recommended that clinical and imaging findings are reviewed and correlated before categorizing a specimen as "Atypical" {463,104}. Clinical signs and symptoms of acute inflammatory conditions can be variable and overlap with many other pathologies, such as pulmonary embolism, interstitial lung disease, cardiac failure, acute respiratory distress syndrome, and malignant tumours {504}. Similarly, the imaging features of benign and neoplastic processes in the lung may overlap.

Definition

Baloch ZW
Raymond WA

A specimen categorized as "Atypical" demonstrates features predominantly seen in benign lesions and minimal features that may raise the possibility of a malignant lesion, but with insufficient features either in number or quality to diagnose a benign or malignant process or lesion.

Discussion and background

Raymond WA
Baloch ZW

The value of an "Atypical" category in a hierarchical system is to maintain a high negative predictive value of a "Benign" category and a high positive predictive value of a "Malignant" category. An "Atypical" categorization is more likely than not to be benign, whereas a "Suspicious for malignancy" categorization is more likely than not to be malignant, and the risk of malignancy increases in a stepwise fashion from "Benign" through "Atypical" to "Suspicious for malignancy" and "Malignant". In the "Atypical" category the cytomorphological findings are mostly benign, but there are some features that are uncommon in benign lesions and which may suggest a malignant lesion. The use of the "Atypical" category should be kept to a minimum, and an institution should regularly audit their indeterminate categories to monitor the use by individual cytopathologists.

The main causes for an "Atypical" categorization include the following:

1. The intrinsic cytomorphological characteristics of the targeted lesion; there may be overlap in the cytopathological features of a reactive process and a neoplastic process
2. The expertise of the operator performing the bronchial wash or bronchial brush procedure or the FNAB, and the level of instruction and assistance given to the patient producing a sputum sample, which impact on the amount and quality of the cellular and background material on the slides
3. Technical issues related to obtaining and preparing the material, particularly the making of direct bronchial brush or FNAB smears
4. The experience of the cytopathologist in interpreting the specimen

Reference(s): {360,723,907,909,464}

Certain pathological processes may produce cytopathological changes that cannot confidently be recognized as a benign process, and which overlap with the cytomorphological criteria of malignant lesions (see Box 5.01, p. 89).

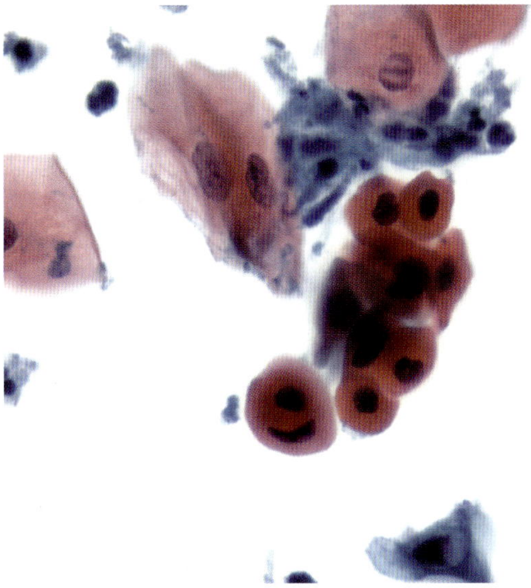

Fig. 5.03 Atypical squamous cells in FNAB. FNAB of an indeterminate-on-imaging lung mass showing atypical squamous cells; a corresponding core needle biopsy showed reactive squamous metaplasia (liquid-based cytopathology, Pap).

Cytomorphological findings that should lead to an "Atypical" categorization can be qualitative or quantitative in nature and include the following:

1. Atypical bronchial or other epithelial cells showing extreme reactive and reparative cellular changes, which may mimic malignancy, occurring in a setting of concurrent inflammatory or infective changes, radiation therapy, or chemotherapy
2. Squamous or other metaplastic changes that cannot be distinguished from a neoplasm; for example, goblet cell hyperplasia, which can mimic mucinous adenocarcinoma

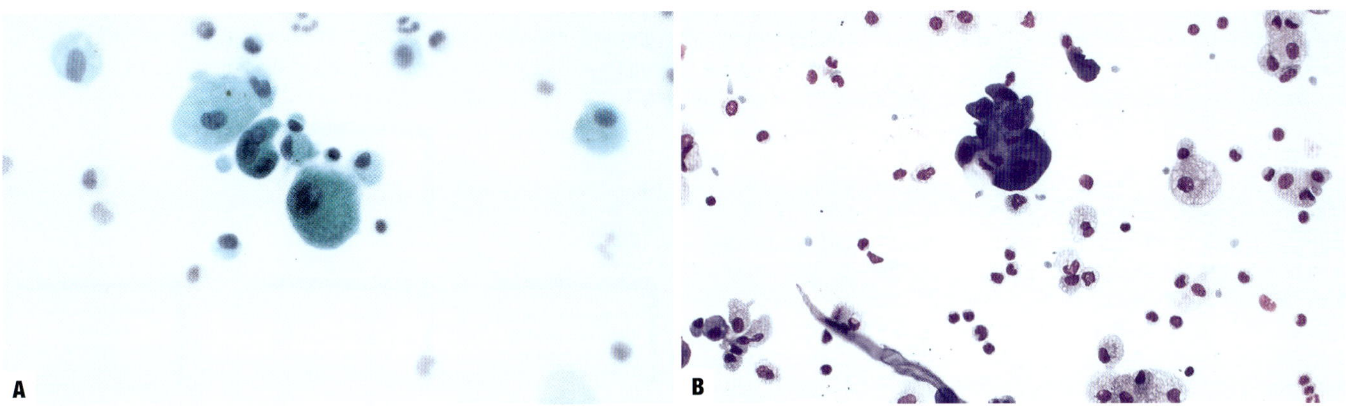

Fig. 5.02 Scant atypical cells secondary to chemotherapy effect. **A** Occasional atypical cells after a history of chemotherapy (Pap). **B** Scant atypical cells in bronchoalveolar lavage (BAL) with a history of chemotherapy (Giemsa).

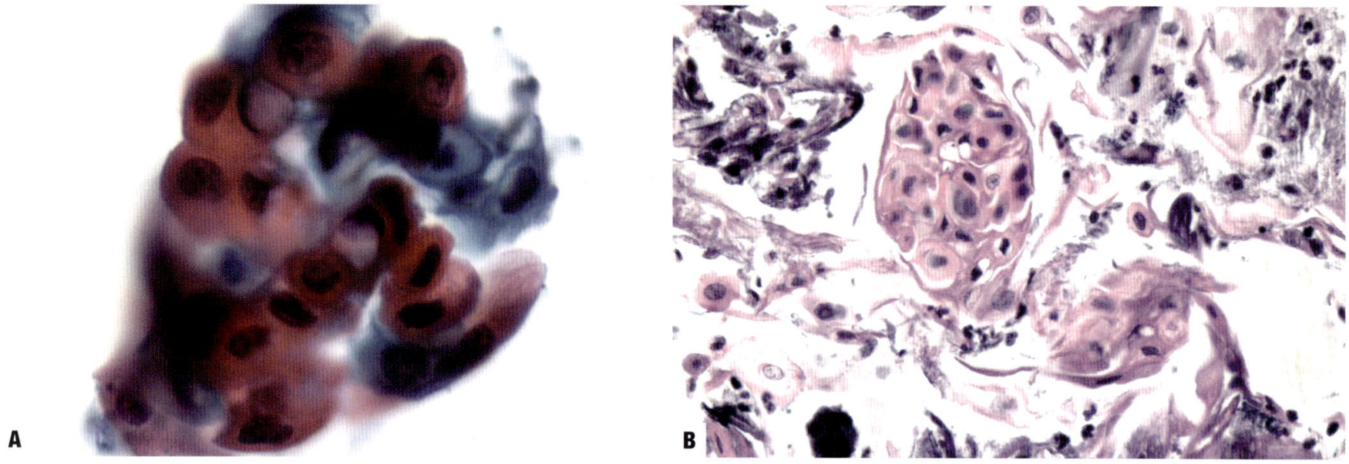

Fig. 5.04 Squamous metaplasia. **A** FNAB of a questionable lung mass showing poorly preserved squamous cells regarded as "Atypical" at initial evaluation. The corresponding core biopsy showed squamous metaplasia (Pap). **B** FNAB of a questionable lung mass showing squamous cells assessed as "Atypical" on cytology. The corresponding core biopsy showed reactive squamous metaplasia (cell block, H&E).

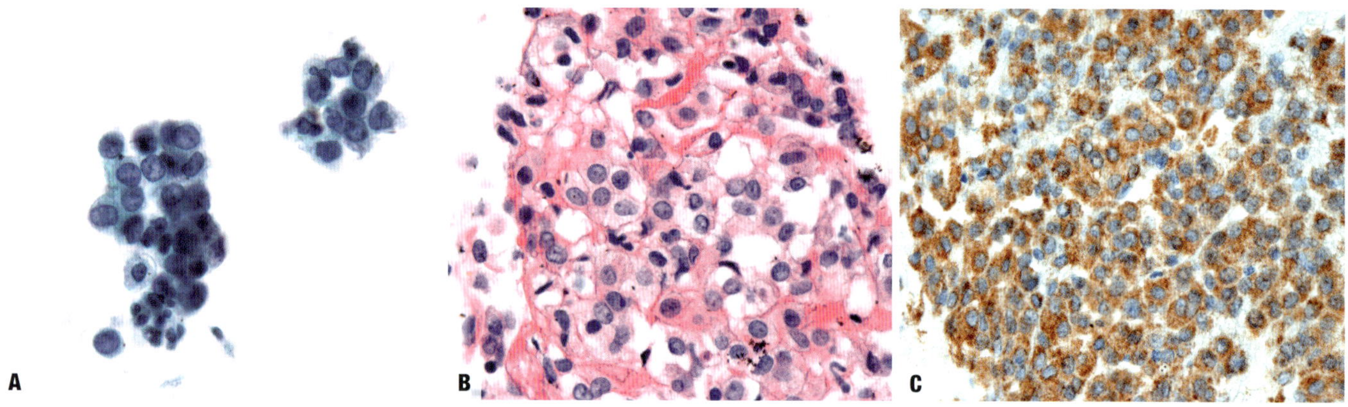

Fig. 5.05 Pulmonary macrophages. **A** Bronchoalveolar lavage (BAL) specimen. Loosely cohesive groups of macrophages, initially difficult to distinguish from neoplastic epithelial cells. **B** These were difficult to distinguish from neoplastic epithelial cells initially and regarded as "Atypical" (cell block, H&E). **C** CD68 immunostain confirms the presence of pulmonary macrophages (cell block).

3. Low cellularity resulting in only scant cells, with some cells showing cytopathological features usually seen in an epithelial malignancy or a lymphoproliferative disorder
4. Specimens with background elements suggestive of a neoplasm, such as necrotic or keratinous debris, thick mucin, or apoptotic cells
5. Spindle cell lesions with bland cytopathology that are likely to be initially assessed as "Atypical" until ancillary tests are able to provide a specific diagnosis

Reference(s): {463,30,1013,93,176}

When reporting atypical features in a pulmonary sample, the salient cytopathological features should be described and the specific atypical features specified, the differential diagnosis discussed, and the most likely diagnosis provided {463,105,338}. The extent to which a detailed cytopathological description is included in a report may vary with local practice, but the aim is to avoid overusing the "Atypical" category as a waste basket, without a clear analysis in each individual case. Inflammatory, degenerative, regenerative, therapy-related, and other reactive conditions, when recognized, should be described as "changes" rather than "Atypical", and the use of such terms as "inflammatory atypia" should be avoided (see *Inflammatory and reactive changes in glandular cells and squamous cells*, p. 61, and Box 5.01). It is important to assess whether the atypical cells represent a distinct cell population, which in general favours a neoplastic lesion, or whether there is a continuum of normal to atypical respiratory epithelial cells, which is likely to be reactive {463,105,106}.

The approach to specimens categorized as "Atypical" is often a two-step process, the first step being the identification of the atypical cells and the second an attempt to resolve the diagnosis by additional workup tests, such as repeating a liquid-based

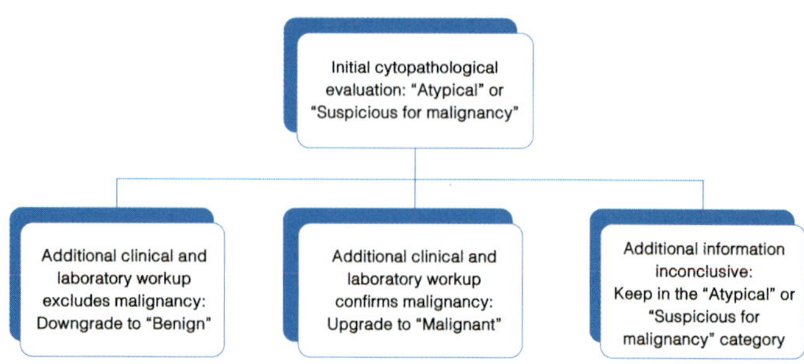

Fig. 5.06 Lung "Atypical" category. Use of "Atypical" and "Suspicious for malignancy" categories in lung cytopathology.

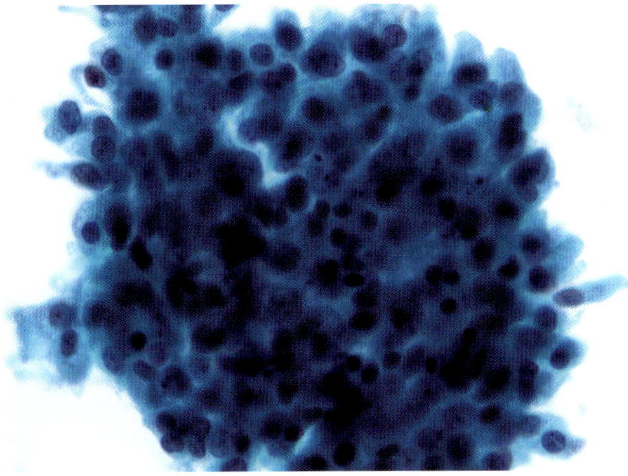

Fig. 5.07 "Atypical". Bronchoalveolar lavage (BAL) specimen showing a group of atypical cells with a glandular morphology. No keratinization is evident. The follow-up biopsy showed a well-differentiated adenocarcinoma (Pap).

preparation or preparing a cell block and performing appropriate ancillary tests. However, performing ancillary tests on FNAB cases with scant atypical cells is not recommended {185,372, 347}. Adequately cellular specimens consisting of atypical lymphoid cells should be submitted for flow cytometric analysis to further characterize the lymphoid population.

If additional laboratory studies resolve the dilemma, the "Atypical" case may be downgraded to "Benign" or upgraded to "Suspicious for malignancy" or "Malignant". If the additional workup is inconclusive owing to a paucity of available material, inherent ambiguous cytopathological features, or equivocal ancillary test results, the case remains categorized as "Atypical". The availability of such ancillary tests in low- and middle-income countries will impact on this process.

Chapter 5

Box 5.01 Atypical features and mimics of malignancy in pulmonary cytopathological preparations {463,30,1013,93,176}

1. **Nonspecific cellular changes due to inflammatory conditions:**
   - Loss of architectural polarity in epithelial tissue fragments associated with nuclear crowding and disorganization
   - Cytomegaly and anisonucleosis within tissue fragments
   - Reactive bronchial cells showing nuclear enlargement and oval nuclei with few minor nuclear membrane irregularities or indentations, although usually showing evenly distributed chromatin and nucleoli; these may lack cilia (ciliocytophthoria); the nuclei tend to show uniform changes, including nucleolar enlargement, across any particular tissue fragment
   - Inflammatory debris mimicking tumour type necrosis; there is usually a prominent inflammatory cell component, varying from predominantly neutrophils to histiocytes or granulomatous epithelioid histiocytes
2. **Reserve cell hyperplasia due to chronic irritation and inflammation:**
   - Usually encountered in bronchoalveolar lavage (BAL) and bronchial brushing specimens
   - Occurs as small cohesive sheets and more 3D tissue fragments of small cells with an increased N:C ratio; hyperchromatic, small, round to mildly pleomorphic nuclei with uniform coarse chromatin and single nucleoli; scant cytoplasm; no cilia are present
   - May mimic neuroendocrine tumours (NETs)
   - Usually cellularity is low, with only a small number of atypical epithelial tissue fragments present in a background of prominent histiocytes
3. **Squamous metaplasia:**
   - Occurs due to chronic irritation and/or infections, including abscesses and fungal or viral infections
   - Round to oval squamous cells with hyperchromatic, round to elongated nuclei and a variable but often low N:C ratio
   - Can be encountered in all types of respiratory cytopathology specimens
   - Can mimic well-differentiated squamous cell carcinoma: difficult differential diagnosis in the setting of possible residual carcinoma after radiotherapy, when need to assess changes related to therapy
   - Associated keratinous debris can mimic tumour necrosis
4. **Postradiotherapy and postchemotherapy changes:**
   - Usually low cellularity with scattered epithelial tissue fragments showing a degree of irregularity in the cell arrangement
   - Readily identifiable cytomegaly with low N:C ratio and vacuolization, nucleomegaly, and nuclear pleomorphism involving all cellular elements of the respiratory tract
   - Hyperchromatic nuclei with varying degrees of blurring of chromatin and vacuoles
   - Foamy histiocytes are seen in amiodarone-associated lung injury
5. **Hyperplasia and reactive changes of type 2 pneumocytes:**
   - Encountered in acute respiratory distress syndrome, chronic obstructive pulmonary disease, and viral infections
   - Enlarged nuclei with vesicular chromatin and prominent nucleoli
   - Crowded tissue fragments (Creola bodies) with a degree of nuclear overlapping, mimicking malignancy
   - Abundant clear cytoplasm, mimicking mucinous adenocarcinoma
6. **Viral infections:**
   - Encountered with herpes simplex virus, CMV, and other viral infections
   - Cytomegaly and enlarged round to oval to mildly pleomorphic nuclei
   - Abnormal nuclear chromatin showing margination and clearing of viral inclusions, and (particularly in herpetic infections) multinucleated epithelial cells; CMV shows classic owl-eye nuclei
   - Bronchial cells with reparative changes including nuclear enlargement, prominent nucleoli, and ciliocytophthoria; nuclei tend to be relatively uniform in size and shape

Risk of malignancy and management recommendations

Raymond WA
Baloch ZW
Navani N
Scagliotti GV

The reported risk of malignancy for the "Atypical" category for all respiratory cytopathology varies from 22% to 62% {464}. This wide variation is partly because not all studies distinguish between the categories of "Atypical" and "Suspicious for malignancy". The risk of malignancy for the "Atypical" category also varies with the procurement method. In recent studies that have included an "Atypical" category, the risk of malignancy was 50–60% for the "Atypical" category and 54–90% for the "Suspicious for malignancy" category {466,105} (see Table 1.04, p. 11, in Chapter 1: *Introduction to the WHO Reporting System for Lung Cytopathology*).

The initial management of cases assigned an "Atypical" category, for all respiratory samples, is correlation with the clinical and imaging findings. If the imaging features are atypical or concerning for malignancy, further investigation is required, either by a repeat cytopathological study or by the use of a more invasive procedure, when available. An "Atypical" sputum sample could be repeated or the patient could progress to bronchial washing/brushing or FNAB (depending on the site of the lesion and presentation), and an "Atypical" bronchial washing/brushing could proceed to endobronchial ultrasound or transthoracic FNAB, with or without transbronchial core needle biopsy if endobronchial ultrasound is used (see Table 1.04, p. 11, in Chapter 1: *Introduction to the WHO Reporting System for Lung Cytopathology*). An "Atypical" FNAB is usually followed by a repeat FNAB or core needle biopsy via endobronchial ultrasound or a transthoracic approach (see Table 1.05, p. 12, in Chapter 1: *Introduction to the WHO Reporting System for Lung Cytopathology*). Additional procedures may also procure adequate tissue for ancillary studies {463}. However, if the atypical cytopathological features correlate with benign imaging and clinical features, then clinical observation for a period of time may be an appropriate option.

Monitoring of "Atypical" case numbers within a pathology department or as reported by individual cytopathologists is essential to assess the quality of a cytopathology service. This may include regular audits of the proceduralists providing the specimens.

Sample reports: Atypical

Field AS
Chandra A
VanderLaan PA

The sample reports provided here are based on the standardized cytopathology report in the *Diagnostic categories and report structure* (p. 8) section of the first chapter. See that section for a discussion on the structure and components.

These are sample reports that include the components required in one possible format; the final report format will depend on local practice and local laboratory information system requirements. For brevity, demographics and information on the macroscopic features and rapid onsite evaluation (ROSE) are not presented here.

Each institution should select a term for the main heading of the diagnostic summary, such as "Diagnostic summary" (as used in the examples below), "Diagnosis", or "Final diagnosis", and use it consistently.

Chapter 5

Sample report 1

Type of specimen:
Sputum sample.

Clinical and imaging information:
30 mm mass in left upper lobe. No definite hilar lymphadenopathy. Smoker.

Diagnostic summary:
Category: Atypical
Diagnosis: Scant atypical glandular cells. See report below.

Microscopic description:
Very occasional small, mildly crowded tissue fragments of epithelial cells with large mildly pleomorphic and minimally indented nuclei, prominent single round nucleoli, and eccentric pale, occasionally vacuolated cytoplasm are present. The nuclei within each tissue fragment show similar changes. These epithelial cells lack cilia and are mixed with plentiful tissue fragments of ciliated bronchial cells in small tissue fragments, along with siderophages, histiocytes, neutrophils, and squamous cells.
Comment: These occasional glandular epithelial tissue fragments are atypical. Correlation with imaging and clinical history is required. Further workup with bronchial brush and FNAB as clinically indicated is recommended.

Sample report 2

Type of specimen:
Bronchial brush.

Clinical and imaging information:
Previous squamous cell carcinoma of lung. Chemotherapy and radiotherapy. Review. Bronchial brush right middle lobe bronchus.

Diagnostic summary:
Bronchial brush right middle lobe bronchus
Category: Atypical
Diagnosis: Occasional atypical squamous cells. See report below.

Microscopic description:
These highly cellular smears show occasional tissue fragments of squamous cells with variable occasionally high N:C ratio, moderately enlarged pleomorphic nuclei with blurred chromatin, and prominent nucleoli in occasional cells. Occasional cells are very large associated with nucleomegaly. Plentiful bronchial epithelial tissue fragments, neutrophils, and histiocytes with some carbon-laden macrophages are also present.

Comment: the features are most likely related to therapy, but residual carcinoma cannot be excluded. Correlation with imaging is required, and FNAB should be considered to provide material for typing, staging, and ancillary tests.

Editorial note:
The diagnostic summary includes the specific information regarding the site of the lesion from the request form and specimen container of any needle-rinsing material.

Sample report 3

Type of specimen:
Endobronchial ultrasound–guided FNAB right upper lobe.

Clinical and imaging information:
FNAB right upper lobe. Poorly defined 30 mm mass. Immunocompromised. Adjacent hilar lymphadenopathy.

Diagnostic summary:
FNAB right upper lobe
Category: Atypical
Diagnosis: Abscess with atypical squamous epithelium. See report below.

Microscopic description:
These moderately cellular smears show considerable pus and debris, with plentiful neutrophils and macrophages, fragments of alveolar septa, occasional small tissue fragments of ciliated bronchial cells, and small tissue fragments of squamous cells with atypical nuclei. No definite fungi are seen on routine stains.
Comment: The features are consistent with an abscess. The squamous epithelium shows atypia, raising a differential diagnosis of metaplastic squamous epithelium or possibly squamous neoplasia. Special stains are underway. Correlation with clinical, imaging, and microbiological findings is required.

Supplementary report 1:
The cell block shows similar material. The methenamine silver stain for fungi is negative, as are the auramine stain for mycobacteria and the Gram stain. Correlation with clinical, imaging, and microbiological findings is required. Consideration should be given to repeat FNAB.

Editorial note:
The diagnostic summary includes the specific information regarding the site of the lesion from the request form and specimen container of any needle-rinsing material.
There has been a supplementary report on special stains for infectious agents for this case performed subsequently on a cell block, and this is included in the single integrated report.

Sample report 4

Type of specimen:
Bronchoalveolar lavage (BAL) right lower lobe; liquid-based cytopathology.

Clinical and imaging information:
74-year-old man with chronic obstructive pulmonary disease (COPD) and chest infection. Started on antibiotics. BAL right lower lobe to exclude malignancy.

Diagnostic summary:
Category: Atypical
Diagnosis: Favour reactive inflammatory changes

Microscopic description:
This liquid-based cytopathology preparation shows numerous alveolar macrophages and occasional 3D tissue fragments of epithelial cells with nuclear enlargement and prominent nucleoli. The changes most likely represent reactive changes; however, well-differentiated adenocarcinoma cannot be excluded on this sample. Further workup with biopsy is recommended.

Sample report 5

Type of specimen:
Endobronchial ultrasound–guided transbronchial FNAB posterior lesion.

Clinical and imaging information:
48-year-old woman with an incidental finding of a poorly defined mass at the lung hilum. ? neoplastic. Endobronchial ultrasound–guided transbronchial FNAB performed.

Diagnostic summary:
Category: Atypical
Diagnosis: Limited material raising the possibility of a schwannoma

Microscopic description:
These smears show limited cellular material with occasional small tissue fragments consisting of small spindle cells with wavy, elongated nuclei. Very occasional single similar spindle cells with small, elongated nuclei are seen in the background. There is no necrosis. Inflammatory cells are scant. Similar spindle cells are seen in the cell block.
Comment: The features may represent a spindle cell neoplasm or possibly a reactive inflammatory proliferation. Ancillary tests are in progress and a supplementary report will follow. Discussion at the lung multidisciplinary meeting recommended.

Supplementary report 1:
Spindle cells in the cell block are positive for S100 and negative for SMA, desmin, and CD34, raising the possibility of a schwannoma. The *SS18*::SSX fusion is negative, excluding synovial sarcoma. Correlation with history and imaging is required. Further biopsy is recommended.

Editorial note:
A preliminary report categorizing the lesion as "Atypical" can be issued and ancillary test results added at a later stage, or some cytopathologists may prefer to wait until the ancillary testing is available before issuing a report. In either situation, only a single integrated final report incorporating the ancillary testing should be made.

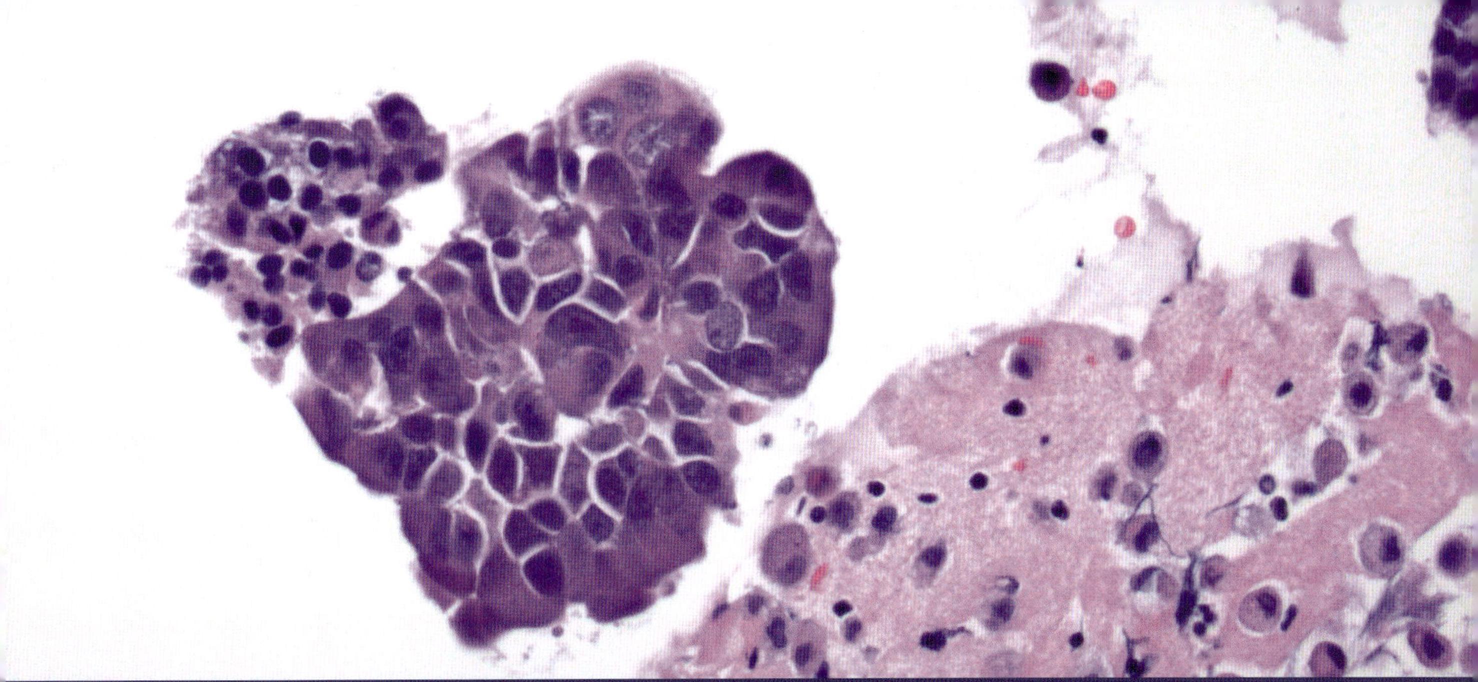

6

Diagnostic category: Suspicious for malignancy

Edited by: Layfield LJ, Schmitt F

Introduction

Moreira AL
Haba R

The category "Suspicious for malignancy" is used in respiratory cytopathology for cases that the cytopathologist assesses as most likely malignant but where there is a degree of uncertainty as to a definitive diagnosis of malignancy {465,338,463}. This category is used when there is insufficient quality or quantity of cellular material in an adequate smear for a definite diagnosis of malignancy. The category remains subjective, with a high rate of interobserver disagreement {468}, because the threshold for the diagnosis of malignancy depends on the cytopathologist's experience, the type of cytopathological preparation, and the degree of cellular atypia. The category is used particularly to avoid a false positive diagnosis of malignancy, which may lead to unnecessary intervention, and so maintain the high positive predictive value of a "Malignant" categorization. The category of "Suspicious for malignancy" should not be used as the sole basis for therapy {463,591,338}. The majority of cases categorized as "Suspicious for malignancy" will have histopathological correlates that are malignant lesions, and the risk of malignancy of the "Suspicious for malignancy" category is approximately 82% (range: 54.5–90%) {465,105,338,466,469}.

Definition

Moreira AL
Haba R

A specimen categorized as "Suspicious for malignancy" demonstrates some cytopathological features suggestive of malignancy but has insufficient features either in number or quality to make an unequivocal diagnosis of malignancy.

Discussion and background

Moreira AL
Haba R

A high degree of accuracy for the diagnosis of malignancy is important in the cytopathology of all body sites, particularly in respiratory cytopathology, where obtaining samples (apart from sputum samples) by bronchoscopy or via the transthoracic approach is relatively invasive, and subsequent unnecessary therapeutic interventions to the chest can be associated with significant morbidity and mortality. Historically, the categories of "Atypical" and "Suspicious for malignancy" have been used to indicate, respectively, a low and a high degree of uncertainty for a diagnosis of malignancy, and to stratify the risk of malignancy (ROM). The category of "Suspicious for malignancy" is used when the cytopathologist encounters an adequate preparation that contains cytopathological features that are inconclusive for an unequivocal diagnosis of malignancy but wants to convey a high degree of concern for the presence of a malignant tumour to the clinical team so that further diagnostic management can be planned. The use of this diagnostic category has been cemented further by studies that applied risk stratification for the final diagnosis of a malignant tumour. Several studies have estimated the ROM for the "Suspicious for malignancy" category to be 75–100% for exfoliative samples and 75–88% for FNAB {465, 105,338,467,469}, whereas the ROM for the "Atypical" category is 62–100% for exfoliative samples and 46–55% for FNAB {105, 466}. Although the ROM is high, the cytopathological categorization should not be used alone as a substitute for a malignant diagnosis, and further biopsy is recommended. However, when this is correlated with suspicious clinical and imaging findings in a multidisciplinary setting, there may be situations where pulmonary multidisciplinary teams proceed to specific treatment.

The "Suspicious for malignancy" category is applicable to a suspicion of any malignant tumour type, including non-small cell carcinoma, neuroendocrine tumours (NETs), small cell carcinoma, large cell neuroendocrine carcinoma (LCNEC), lymphoma, sarcoma, and metastatic carcinomas, and the type of tumour or a differential diagnosis of the suspected tumour types should always be stated in the cytopathology report. The category is equally applicable to any cytopathological study, i.e. sputum sampling, bronchial wash, bronchoalveolar lavage (BAL), bronchial brush, CT-guided transthoracic FNAB, and endobronchial ultrasound–guided transbronchial FNAB.

The "Suspicious for malignancy" category is usually applied in cases where there is significant cytopathological atypia (including nuclear enlargement; anisonucleosis; irregular nuclear membrane; coarse or hyperchromatic chromatin; and prominent, often large or irregular nucleoli) along with loss of architectural orientation or polarity, nuclear crowding and moulding, and variability in cell size and shape, but where there are only a small number of cells showing these features or the qualitative features are not definitive for a diagnosis of malignancy. Rapid onsite evaluation (ROSE) has been shown to reduce the rate of "Suspicious for malignancy", but limiting factors related to the intrinsic cytopathological characteristics of the tumour and technical problems remain {306,372,568}.

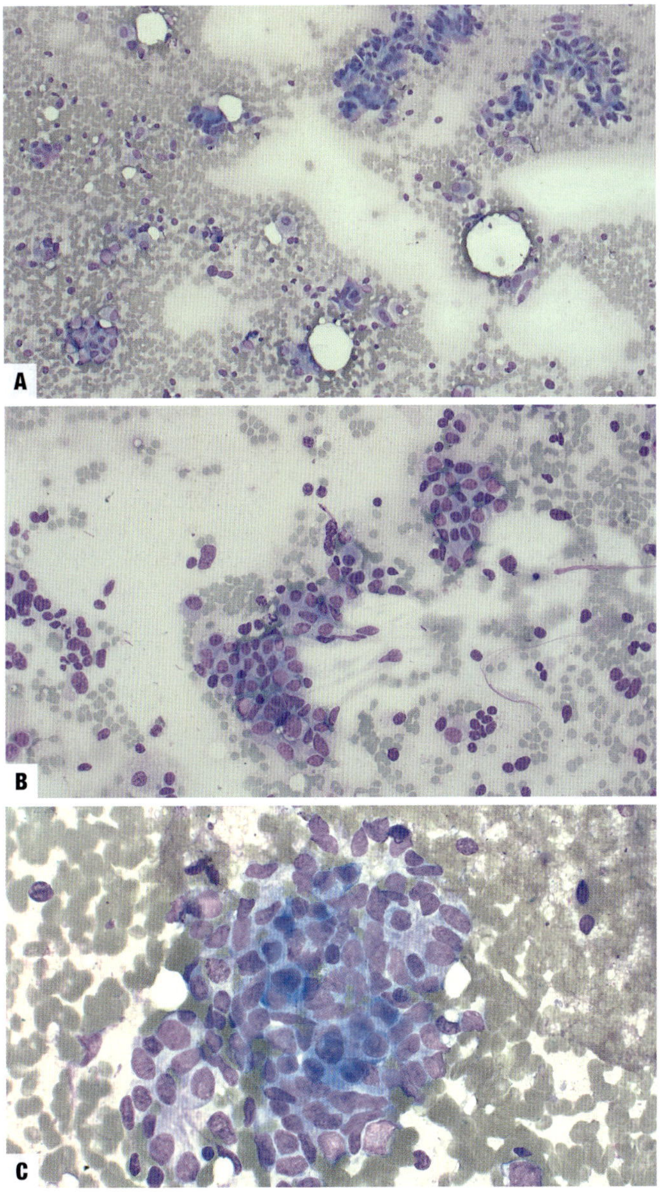

Fig. 6.01 Incidental right lower lobe nodule in a 60-year-old woman. PET-negative, increasing in size. Non-smoker. Category: "Atypical". **A** Smear of atypical cells, both as cohesive tissue fragments and as dispersed single cells (lower left of field). Contrast with normal bronchial epithelial cells (top right) (Giemsa). **B** Smear of atypical cells with oval nuclei; bland, fine, evenly dispersed chromatin; and a moderate amount of cytoplasm. Some nuclei are stripped of cytoplasm (Giemsa). **C** Higher magnification shows mild to moderate anisonucleosis and a single mitosis. Some cells have a higher N:C ratio but no coarse chromatin (Giemsa).

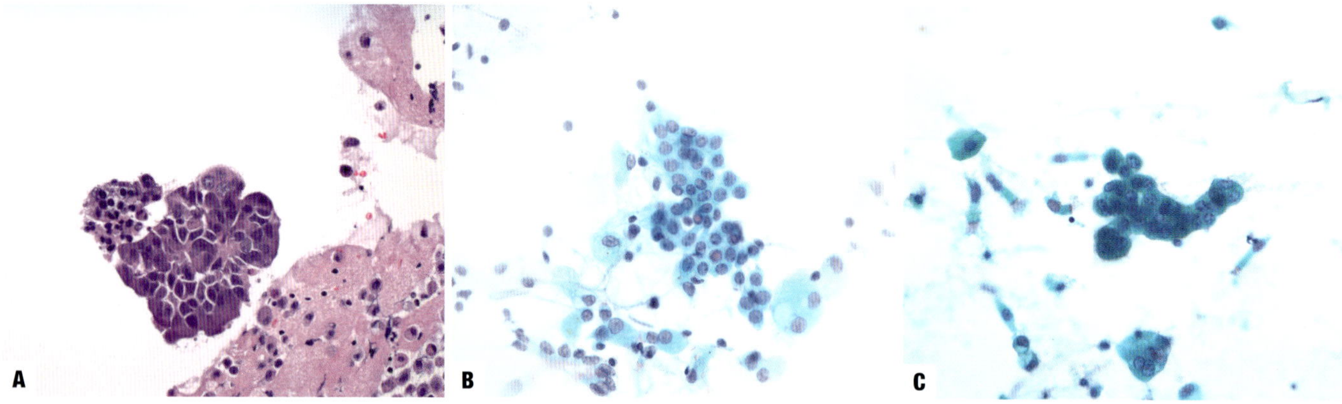

Fig. 6.02 "Suspicious for malignancy". **A** Tissue fragment of epithelial cells lacking cilia and showing a low N:C ratio and a degree of columnar orientation, but with hyperchromatic nuclei and pleomorphic nuclei, with necrosis in the background (cell block, H&E). **B** Suspicious for well-differentiated adenocarcinoma. Flat, cohesive sheet of cells lacking cilia, showing mild nuclear enlargement, fine chromatin, occasional nuclear grooves, and occasional nuclear pseudoinclusions, in a background of foamy macrophages and ciliated bronchial epithelium. The lack of overtly malignant characteristics leads to the categorization of "Suspicious for malignancy" (Pap). **C** After radiation therapy. Cohesive crowded tissue fragment of atypical cells categorized as "Suspicious for malignancy" in a bronchial brushing of a patient with a prior history of surgery and radiation therapy (bronchial brushing, Pap).

Necrotic tumours that yield limited intact cell numbers, dense obscuring inflammatory backgrounds, obscuring granulomatous reactions, and tumours with a prominent fibrotic component are examples of intrinsic tumour characteristics that may produce highly atypical samples with scant cellularity independent of the number of FNAB passes or ROSE. There may be overlap of cytopathological features between inflamed reactive epithelium and the sheets of cells with low nuclear atypia found in well-differentiated adenocarcinoma of the lung, which may be categorized as "Suspicious for malignancy" owing to a lack of overtly malignant nuclear characteristics. Prior radiation and or chemotherapy, particularly for lung carcinomas, may result in significant atypia in a sample with low cellularity, which mimics and cannot be distinguished from previous carcinoma, and the "Suspicious for malignancy" category is appropriate. The size of the tumour (particularly those measuring < 20 mm), the location of the targeted nodule, and the experience of the interventionalist procuring the biopsy may result in low cellularity and an inability to give an unequivocal diagnosis of malignancy {656,815,1021,753}.

Ancillary techniques, particularly ICC, can assist in making a malignant diagnosis, for example where ICC can confirm metastatic and neuroendocrine carcinomas. But in many cases the quality and quantity of the suspicious cells on direct smears and in cell blocks may prevent further definition of the diagnosis, and a "Suspicious for malignancy" categorization and a statement regarding the type of carcinoma suspected should be included in the report. For example, positive ICC for neuroendocrine markers on a small amount of extensively crushed material in a cell block from a lung FNAB may favour a NET and exclude lymphoma, but there may be insufficient tumour for the proliferation marker Ki-67 to define the tumour grade {1000,903}. Thyroid transcription factor 1 (TTF1) as a marker of lung adenocarcinoma and p40 as a marker of squamous differentiation are often used for further classification of non-small cell carcinomas. However, these markers are also expressed in reactive cells and do not separate benign from malignant.

Risk of malignancy and management recommendations

Moreira AL
Haba R

The risk of malignancy for the "Atypical" category is 62–100% for exfoliative samples and 46–55% for FNAB, and for the "Suspicious for malignancy" category, 75–100% for exfoliative samples and 75–88% for FNAB {466,105}. The use of the category "Suspicious for malignancy" has a high rate of interobserver variability, so consultation with more experienced cytopathologists is recommended when assessing cases with a limited cellularity, obscuring or technical problems, or cytopathological features that may be shared by inflammatory reactive epithelium and malignancies. It is mandatory to review the clinical presentation and any imaging that is available, ideally in a multidisciplinary setting, before proceeding to further diagnostic steps or definitive management.

If a sputum sample is "Suspicious for malignancy", it can be repeated, or the patient can proceed to bronchoscopy with bronchial washings and brushings or endobronchial ultrasound-directed transbronchial FNAB with or without core needle biopsy. Transthoracic FNAB is an option for peripheral lesions or where bronchoscopy is not available in low- and middle-income countries. If the bronchial washings/brushings and/or FNAB are "Benign" and correlate with benign clinical and imaging findings, routine follow-up with imaging at 3–6 months can be recommended. If the cytopathology remains "Suspicious for malignancy" and the clinical and imaging are suspicious, repeat FNAB (preferably with rapid onsite evaluation [ROSE]) is recommended and core needle biopsy can be added, although proceeding to surgical biopsy with or without frozen sectioning should be considered on the basis of the overall findings.

The categorization of a case as "Suspicious for malignancy" is not equivalent to a final diagnosis of malignancy. It is imperative to have good communication with the members of the clinical team (with review of all relevant clinical and imaging information) for the determination of a management plan, in order to avoid unnecessary additional risks and costs.

Sample reports: Suspicious for malignancy

Field AS

The sample reports provided here are based on the standardized cytopathology report in the *Diagnostic categories and report structure* (p. 8) section of the first chapter. See that section for a discussion on the structure and components.

These are sample reports that include the components required in one possible format; the final report format will depend on local practice and local laboratory information system requirements. For brevity, demographics and information on the macroscopic features and rapid onsite evaluation (ROSE) are not presented here.

Each institution should select a term for the main heading of the diagnostic summary, such as "Diagnostic summary" (as used in the examples below), "Diagnosis", or "Final diagnosis", and use it consistently.

Sample report 1

Type of specimen:
Sputum sample.

Clinical and imaging information:
30 mm mass in left upper lobe. No definite hilar lymphadenopathy. Smoker.

Diagnostic summary:
Category: Suspicious for malignancy
Diagnosis: Atypical glandular cells. See report below.

Microscopic description:
Very occasional small, crowded tissue fragments of epithelial cells with large, mildly pleomorphic, occasionally indented nuclei with prominent single round nucleoli and eccentric pale, occasionally vacuolated cytoplasm are present. These epithelial cells lack cilia, and they are mixed with small tissue fragments and sheets of bronchial cells, along with siderophages, histiocytes, neutrophils, and squamous cells.
Comment: These scattered glandular epithelial tissue fragments are suspicious for adenocarcinoma. Correlation with imaging and clinical history is required. Further workup with bronchial brush and FNAB, as clinically indicated, is recommended.

Sample report 2

Type of specimen:
Bronchial brush.

Clinical and imaging information:
Previous squamous cell carcinoma of lung. Chemotherapy and radiotherapy. Review. Bronchial brush right middle lobe bronchus.

Diagnostic summary:
Bronchial brush right middle lobe bronchus
Category: Suspicious for malignancy
Diagnosis: Atypical squamous cells suspicious for residual squamous cell carcinoma

Microscopic description:
These highly cellular smears show plentiful bronchial epithelial tissue fragments, neutrophils, and histiocytes, with some carbon-laden macrophages. In addition, there are a small number of squamous cells with variable (occasionally high) N:C ratios and moderately enlarged, pleomorphic nuclei with coarse chromatin and prominent nucleoli. There are also large cells with large, sometimes vacuolated nuclei, some of which have blurred chromatin. There is a background of debris but no definite keratinous material or necrosis.

Comment: The features are suspicious for residual squamous cell carcinoma, although therapy-related changes are also present. Correlation with imaging is required, and FNAB should be considered to provide material for typing, staging, and ancillary tests.

Editorial note:
The diagnostic summary includes the specific information regarding the site of the lesion from the request form and specimen container of any needle-rinsing material.

Sample report 3

Type of specimen:
Endobronchial ultrasound–guided FNAB right upper lobe.

Clinical and imaging information:
FNAB right upper lobe. Poorly defined 30 mm mass. Immunocompromised. Adjacent hilar lymphadenopathy.

Diagnostic summary:
FNAB right upper lobe
Category: Suspicious for malignancy
Diagnosis: Necrosis with scant atypical squamous epithelium suspicious for keratinizing squamous cell carcinoma. See report below.

Microscopic description:
There is considerable necrotic material and keratinous debris, as well as two minute tissue fragments of keratinized cells with small pyknotic, hyperchromatic nuclei and a low to moderate N:C ratio. Occasional macrophages are also present. No definite fungi are seen on routine stains.
Comment: The features are suspicious for keratinizing squamous cell carcinoma. Special stains are underway. Correlation with clinical, imaging, and microbiological findings is required.

Supplementary report 1:
The cell block shows similar necrotic and keratinous debris, with no viable epithelium present. The methenamine silver stain for fungi is negative, as are the auramine stain for mycobacteria and the Gram stain. Correlation with clinical, imaging, and microbiological findings is required. Consideration should be given to repeat FNAB.

Editorial note:
The diagnostic summary includes the specific information regarding the site of the lesion from the request form and specimen container of any needle-rinsing material.
There has been a supplementary report on special stains for infectious agents for this case performed subsequently on a cell block, and this is included in the single integrated report.

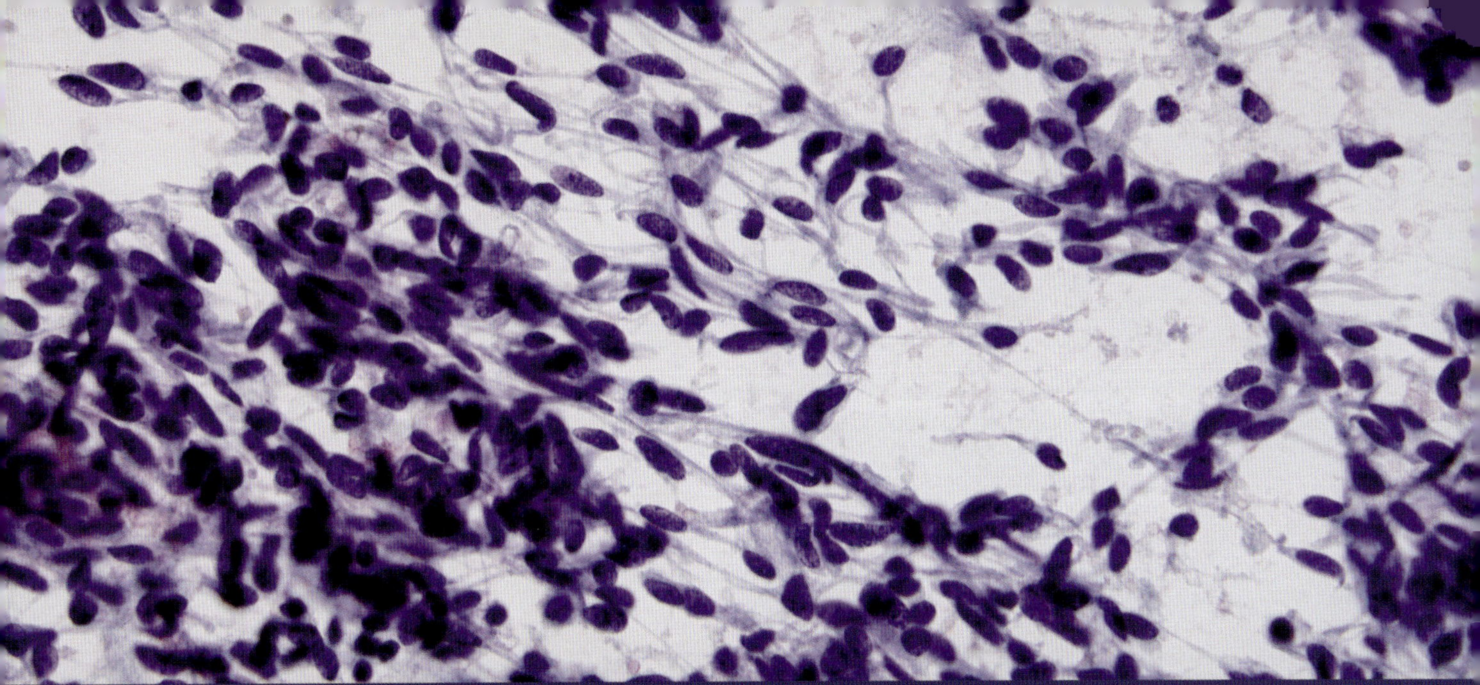

7

Diagnostic category: Malignant

Edited by: Bubendorf L, Engels M, Field AS, Hiroshima K, Layfield LJ, Osamura RY, Pitman MB, Satoh Y, Schmitt F, Zakowski MF

Introduction

Bubendorf L
Baloch ZW

Most carcinomas of the lung present at an advanced stage, and the majority of advanced lung cancers are diagnosed utilizing limited tissue samples, including cytopathology and forceps or core needle biopsy {916}. The cytopathology specimens employed for the diagnosis of lung malignancies include FNAB and exfoliative specimens, including sputum samples, bronchial washing, bronchial brushing, and (rarely) bronchoalveolar lavage (BAL). The FNAB of mass lesions can be guided by endobronchial ultrasound or CT. Rapid onsite evaluation (ROSE) allows for ensuring specimen adequacy during the procedure, helps to avoid the need for repeat tissue sampling, and allows for best practice and cost-effective triaging of specimens {812,94,736,378}.

Precise characterization of malignancies is essential because patient management with targeted therapy is based on the WHO classification tumour type and molecular biomarker profile. This has been driven by major advances in the personalized treatment of advanced non-small cell lung cancer with various tyrosine kinase inhibitors for tumours with sensitizing genetic alterations of *EGFR*, *ALK*, *ROS1*, *RET*, *NTRK*, *BRAF*, and *MET*, as well as the recent addition of immune checkpoint inhibitors {915,701,437,733}. Attaining this goal of a precise diagnosis may be challenging in limited tissue samples of primary or metastatic lung tumours because of the small amount of tumour or the low neoplastic cell fraction in small samples and/or poor tumour differentiation. Therefore, it is important to employ a multidisciplinary strategy to obtain adequate tumour cellularity for pathological diagnosis, to confirm histopathological type by a limited panel of ICC markers and then perform molecular biomarker testing {93,1000}. Molecular testing including next-generation sequencing can be successfully performed on cytopathology samples {736,924,699}. Obtaining multiple biopsy and cytopathology samples during the same procedure helps in prioritizing and optimizing the use of different tissue samples for ancillary testing.

A classification for lung cancer diagnosis in non-resection specimens, which are mostly cytopathology and core needle biopsy specimens, was recommended in the 2015 WHO classification and updated in the 2021 edition. This has provided a workflow for managing small biopsy and cytopathology samples to make a specific diagnosis of primary lung adenocarcinoma by ICC and molecular testing {916}. It is recommended to limit the use of ICC and/or mucin stains to diagnose and subtype non-small cell lung cancer, so as to preserve tumours cells for subsequent molecular analysis.

Definition

Baloch ZW
Savic Prince S

A specimen categorized as "Malignant" demonstrates unequivocal cytopathological features of malignancy.

Discussion and background

Baloch ZW
Savic Prince S

Malignant neoplasms involving the lungs include both primary and secondary tumours. These can occur confined to the pulmonary parenchyma, or as pleural-based lesions with minimal parenchymal involvement, or as small or imaging-occult pulmonary lesions with extensive mediastinal lymph node involvement giving rise to a hilar mass {463,915,731,161}. It is important to be aware of the limitations of cytopathology samples due to qualitative and quantitative issues {212,50,153}. Therefore, a "Malignant" categorization and, wherever possible, a specific tumour type diagnosis should be rendered only in specimens

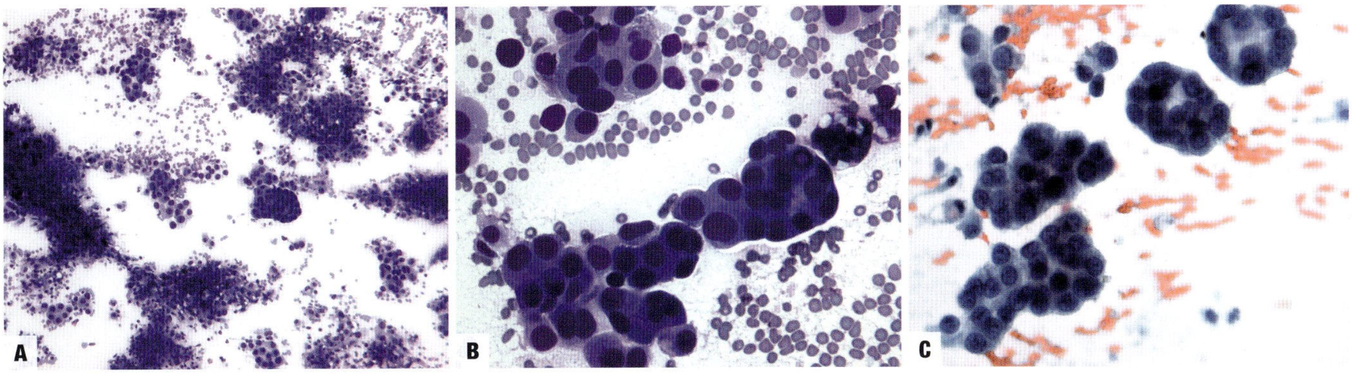

Fig. 7.01 Lung adenocarcinoma. **A** Adenocarcinoma showing 3D tissue fragments consisting of pleomorphic tumour cells with eccentric cytoplasm (Giemsa). **B** 3D tissue fragments with a suggestion of an acinar arrangement made up of pleomorphic tumour cells with rounded nuclei and eccentric cytoplasm (Giemsa). **C** Crowded, relatively cohesive 3D tissue fragments, some showing acinar or glandular architecture and consisting of cells with rounded nuclei and eccentric cytoplasm (Pap).

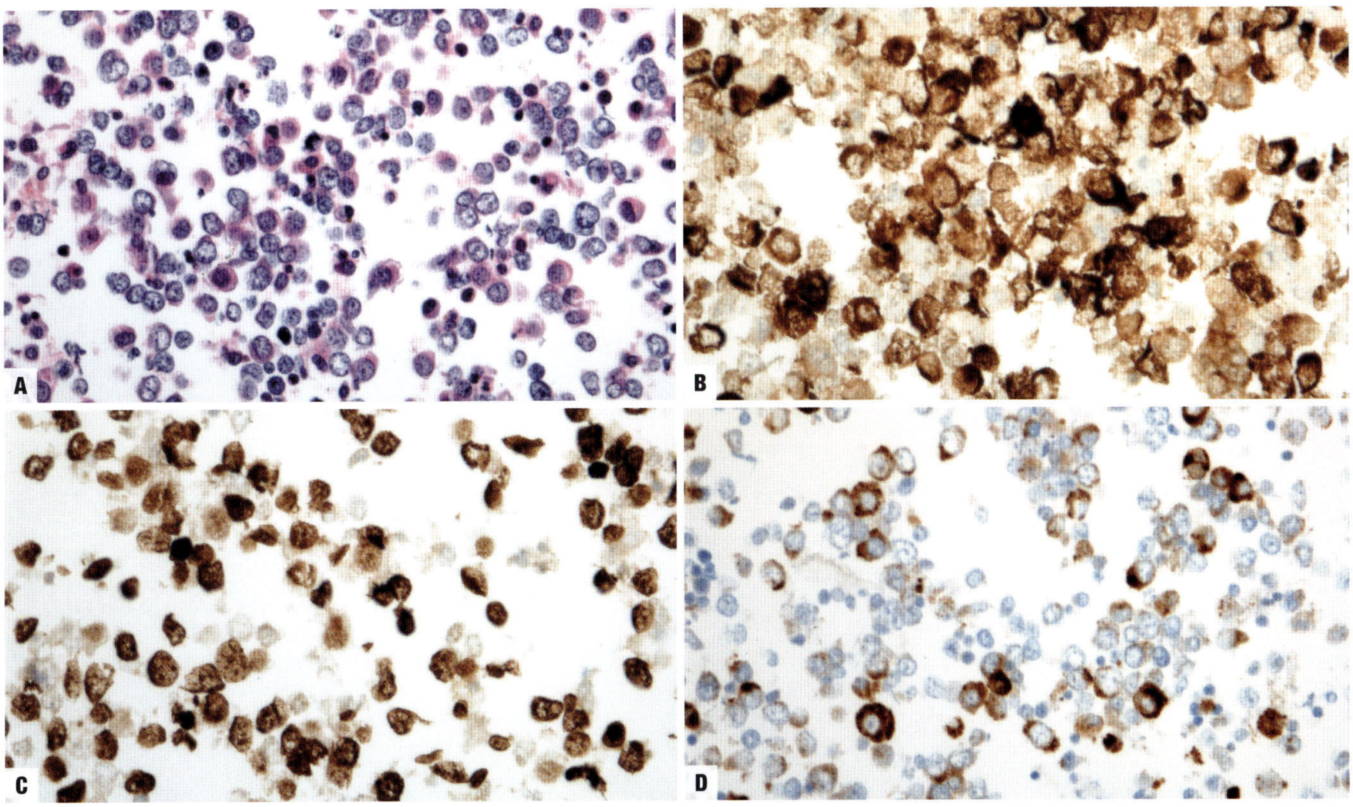

Fig. 7.02 Lung adenocarcinoma. **A** Single dispersed cells with highly pleomorphic nuclei and eccentric cytoplasm (cell block, H&E). **B** Adenocarcinoma showing positive cytoplasmic staining for CK7 (cell block). **C** Adenocarcinoma showing positive nuclear expression of thyroid transcription factor 1 (TTF1), confirming the carcinoma as an adenocarcinoma (cell block). **D** Adenocarcinoma showing positive cytoplasmic expression of napsin A, confirming a primary lung adenocarcinoma (cell block).

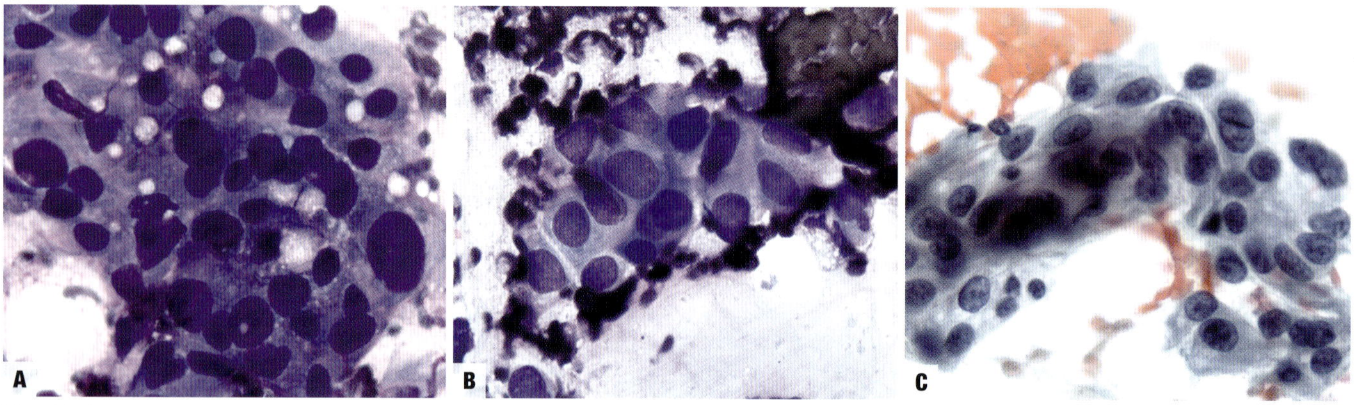

Fig.7.03 Squamous cell carcinoma. **A** This tissue fragment shows tumour cells with pleomorphic nuclei and relatively dense cytoplasm (Giemsa). **B** Tissue fragment of pleomorphic tumour cells with relatively dense cytoplasm and defined cytoplasmic borders and with pleomorphic nuclei that tend to be centrally placed (Giemsa). **C** Cohesive tissue fragment of large tumour cells with round to oval pleomorphic nuclei that tend to be central in relatively dense cytoplasm with well-defined margins. Some tumour cells are elongated. Nucleoli are not prominent (Pap).

with adequate cellularity demonstrating definitive key diagnostic cytopathological criteria for malignancy {606}.

On the basis of cytomorphology, good accuracy (> 70%) can be achieved in differentiating between non-small cell (lung) carcinoma, which is most commonly adenocarcinoma or squamous cell carcinoma (SCC), and small cell neuroendocrine carcinoma (SCNEC). A diagnosis of adenocarcinoma can be made without a need for special stains if there is distinct glandular morphology with or without intracellular or extracellular mucin production, and a diagnosis of SCC can be made if there is keratinization, although thyroid transcription factor 1 (TTF1) staining may be required to confirm lung origin in adenocarcinomas. However, with the advent of targeted therapies, exact classification of the cancer as adenocarcinoma or SCC is essential and the current standard of care {470,998}. This can be achieved using a limited ICC panel consisting of TTF1, p40, and napsin A {470, 998,636,680}. Dual stains such as napsin A / p40 are especially helpful in preserving tissue in very scant samples {635}. In cases of poorly differentiated carcinomas lacking overt glandular or squamous differentiation but displaying a clear immunophenotype of TTF1 positivity and p40 negativity, a diagnosis of poorly differentiated adenocarcinoma can be rendered with confidence. The diagnostic designation of non-small cell carcinoma NOS is appropriate for poorly differentiated carcinomas lacking adenocarcinoma or SCC differentiation both by cytopathology and ICC (if available).

It is also important to be aware of the diagnostic pitfalls associated with ICC stains, especially in cases of common secondary malignancies of the lung; for example, TTF1 positivity can be seen in metastatic thyroid carcinoma, and further specific ICC may be required {470,636,134}.

The "Malignant" category also includes salivary gland–type carcinomas, adenosquamous carcinoma, pleomorphic carcinoma, pulmonary blastoma, carcinosarcoma, NUT carcinoma, thoracic SMARCA4-deficient undifferentiated tumour, low-grade neuroendocrine tumour (NET) (previously known as "carcinoid" and "atypical carcinoid"), lymphoproliferative malignancies, mesenchymal tumours, mesothelioma, angiosarcoma, and metastatic malignancies. Once a case has been categorized as "Malignant", the cytopathologist should attempt, wherever possible, to give as specific a tumour diagnosis as possible.

A "Malignant" cytopathology report of a lung lesion requires the WHO Reporting System category and a clear statement, if at all possible, of the specific diagnosis classified by the WHO classification of thoracic tumours, and if this is not possible, then the presentation of a brief differential diagnosis is required. Some cytopathologists may want to add a statement that the material received was adequate, whereas others may want to

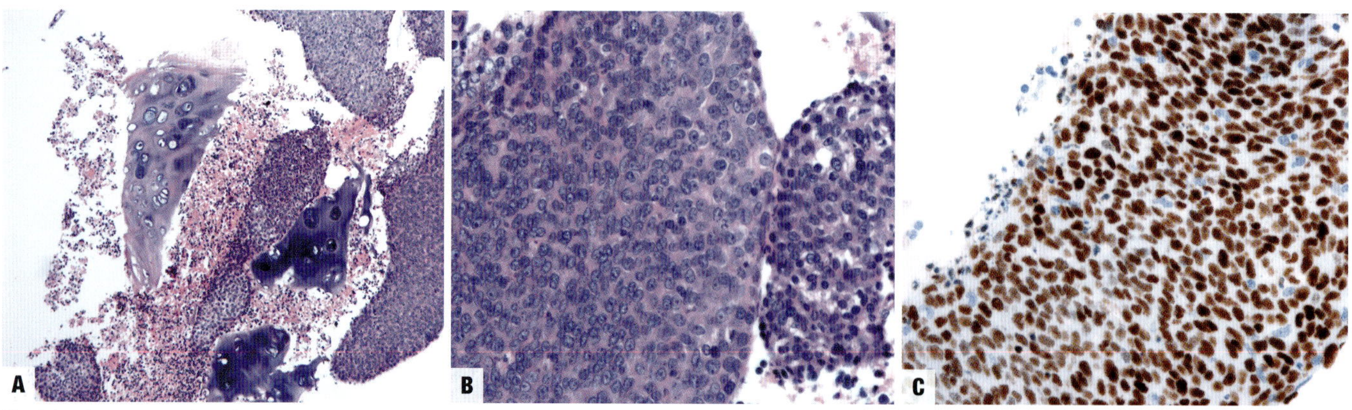

Fig. 7.04 Squamous cell carcinoma. **A** Tissue fragments of non-keratinizing squamous cell carcinoma among fragments of benign cartilage and cellular debris (cell block, H&E). **B** Non-keratinizing squamous cell carcinoma forming crowded tissue fragments with highly pleomorphic nuclei with single prominent nucleoli and considerable eosinophilic cytoplasm but no keratinization (cell block, H&E). **C** An example showing nuclear staining for p40 by ICC, confirming the diagnosis of squamous cell carcinoma (cell block).

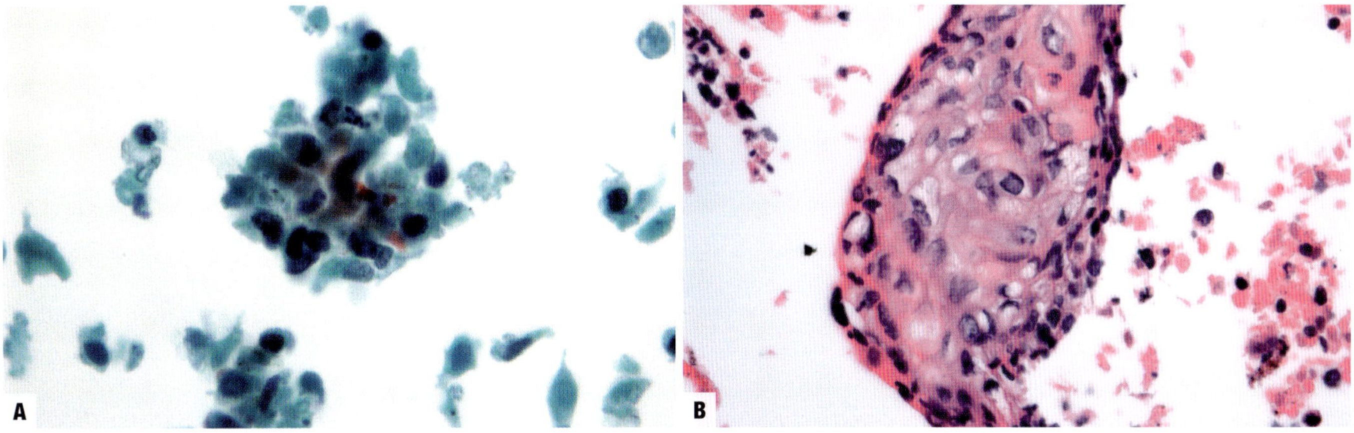

Fig. 7.05 Squamous cell carcinoma. **A** Squamous cell carcinoma showing hyperchromatic nuclei, poorly preserved cytoplasm, and tumour necrosis (liquid-based cytopathology, Pap). **B** Keratinizing well-differentiated squamous cell carcinoma tissue fragment consisting of large cells with highly pleomorphic, hyperchromatic nuclei and considerable eosinophilic keratinized cytoplasm with well-defined margins in a background of necrotic debris (cell block, H&E).

state the degree of cellularity and provide a clear and concise microscopic description of the key diagnostic cytopathological features present. In institutions routinely using molecular ancillary testing, the report should state, if possible, the tumour fraction of both the direct smears and the cell block. It is essential that any subsequent ancillary testing results (including ICC, molecular studies, and flow cytometry) are incorporated into a final integrated cytopathology report.

Risk of malignancy and management recommendations

Bubendorf L
Satoh Y
Savic Prince S
Scagliotti GV

The reported risk of malignancy for a sputum sample categorized as "Malignant" is 100%; however, the sensitivity of sputum sample cytopathology is as low as 5%, particularly for more peripheral lung cancers {292,599} (see Table 1.04, p. 11, in Chapter 1: *Introduction to the WHO Reporting System for Lung Cytopathology*). If a sputum sample is categorized as "Malignant", the next step should be bronchoscopy to identify central lesions, and imaging including CXR and CT for peripheral lesions {791}. Lesions detected can then undergo endobronchial ultrasound–guided transbronchial FNAB or transthoracic FNAB depending on their site and the available biopsy expertise. Supplementing bronchoscopy, autofluorescence bronchoscopy has improved the detection of preinvasive and malignant endobronchial lesions, and narrow-band imaging is useful for detecting the microvascular network of bronchial mucosa {362, 838}. If these further procedures are negative, close follow-up of initially undetectable cases with repeat sputum sample studies and imaging is required to localize carcinoma in cases with positive sputum sample cytopathology.

The reported risk of malignancy for exfoliative cytopathology, i.e. bronchial wash and bronchial brush, is 94–100% (see Table 1.04, p. 11, in Chapter 1: *Introduction to the WHO Reporting System for Lung Cytopathology*). A bronchial brush, bronchial wash, or bronchoalveolar lavage (BAL) is typically performed for the evaluation of peripheral lung lesions, which are usually small in size, solitary, and not visible on bronchoscopy {754}. For a peripheral non-small cell lung carcinoma without evidence of distant metastasis, further management is dependent on imaging: a small primary tumour (< 30 mm) without evidence of mediastinal lymph node involvement can directly undergo surgical resection if not contraindicated by poor lung function or comorbidities.

Mediastinal staging by endobronchial ultrasound–guided transbronchial FNAB is indicated in cases where there are enlarged mediastinal or hilar lymph nodes measuring > 10 mm in their short axis on CT or there is uptake on PET, or where the primary tumour is > 30 mm {709}. If the FNAB does not yield a diagnosis, transthoracic FNAB and/or core needle biopsy or surgical resection (depending on the site and size of the lesion) are recommended.

The reported risk of malignancy for FNAB specimens categorized as "Malignant" at endobronchial ultrasound is 87–100% {466,76,105} (see Table 1.05, p. 12, in Chapter 1: *Introduction to the WHO Reporting System for Lung Cytopathology*). The cytopathology specimen frequently provides material for further specific diagnostic testing using ICC, FISH, and next-generation sequencing performed on cell block and direct smear slide scrapings. If there is correlation between the clinical, imaging, and cytopathology findings, the decision to proceed to definitive treatment may be made. If there is insufficient material for ancillary testing or if there is no correlation that the lesion is malignant, then repeat FNAB with or without core needle biopsy should be considered. Each case should, as far as possible, be reviewed with full correlation and discussion in a multidisciplinary setting to establish a management plan.

Adenocarcinoma of the lung

Geisinger KR
Bubendorf L
Kholova I
Michael CW

Definition

Adenocarcinoma is an epithelial neoplasm with glandular differentiation and is the most common type of primary lung malignancy.

Clinical features and imaging

At presentation, the vast majority of patients are middle-aged and older adults. Common presenting symptoms are not specific and include cough, dyspnoea, chest pain, and haemoptysis. Relatively commonly, patients present with clinical manifestations related to distant metastases. Most patients are current or prior smokers, but a significant minority are non-smokers.

On imaging, a single peripherally located mass is most often detected, but other presentations include multiple unilateral or bilateral nodules or masses, a miliary pattern, or lung consolidation resembling pneumonia. With CT scans, in general, nodules may be classified as pure ground-glass or non-solid, pure solid, and mixed partly solid partly non-solid, with solid appearances commonly corresponding to invasive tumour. Pleural effusions are present in some patients.

Histopathology

Adenocarcinomas show varying degrees of glandular differentiation, from well to poorly differentiated. The glandular differentiation may include acini, papillae, and micropapillae, whereas other growth patterns include solid, lepidic, and cribriform. With solid growth, the neoplastic cells show glandular differentiation via mucin histochemistry or ICC. The vast majority of resected tumours show heterogeneity with a mix of the architectural patterns, and for prognostic purposes grading is based on the predominant pattern. In addition to the histopathological pattern, lung adenocarcinoma may be classified as mucinous, characterized by tumour cells with clear-cut cytoplasmic and (at times) extracellular mucin, or more frequently as non-mucinous, showing no obvious cytoplasmic mucin production. The cells may be

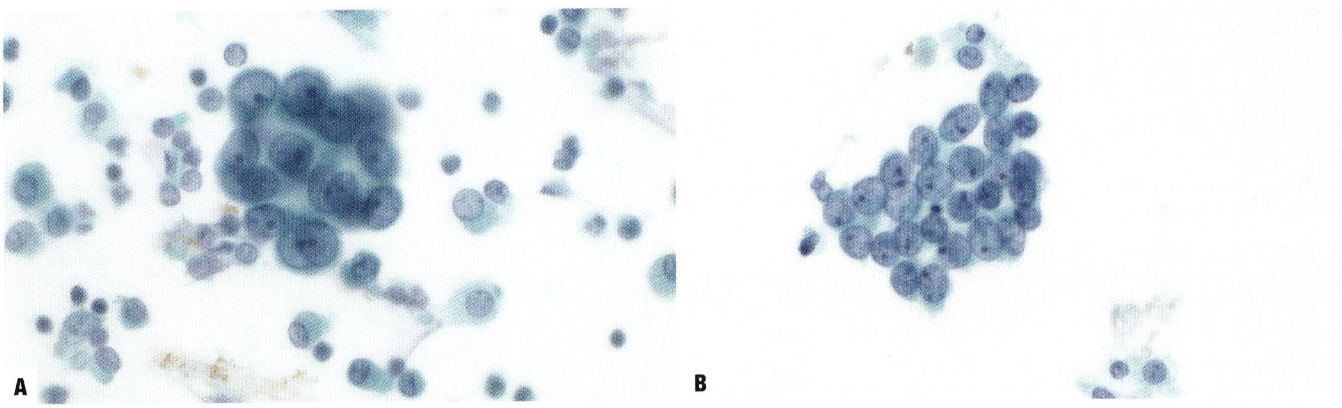

Fig. 7.06 Well-differentiated adenocarcinoma. **A** 3D rounded tissue fragment of adenocarcinoma cells with peripherally located nuclei showing perinucleolar clearing and prominent nucleoli, and with delicate cytoplasm (bronchoalveolar lavage [BAL], Pap). **B** Round to oval nuclei with mild variation in size and regular nuclear membranes, high N:C ratio, only mild chromatin abnormality, and small nucleoli. Histopathology showed a predominant lepidic architecture (transbronchial FNAB, Pap).

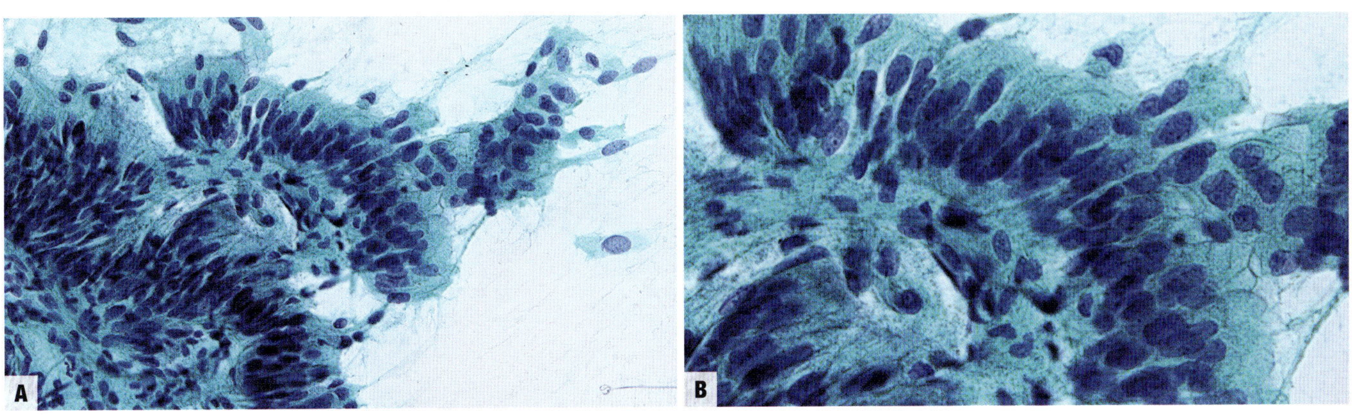

Fig. 7.07 Well-differentiated adenocarcinoma. **A** Well-oriented columnar cells with mainly basal, crowded nuclei, arranged along fibrovascular stroma suggestive of alveolar septa and lepidic architecture (Pap). **B** High-power view, showing columnar cells with crowded moderately enlarged and atypical nuclei arranged along a fibrovascular strand suggestive of an alveolar septum and lepidic architecture (Pap).

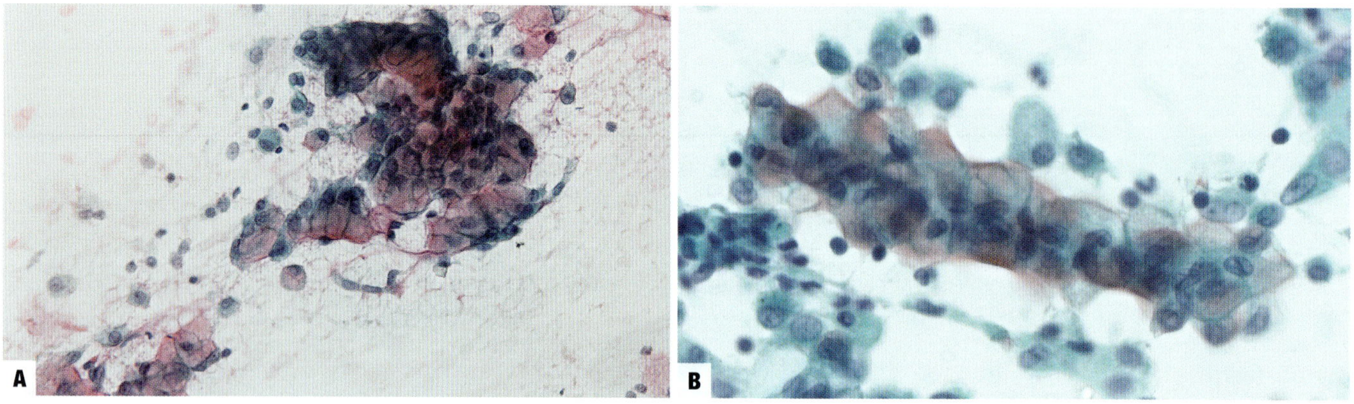

Fig. 7.08 Mucinous adenocarcinoma. **A** Tissue fragments of oriented large cells with large eccentric single eosinophilic mucin vacuoles and basal mildly enlarged and pleomorphic nuclei (Pap). **B** Strand of carcinoma cells with abundant eccentric intracytoplasmic eosinophilic mucin and irregular, indented, wrinkled nuclei with open chromatin. This tumour was negative for thyroid transcription factor 1 (TTF1), and *KRAS* was mutated (bronchoalveolar lavage [BAL], Pap).

columnar or goblet cells, typically with distinct cell borders. The nuclei are often oval and vary in size, and the N:C ratio is often low, owing to the abundant eccentric mucinous cytoplasm. Rare histopathological variants include colloid, fetal, and enteric.

Key diagnostic cytopathological features

- Variable cellularity, largely related to specimen type: low in sputum samples and usually high in brushings and FNAB
- Variable proportions of tumour cells varying with specimen type: low in sputum samples and high in brushings and FNAB
- Varying numbers of cohesive tissue fragments and dispersed single cells
- Tissue fragments include flat sheets; spheres; papillae with true fibrovascular cores, acini, and glands; pseudopapillae; and micropapillae, which present as floret-like tissue fragments
- Glandular and acinar tissue fragments show peripheral or basal nuclei and more-centrally located cytoplasm; small, less cohesive tumour cells exfoliate from the surface of tissue fragments
- Sheets show subtle to prominent loss of polarity and may contain acini that resemble rosettes with central cytoplasm or show a true central luminal space
- Tumour cells are cuboidal to columnar with moderate to abundant cytoplasm, which varies from homogeneous to granular to foamy to clearly vacuolated, with fine vacuoles more frequent than large vacuoles containing mucin droplets
- Goblet cells are present in mucinous and enteric variants
- Solitary, large, round to oval nuclei with fine to coarse chromatin, which varies in staining intensity but often is not highly hyperchromatic
- Nuclear membranes often show minor irregularities, and pseudoinclusions and grooves occur, especially in well-differentiated tumours, whereas poorly differentiated adenocarcinomas may show marked pleomorphism of nuclear shape and chromatin
- One or more large and prominent nucleoli
- Background may include necrotic debris, which is seen particularly in high-grade carcinomas, as well as mucin and psammoma bodies

Less common defined types

- Fetal adenocarcinoma: uniform cells with small nuclei and subnuclear glycogen-rich vacuoles best appreciated by Giemsa, and occasional squamoid morules, seen best in Pap-stained preparations
- Colloid carcinoma: low cellularity; tumour cells in tissue fragments and as single cells, often resembling histiocytes, suspended in thick extracellular mucin pools
- Mucinous carcinoma: flat sheets with irregular nuclear arrangement with typical columnar or goblet cells with voluminous vacuolated cytoplasm and bland nuclei with finely granular chromatin pattern

Discussion and differential diagnosis

One limitation of cytopathological specimens is that the tissue fragment architecture seen may not predict the often mixed histopathological patterns seen in resected specimens. However, histopathological grade does correlate with cytopathological nuclear features (which include size, contour, chromatin

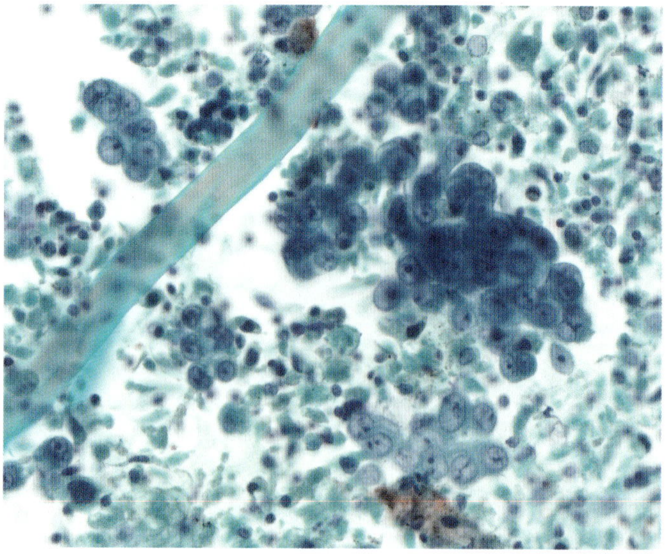

Fig. 7.09 Poorly differentiated adenocarcinoma. Poorly differentiated adenocarcinoma with irregularly shaped, crowded tissue fragments, with loss of polarity, prominent nucleoli, and necrotic debris in the background (transbronchial FNAB, Pap).

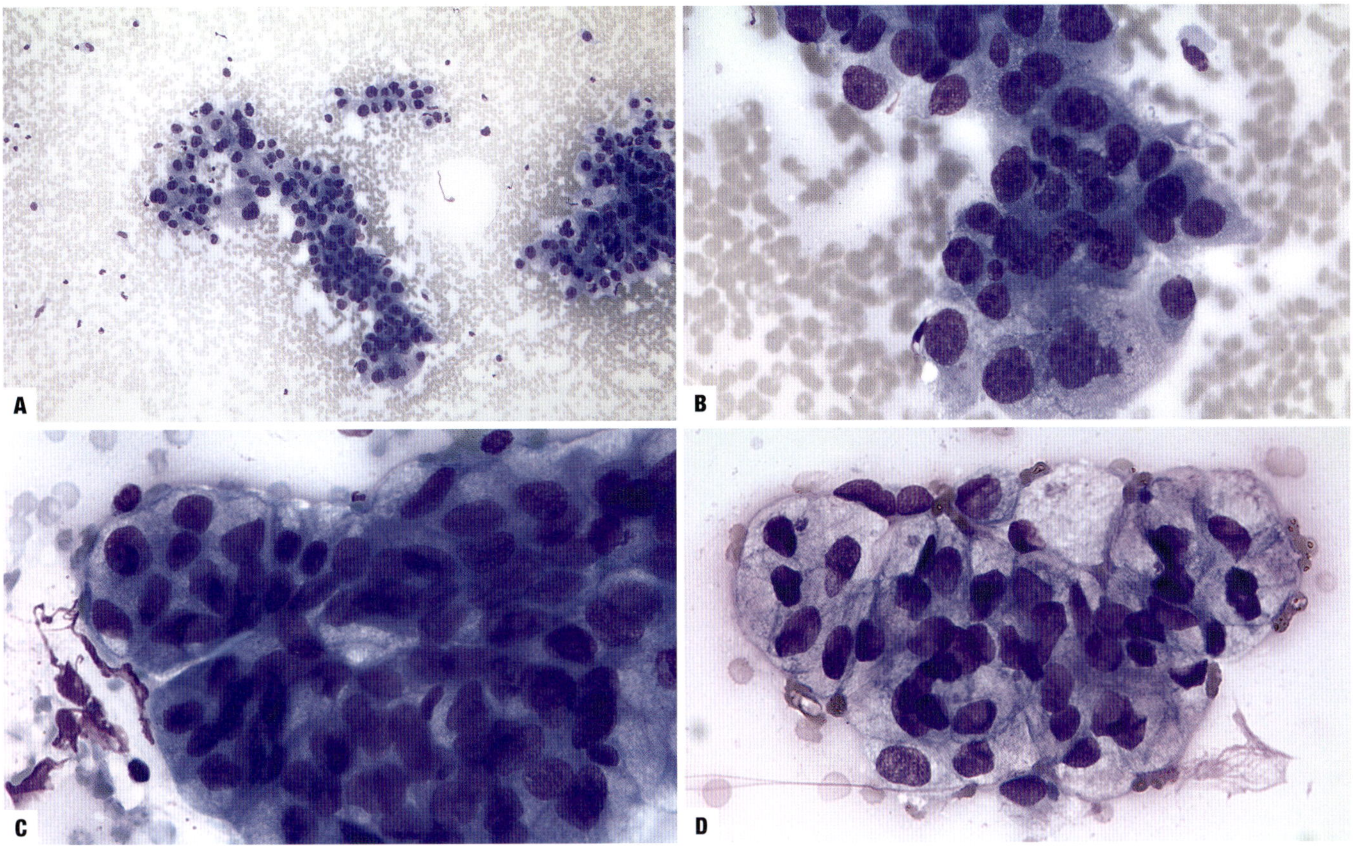

Fig. 7.10 Adenocarcinoma. **A** Irregular tissue fragments varying in size, consisting of tumour cells with enlarged, hyperchromatic nuclei and some cells with abundant cytoplasm (transbronchial FNAB, Giemsa). **B** At higher power: tumour cells with enlarged, hyperchromatic nuclei; a coarse chromatin pattern with large nucleoli; and abundant foamy cytoplasm in some cells (transbronchial FNAB, Giemsa). **C** This case, which was subsequently shown to be *KRAS* mutant, shows a cohesive crowded tissue fragment with enlarged cells, hyperchromatic nuclei, large nucleoli, and abundant eccentric cytoplasm containing mucus (transbronchial FNAB, Giemsa). **D** Small cohesive tissue fragment of tumour cells with enlarged, hyperchromatic nuclei and abundant eccentric cytoplasm, filled with foamy mucus. Subsequent histopathology showed a lepidic adenocarcinoma (bronchial brushing, Giemsa).

patterns, and nucleoli), and nuclear grading may have prognostic value {851,611}.

The distinction between adenocarcinoma in situ, minimally invasive adenocarcinoma, and invasive adenocarcinoma of lepidic and related types is not highly accurate in small samples from FNAB and core needle biopsy, and it should be restricted to the assessment of resection specimens.

Poorly differentiated carcinomas are challenging to subclassify by cytomorphology alone, and ICC and molecular studies are recommended {375}.

The differential diagnosis of mucinous versus non-mucinous adenocarcinoma of the lung rests on the recognition of malignant mucin-containing cells. Intracellular mucin is seen as single vacuoles containing mucin droplets or fine vacuolation or fine

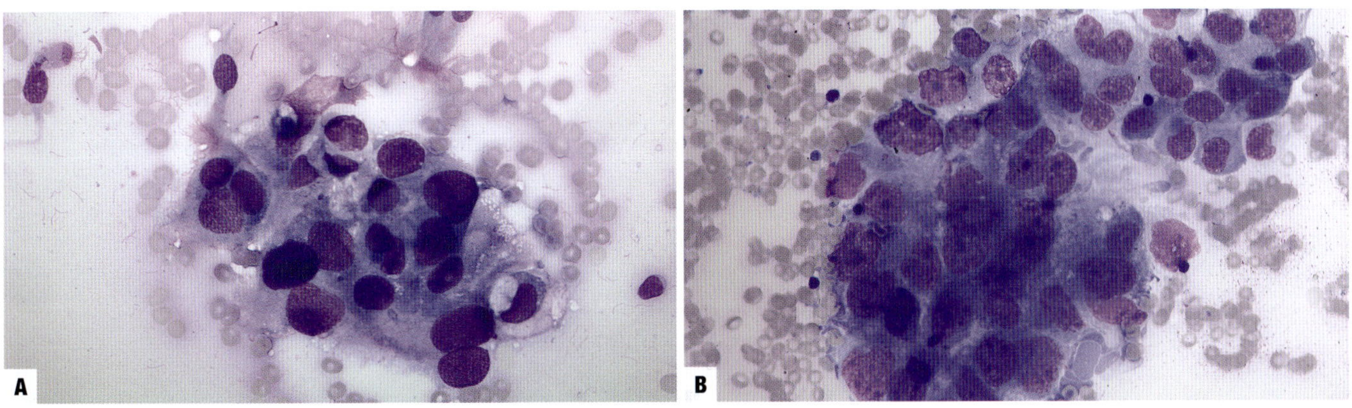

Fig. 7.11 Adenocarcinoma. **A** Pulmonary adenocarcinoma. Small irregular tissue fragment of tumour cells with enlarged, hyperchromatic nuclei and partially vacuolated cytoplasm. In the upper part of the image, two normal ciliated respiratory epithelial cells are present (bronchial brushing, Giemsa). **B** Crowded tissue fragment of poorly differentiated adenocarcinoma lacking glandular architecture, with enlarged and irregular nuclei, coarse chromatin, occasional large nucleoli, and variable (sometimes abundant) foamy cytoplasm (transbronchial FNAB, Giemsa).

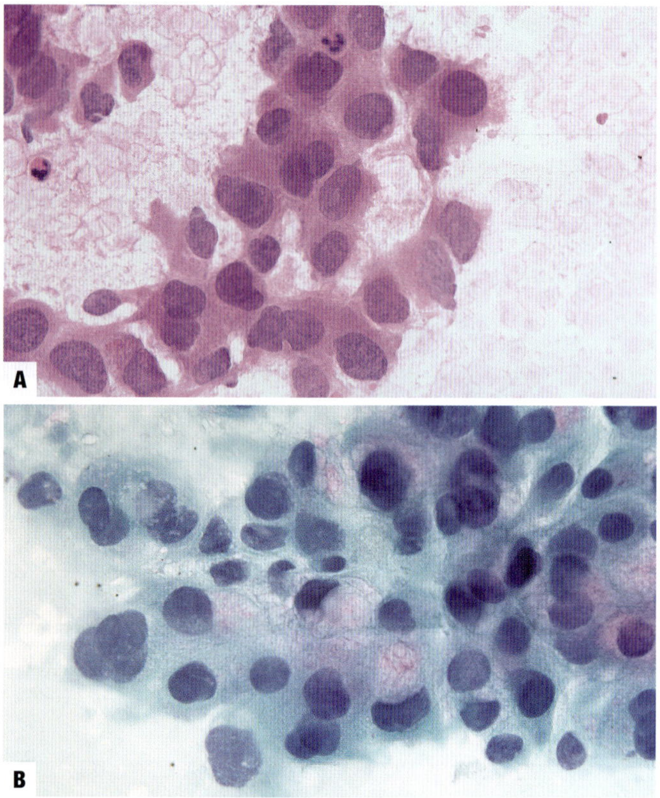

Fig. 7.12 Adenocarcinoma. **A** Loosely cohesive tissue fragment of large tumour cells with enlarged and irregular nuclei, coarse chromatin, occasional large nucleoli, and eccentric cytoplasm. Note the intracytoplasmic neutrophil, a feature of adenocarcinoma with mucinous cytoplasm (transbronchial FNAB, H&E). **B** Sheet of tumour cells with enlarged and irregular hyperchromatic nuclei showing marked anisonucleosis, and some goblet cells with large mucus-filled single vacuoles often indenting the nucleus (transbronchial FNAB, Pap).

magenta granules (Giemsa) in the eccentric cytoplasm, and it must be present, because extracellular mucin in the background alone is insufficient to make this distinction. When these mucinous carcinoma cells are present in sheets, the nuclear arrangement will show irregularities with focal displacement of nuclei representing the drunken-sailor or irregular honeycomb pattern. Mucin must be distinguished from other vacuoles in the cytoplasm that may push the nucleus to an eccentric position and represent degenerative changes. A mucin stain such as mucicarmine or PASD can be helpful if there is a cell block. The background of both mucinous and non-mucinous tumours is usually clean, with the exception of the fine mucin threads that may be present. This is in contrast to metastatic tumours from the gastrointestinal tract, such as colorectal cancer, that often have a necrotic and inflamed background with a prominent mucinous component {657}.

Benign inflammatory processes that are in the differential diagnosis of well-differentiated adenocarcinoma include acute inflammation, granulomatous inflammation, diffuse alveolar damage, oxygen toxicity, fibrosing alveolitis, pulmonary infarcts, and particularly chemotherapy and/or radiotherapy. Features favouring a benign process include low cellularity with few atypical tissue fragments, preservation of cellular cohesion and nuclear polarity in tissue fragments that are often flat and small, and a low number of atypical cells. Macronucleoli in the absence of hyperchromasia, nuclear membrane irregularities, and denser cytoplasm also support a reactive process. The following favour well-differentiated adenocarcinoma: high cellularity including a large number of atypical tissue fragments showing loss of polarity; a papillary, micropapillary, or distinctly glandular or acinar architecture; and nuclear pleomorphism with indentations, grooves, and pseudoinclusions.

One benign tumour that may closely mimic adenocarcinoma in FNAB smears is the sclerosing pneumocytoma {790,441}. Arranged in sheets and papillae, the cuboidal tumour cells have single bland nuclei with grooves, pseudoinclusions, and single nucleoli.

The distinction from squamous cell carcinoma can generally be made on a constellation of features: adenocarcinoma cells have more translucent eccentric cytoplasm with fine or sometimes larger vacuoles, oval and often less pleomorphic nuclei with relatively smooth membranes, finer chromatin, and prominent nucleoli. However, poorly differentiated carcinomas cannot be distinguished and require ICC and molecular studies on cell blocks.

Ancillary testing

It is imperative to preserve as much of a small sample as possible for molecular analyses, so ICC should be minimized on cell block material, although cellular material can be scraped from Pap-stained and Giemsa-stained smears for molecular

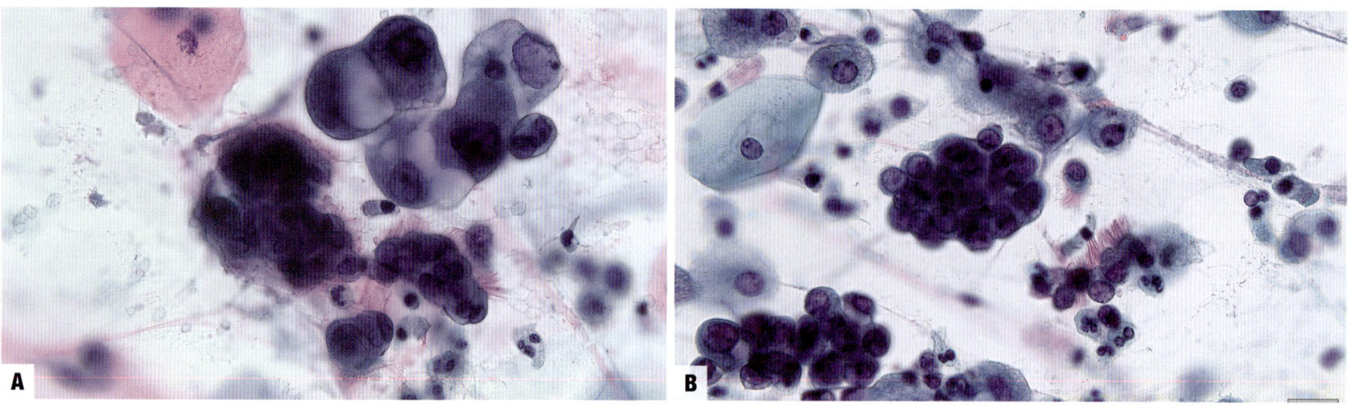

Fig. 7.13 Adenocarcinoma. **A** Minute tissue fragment of very large tumour cells with large, often hyperchromatic nuclei and eccentric cytoplasm containing single clear mucin vacuoles. In the background, dense tissue fragments of normal ciliated epithelium are present for comparison of size (bronchial washing, Pap). **B** Two cohesive dense tissue fragments of tumour cells with enlarged, round, hyperchromatic nuclei, often with a centrally located macronucleolus. In the background are benign ciliated cells, alveolar macrophages, and benign squamous cells of the upper respiratory tract (bronchial washing, Pap).

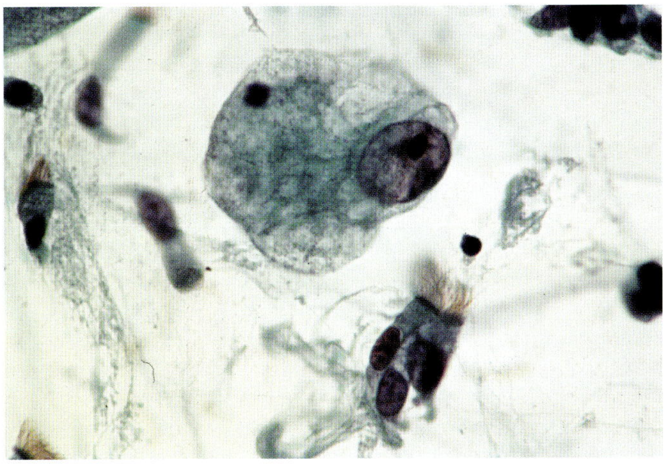

Fig. 7.14 Adenocarcinoma. Single very large tumour cell with eccentric abundant vacuolated cytoplasm and a large nucleus with pale chromatin and two large nucleoli. Note the benign ciliated cells in the background for comparison of the size (bronchial washing, Pap).

next-generation sequencing. The majority of adenocarcinomas are positive for thyroid transcription factor 1 (TTF1) and napsin A and negative for p40; TTF1 and p40 are usually sufficient. Regardless of whether TTF1 is positive or not, if neuroendocrine differentiation is suspected cytopathologically, synaptophysin, chromogranin, or INSM1 should be added, although focal positivity with one or more of these markers does not negate the diagnosis of adenocarcinoma {916}.

ICC stains may be confusing in primary mucinous adenocarcinoma of the lung, which may not stain for TTF1 (although it usually is positive for napsin A) and instead may have markers suggesting a gastrointestinal primary. In such cases, the diagnostic terminology should include a statement that the tumour is acceptable as a lung primary if other sites of disease have been ruled out. Mucinous adenocarcinoma of lung is almost never positive for *EGFR* mutations but shows *KRAS* mutations {456,395,304}.

If there is a history of a specific malignancy and a metastasis is considered, such as from a breast or colon primary, then specific ICC should be considered on the cytopathology material.

Squamous cell carcinoma

Schmitt F
Bubendorf L
Chandra A
Jain D
Lloveras B

Definition

Squamous cell carcinoma is a malignant epithelial tumour characterized by the presence of keratinization and intercellular bridges or, if non-keratinizing, by immunocytochemical markers of squamous cell differentiation.

Clinical features and imaging

The signs and symptoms of squamous cell carcinoma (SCC) are similar to those of other non-small cell lung carcinomas but are generally related to the tumour location, which is more commonly central, causing endobronchial obstruction, leading to haemoptysis, cough, and recurrent pneumonitis. SCC tends to be locally aggressive, with progressive involvement of peribronchial structures through direct invasion, but distant metastases and related symptoms occur similarly to other non-small cell lung carcinomas. With central tumours, the proximity to the carina is a crucial factor for planning surgical treatment {915}. Peripherally located SCC may show necrosis and cavitation with superimposed fungal and bacterial infections {460}.

Histopathology

Keratinizing, non-keratinizing, and basaloid SCC subtypes are recognized, with the same histopathological features as SCC in other anatomical regions. All histopathological subtypes of SCC can show a variety of unusual patterns, including spindle and clear cell changes, as well as papillary, pseudovascular, or alveolar-filling patterns. Defining histopathological features include the presence of keratinization and/or intercellular bridges, but other tumours may be non-keratinizing or poorly differentiated. Keratinizing SCC is often associated with a granulomatous reaction.

Key diagnostic cytopathological features

Well-differentiated keratinizing SCC

- Usually high cellularity

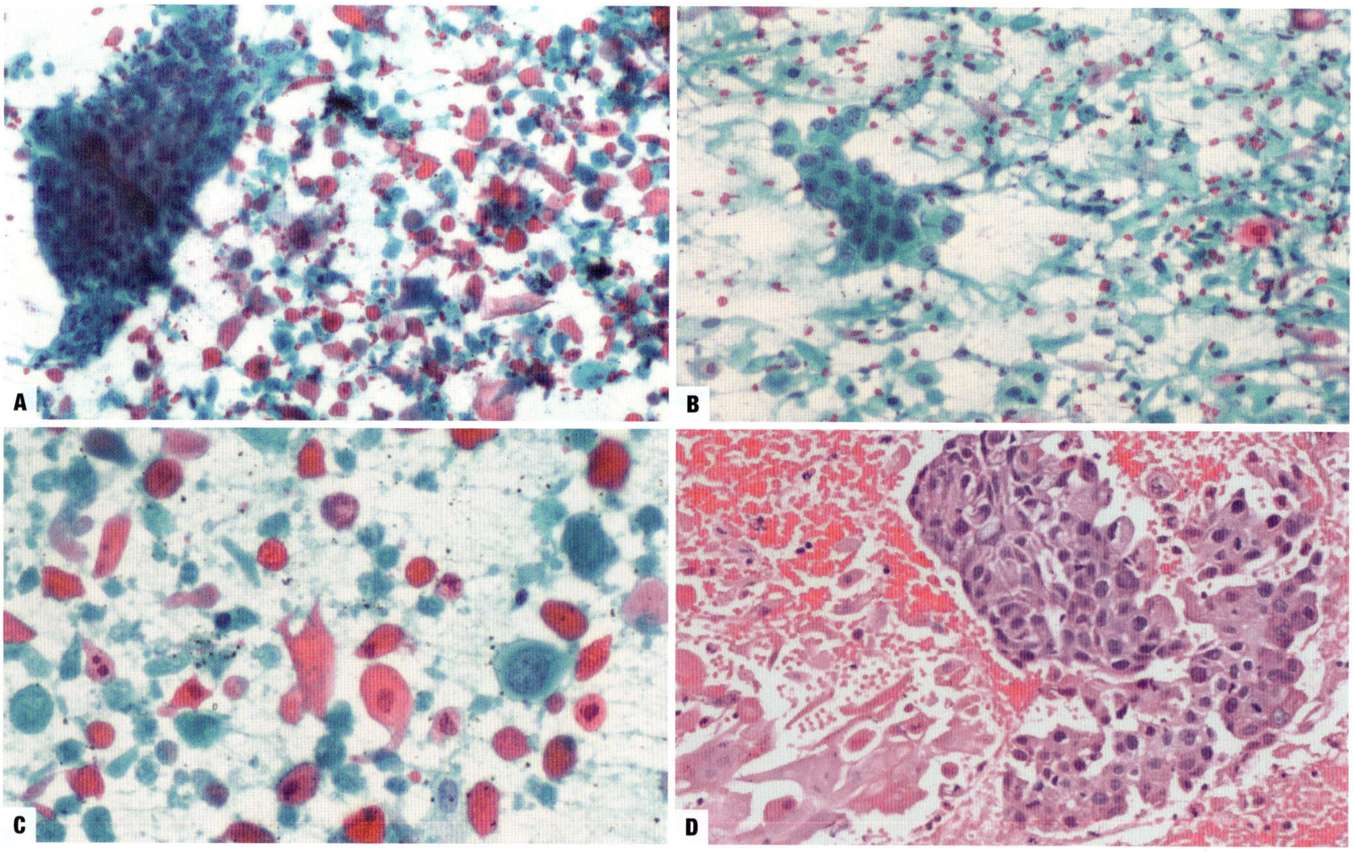

Fig. 7.15 Squamous cell carcinoma. **A** Endobronchial ultrasound–guided transbronchial FNAB (EBUS-TBFNAB) specimen showing mainly dispersed necrotic keratinized squamous cells, with a rare cohesive tissue fragment of tumour cells (Pap). **B** Pap-stained smear from EBUS-TBFNAB showing dispersed keratinized squamous cells with a cohesive tissue fragment of tumour cells. **C** Photomicrograph of EBUS-TBFNAB specimen showing mainly dispersed necrotic keratinized squamous cells, with a rare cohesive tissue fragment of tumour cells (Pap). **D** Cell block from EBUS-TBFNAB shows features of squamous cell carcinoma (H&E).

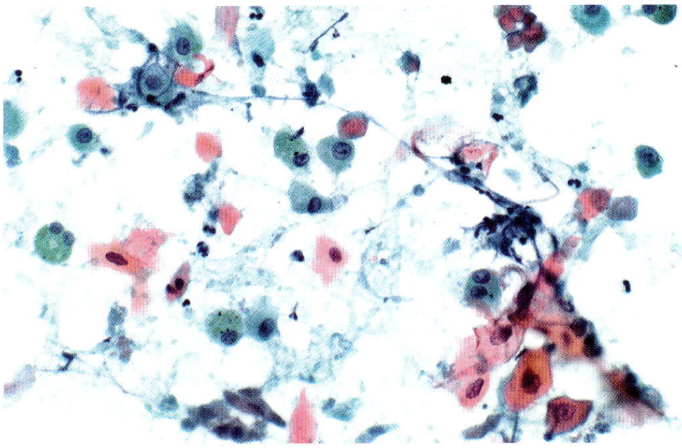

Fig. 7.16 Squamous cell carcinoma. Dispersed keratinizing squamous cells and some macrophages (bronchial washing, Pap).

- Single keratinized cells and relatively cohesive small to larger tissue fragments, including flat sheets
- Dense, sharply defined cytoplasm with well-demarcated margins
- Orangeophilic or eosinophilic (Pap) or light sky-blue (Giemsa) cytoplasm
- Centrally located nuclei, usually large, which may show angular contours and hyperchromatic, irregularly distributed clumped chromatin
- Polygonal, rounded, elongated, or bizarre cells that can be tadpole-, spindle-, or fibre-shaped or show pseudopodia
- Foci of keratinization (keratin pearls) in cohesive tissue fragments may be present
- Keratinized cells frequently show degenerative pyknotic dense nuclei, making it very difficult to examine nuclear details, or they may be anucleate
- Inconspicuous nucleoli except in basal or non-keratinizing cells
- Dirty background with necrotic debris, particularly in FNAB samples, due to central necrosis and cavitation
- Acute inflammation with abundant neutrophils or a granulomatous reaction with multinucleated giant cells and epithelioid histiocytes can be associated with necrosis and keratinous debris

Poorly differentiated non-keratinizing SCC, including basaloid SCC

- Usually high cellularity with necrotic debris in the background, particularly in FNAB material, and less cellularity in sputum samples

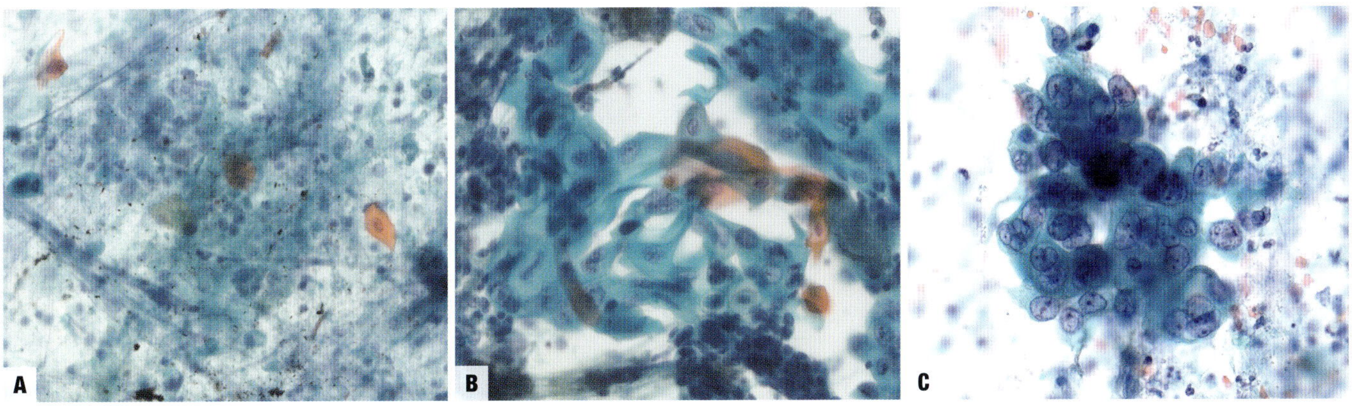

Fig. 7.17 Squamous cell carcinoma. **A** Necrotic debris with few keratinized tumour cells (transbronchial FNAB, Pap). **B** From the same case: tumour cells with polymorphic nuclei, waxy cytoplasm, and focal keratinization (transbronchial FNAB, Pap). **C** Squamous cell carcinoma with pleomorphic nuclei and waxy, dense cytoplasm. Intercellular bridges are not as obvious as in the core needle biopsy (bronchial washing, Pap).

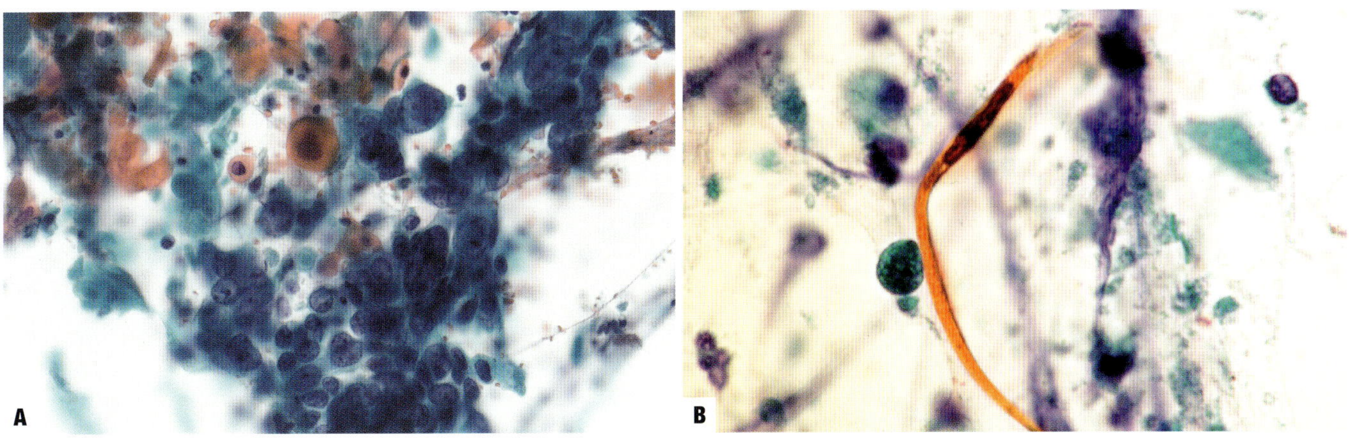

Fig. 7.18 Squamous cell carcinoma. **A** Tumour cells with hyperchromatic nuclei, focal keratinization, and some necrotic cells (bronchial brushing, Pap). **B** One long, highly atypical keratinized tumour cell with a dark nucleus and elongated cytoplasm (fibre cell) (bronchial washing, Pap).

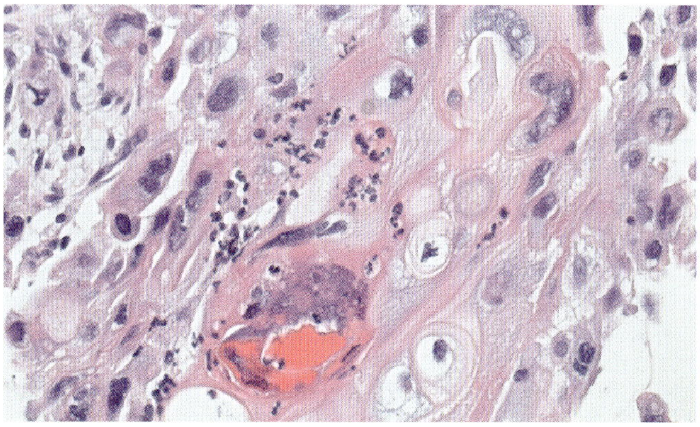

Fig. 7.19 Squamous cell carcinoma. Squamous cell carcinoma with focal keratinization, well-defined abundant cytoplasm, and intercellular bridges (core needle biopsy, H&E).

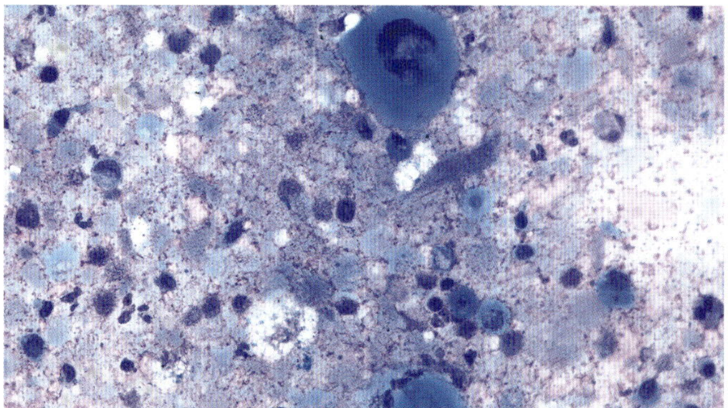

Fig. 7.20 Squamous cell carcinoma. One large, keratinizing tumour cell with a large, dark nucleus and abundant dense cytoplasm, in a background of necrosis and degenerating inflammatory cells. In the lower part of the image, an anucleate keratinized ghost cell is present, representing a degenerating keratinized tumour cell (transbronchial FNAB, Giemsa).

- Tissue fragments are cohesive, often flat sheets or more 3D, with a variable number of dispersed single cells
- Cells have well-defined, often dense cytoplasm, which is frequently elongated or spindle, but lacks keratinization and/or intercellular bridges; occasional keratinized cells may be present
- Nuclei are usually centrally placed, elongated, or pleomorphic, with irregular dense chromatin and prominent nucleoli
- Basaloid subtype shows predominantly cohesive sheets or irregular tissue fragments with variable palisading at their margins, consisting of small to medium-sized cells with a high N:C ratio, round to oval to variably angulated nuclei with dense and coarsely granular chromatin, usually inconspicuous nucleoli, and a scant rim of cytoplasm; focal nuclear moulding may be seen
- Basaloid subtype may show pseudoglandular spaces, palisades of nuclei or pseudorosettes, necrosis, nuclear crushing, and stromal hyaline basement membrane–like material wrapping the epithelial tissue fragments

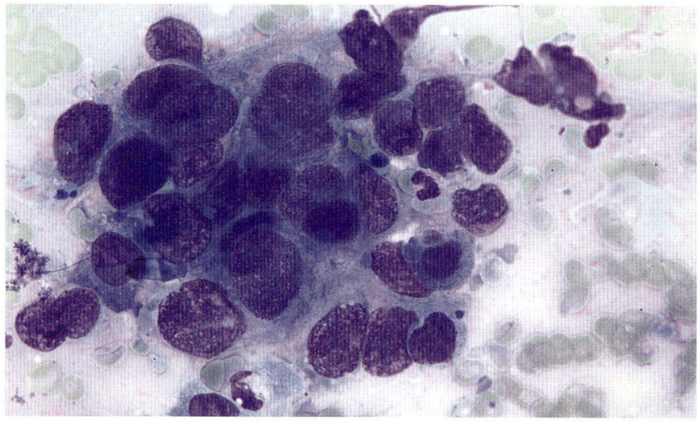

Fig. 7.22 Squamous cell carcinoma. Tissue fragment of crowded non-keratinizing tumour cells with hyperchromatic nuclei, coarse irregular chromatin pattern, and large nucleoli. There is blood in the background (bronchial brushing, Giemsa).

Reference(s): {360,523,175,536,229}

Discussion and differential diagnosis

SCC of the lung can be diagnosed in cytopathological samples when keratinization is present, or when the less common intercellular bridges are visible. Poorly differentiated or non-keratinizing SCC usually requires additional stains to confirm squamous differentiation {982}.

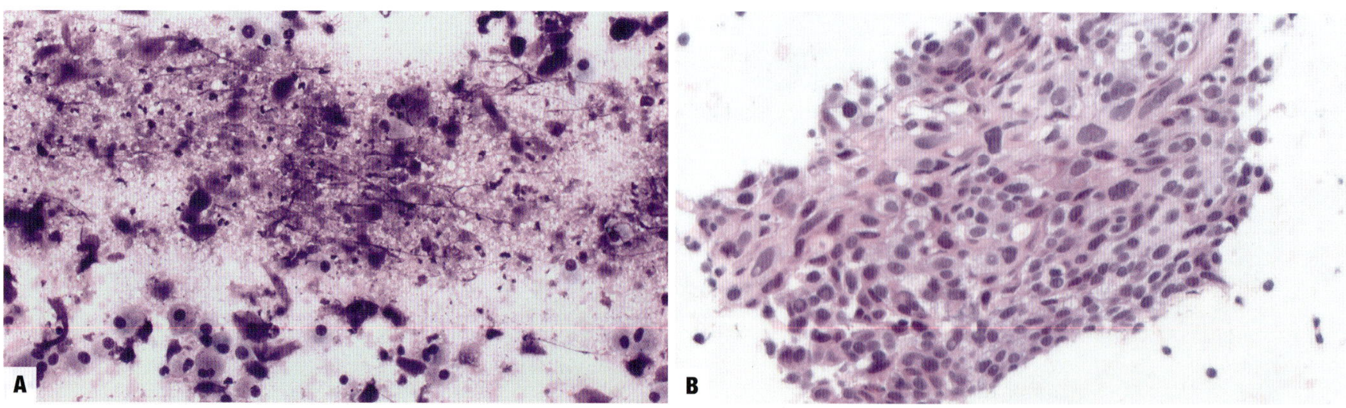

Fig. 7.21 Squamous cell carcinoma. **A** Giemsa-stained smears from lung FNAB show mainly dispersed necrotic keratinized squamous cells. **B** Non-keratinizing squamous cell carcinoma. Cell block corresponding to the smear shown in Panel A (H&E).

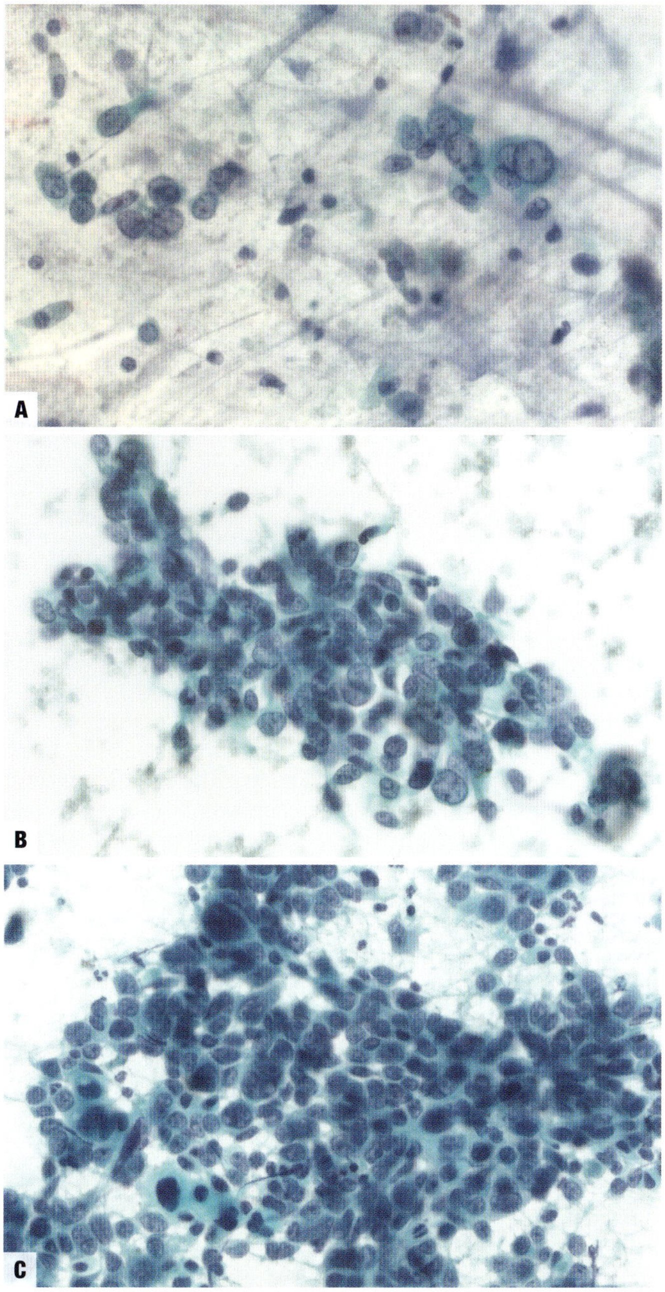

Fig. 7.23 Non-keratinizing squamous cell carcinoma. **A** Some tumour cells show dense, waxy cytoplasm (bronchial washing, Pap). **B** 3D tumour cell tissue fragment. Some of the neoplastic cells have hyperchromatic nuclei. The nucleoli are inconspicuous. The cytoplasm is relatively dense (bronchial brushing, Pap). **C** Numerous cohesive carcinoma cells with hyperchromatic nuclei and often dense, waxy cytoplasm (transbronchial FNAB, Pap).

Distinguishing well-differentiated metastatic SCC from primary pulmonary SCC is not possible either in cytopathology or in core needle biopsy. HPV positivity in head and neck primaries and clinical and imaging correlation offer the most significant assistance, including p16 ICC and HPV probes {67, 1027,942}.

Squamous in situ lesions sampled in sputa and in bronchial brush and wash preparations are difficult to distinguish from invasive SCC, although invasive tumours usually exfoliate a large number of neoplastic cells with a greater degree of nuclear atypia. Similarly, reactive, metaplastic, and dysplastic squamous cells may show overlapping nuclear features, hence clinical and imaging correlation is mandatory to avoid overcalling these cases as malignant {360,785}.

In regard to distinguishing less differentiated SCC from poorly differentiated adenocarcinomas, adenocarcinomas have delicate, finely or coarsely vacuolated, and often eccentric cytoplasm; more oval nuclei with less marked nuclear irregularities; prominent, often single large nucleoli with perinucleolar clearing (vesicular in Pap-stained preparations); and intracytoplasmic and/or extracellular mucin. On the other hand, the squamous phenotype is characterized by dense cytoplasm, well-defined cytoplasmic margins, and coarser nuclear chromatin. In many cases, the two carcinomas cannot be differentiated and the report will be that of non-small cell carcinoma, where ICC is required {375}.

Basaloid SCC closely resembles small cell neuroendocrine carcinoma (SCNEC) but lacks the predominantly discohesive cell pattern, extensive nuclear moulding, dark and light (salt-and-pepper when Pap-stained) finely granular chromatin, marked nuclear irregularity, chromatinic smearing, and apoptotic debris of SCNEC {523}. The distinction is particularly difficult in sputum samples. Owing to peripheral palisading and large cohesive tumour cell tissue fragments, SCC and its basaloid subtype can also be difficult to distinguish from large cell neuroendocrine carcinoma (LCNEC).

NUT carcinomas show remarkable similarity to basaloid and poorly differentiated SCC, but show predominantly discohesive, monotonous, primitive, basaloid tumour cells with a high N:C ratio and prominent nucleoli {235}. ICC is required.

The presence of thick basement membrane material wrapping around tissue fragments of basaloid carcinoma can be mistaken for hyaline globules of adenoid cystic carcinoma, and ICC is required.

Ancillary testing

Diffuse positive staining with a marker for SCC and negative staining for thyroid transcription factor 1 (TTF1) is used to confirm the diagnosis of SCC, although some markedly keratinized tumours may show a lack of staining with squamous cell markers. In SCC, the percentage of tumour cells staining positive for p40 should be > 50% {1000}. p40 is considered the most specific marker for SCC, whereas high-molecular-weight cytokeratins (CK5/6, CK14, 34βE12), desmocollin, desmoglein, and p63 are less specific {773,688,1000}. Diffuse p40 expression and largely negative neuroendocrine markers favour a diagnosis of basaloid carcinoma and exclude SCNEC and LCNEC, which are positive for TTF1. NUTM1 ICC is required for the diagnosis of NUT carcinomas {235}. Adenoid cystic carcinoma can be differentiated from basaloid SCC by the dual staining of epithelial and myoepithelial markers, i.e. CK7 and p63, and by the more specific *NFIB* or *MYBL1::NFIB* fusions detected by FISH in a subset of cases.

Predictive PDL1 testing, if available, should be done for all advanced SCCs {102}. *EGFR* mutation or *ALK* rearrangement can occur in lung SCC. Therefore, testing should be considered in young, never-smoking patients {495,993,739,559}. *EGFR* mutations are also common in adenosquamous carcinomas that can appear as SCC in small biopsy and cytopathology specimens due to limited sampling {140,439}.

Non-small cell carcinoma NOS

Bubendorf L
Roy-Chowdhuri S

Definition

The diagnosis of non-small cell carcinoma NOS (NSCC-NOS) is only used for small biopsies and cytopathological specimens that show poorly differentiated carcinoma, lack adenocarcinoma or squamous cell carcinoma differentiation by morphology and mucin staining, and have indeterminate or negative ICC – including negative thyroid transcription factor 1 (TTF1) and p40.

Clinical features and imaging

The signs and symptoms of NSCC-NOS are similar to those of other non-small cell lung carcinomas. Presenting symptoms include cough, pain, haemoptysis, and dyspnoea. Because "NSCC-NOS" is used for poorly differentiated forms of adenocarcinoma, squamous cell carcinoma, and less common histopathological subtypes, the imaging appearance varies according to the underlying histopathological subtype {892}. Imaging and clinical features should be consistent with a primary lung origin.

Histopathology

NSCC-NOS is defined by a lack of morphological and ICC features of adenocarcinoma or squamous cell carcinoma. Histopathology shows poorly differentiated, solid or diffuse infiltrates of NSCC with a lack of unequivocal glandular or squamous differentiation and variable degrees of cellular pleomorphism and nuclear enlargement and atypia in cases with the clinical features and imaging of primary lung tumours.

Key diagnostic cytopathological features

- Highly cellular smears
- Mix of tissue fragments and dispersed large single cells
- Tissue fragments are crowded and lack diagnostic cytopathological features of glandular or squamous differentiation, including a lack of acinar, glandular, or papillary architecture; intracellular or extracellular mucin; delicate vacuolated cytoplasm or keratinization; intercellular bridges; and denser well-defined cytoplasm
- Dispersed single cells are highly pleomorphic and usually large, with enlarged pleomorphic nuclei, variable chromatin, and prominent nucleoli
- Often necrotic background lacking mucin or keratinous debris

Discussion and differential diagnosis

The appearance of the lung lesion on imaging should be that of a lung primary. The use of ICC for subtyping NSCC in small biopsies and cytopathological specimens has markedly reduced the proportion of unclassified NSCC-NOS, from 25–47% to 7–14% {505,749,750,956}. It is important in such cases to perform an additional limited ICC workup to confirm that the tumour is a carcinoma, such as pankeratin and lymphoid markers, and to exclude common possible metastatic tumour types, if it can be done without compromising molecular testing. The choice of which stains to perform is dependent upon cytomorphology and clinical circumstances. If the diagnosis of carcinoma is confirmed and a metastatic tumour appears to be excluded, the diagnosis of NSCC-NOS can be made. It may be useful to mention in the report that although these findings are consistent with a primary carcinoma of the lung, they are not specific. In some cases, when poorly differentiated carcinomas are encountered without any cell block material or cytopathological slides for further workup, the diagnosis of NSCC-NOS can be made, but the

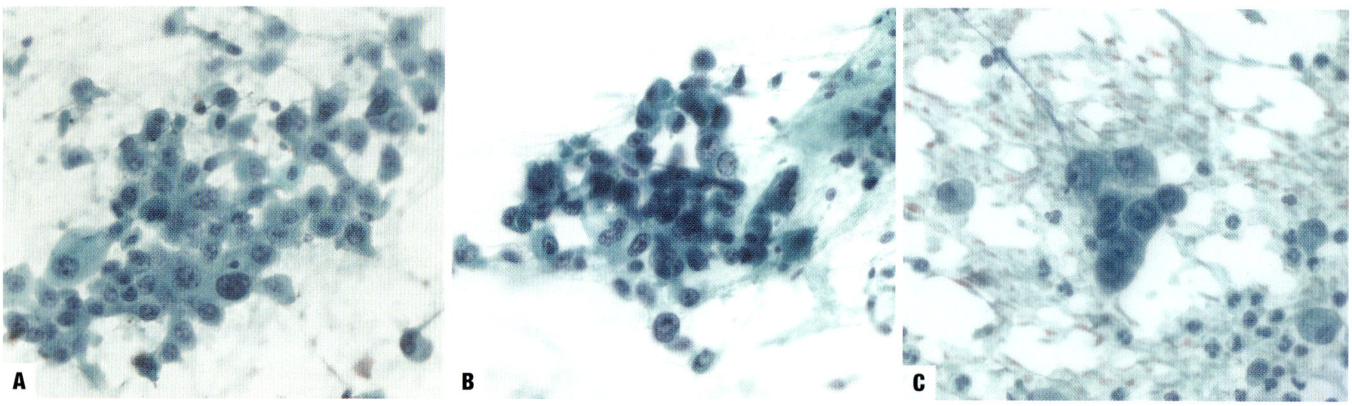

Fig. 7.24 Non-small cell carcinoma NOS. **A** Loosely cohesive tissue fragment of large cells with highly pleomorphic and hyperchromatic nuclei and no glandular or squamous differentiation; subsequent thyroid transcription factor 1 (TTF1) and p40 ICC was negative (Pap). **B** Large cells in a crowded, discohesive tissue fragment with highly pleomorphic nuclei, abnormal dark and unevenly distributed chromatin, and dense cytoplasm, with no distinct features of glandular or squamous differentiation; subsequent TTF1 and p40 were negative. There was *MET* amplification and *TP53* mutation present on molecular testing (Pap). **C** Crowded tissue fragment made up of cells with pleomorphic nuclei with perinucleolar clearing and coarse chromatin, and delicate cytoplasm; subsequent TTF1 and p40 were negative (Pap).

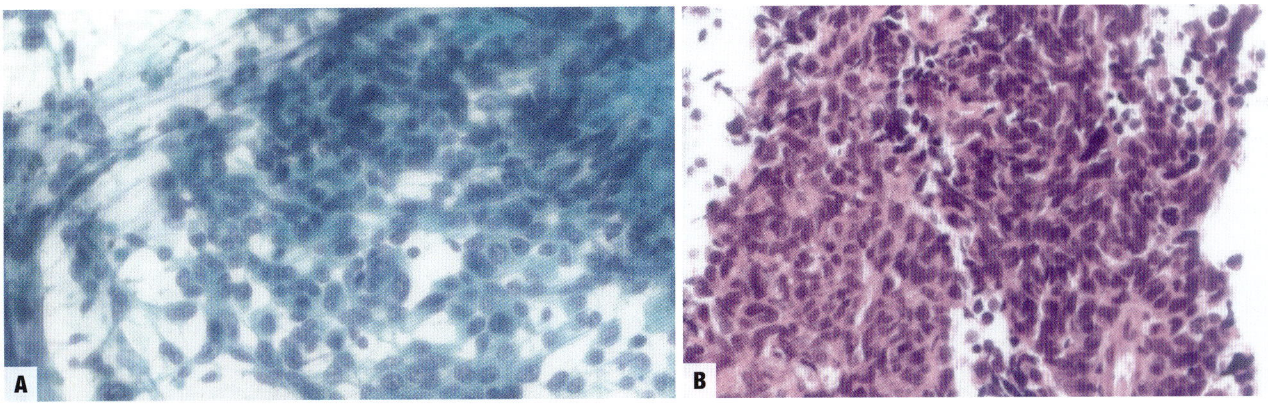

Fig. 7.25 Non-small cell carcinoma NOS. **A** Large tissue fragments of tumour cells with moderately polymorphic nuclei, chromatin abnormalities, inconspicuous nucleoli, and delicate cytoplasm. No clear features of glandular or squamous differentiation. Thyroid transcription factor 1 (TTF1) and p40 were negative (not shown) (transbronchial FNAB, Pap). **B** Tumour cells from the same case appear more polymorphic in this cell block specimen than on the smears (cell block, H&E).

report should state that this is being done only because material is not available for further workup {916}.

Ancillary testing

If available, TTF1 and p40 ICC should be applied before diagnosing NSCC-NOS, along with napsin A if the TTF1 is negative. A PASD or mucicarmine stain can be used to demonstrate mucin production, but if molecular testing is available, then care should be taken to leave sufficient material for predictive molecular biomarker studies. Patients diagnosed with advanced NSCC-NOS should be tested for the same predictive molecular biomarkers as those tested for adenocarcinoma or non-small cell lung carcinoma, favour adenocarcinoma {437}.

Salivary gland–type carcinomas

Baloch ZW
Maleki Z

Definition

Pulmonary salivary gland–type carcinomas are neoplasms that are believed to originate from the seromucinous glands of the central airways and that closely resemble their counterparts in the salivary glands.

Clinical features and imaging

Primary pulmonary salivary gland–type tumours (PSGTs) account for 0.1–0.2% of all pulmonary neoplasms (see Table 7.01) {584,580,717,346,281,744,1029,239}, and the great majority are malignant {315,717}. Mucoepidermoid carcinoma (MEC) of either low or high grade is the most common, followed by adenoid cystic carcinoma (AdCC), with fewer reports of epithelial-myoepithelial carcinoma (EMC), acinic cell carcinoma, and other rare neoplasms. EMC is a low-grade malignant tumour {584,580,446}.

The clinical symptomatology associated with PSGT includes cough, dyspnoea, wheeze, chest pain, hoarseness, pneumonia, and haemoptysis {315,717}.

Both CT and MRI are useful. Pulmonary MEC on CT appears as one or more well-defined tumour nodules involving the segmental or lobar bronchi. Usually AdCCs are infiltrative and occur in the inferior portion of the trachea or mainstem bronchi, leading to circumferential thickening of the airway wall with or without intraluminal or extraluminal thickening. The pulmonary EMC presents as an endobronchial mass on imaging {315,39,416}.

Lymph node metastases are rare; however, tumour recurrence and distant metastasis have been reported with AdCC {584,717}.

Histopathology

MEC can be low-grade and show cystic architecture with minimal or no invasive growth into the lung parenchyma, and it consists of a varying proportion of mucin-containing cells, squamous (epidermoid) cells, and intermediate cells. High-grade carcinomas show a solid growth pattern with infiltration into the surrounding lung parenchyma and consist of a varying number of mucus-secreting squamous and intermediate cells, with frequent necrosis and mitoses.

Adenoid cystic carcinoma can show (most commonly) cribriform and (on occasion) tubular or solid architecture, with infiltrative growth at the edges of the tumour and without associated tumour necrosis. The cribriform architecture shows a readily identifiable mucinous-type matrix filling the luminal spaces. The cells are basaloid with minimal nuclear pleomorphism and scant mitoses.

EMC is a biphasic tumour consisting of cuboidal epithelial cells with eosinophilic cytoplasm in the inner luminal layer of tubules, and myoepithelial cells (which are round or spindle with eosinophilic or clear cytoplasm) at the outer margin of the epithelial cells and in solid nests {584,446,248,398}.

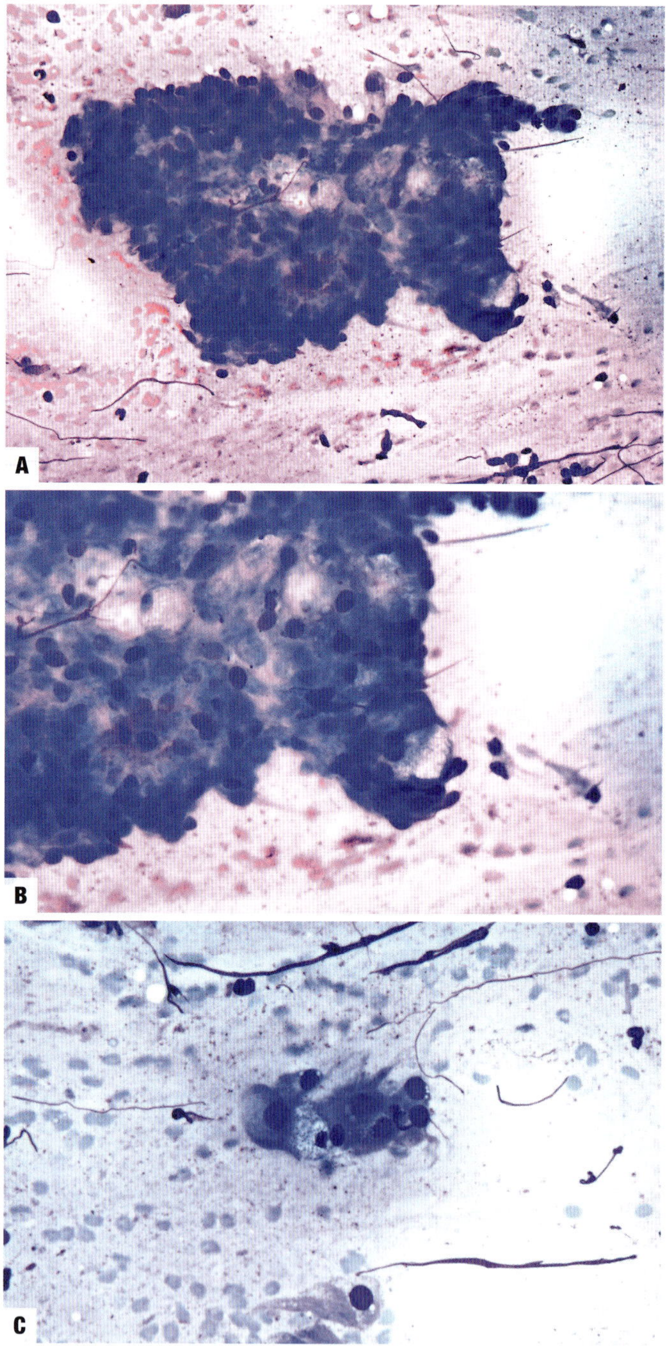

Fig. 7.26 Mucoepidermoid-like carcinoma of the lung. **A,B** Mucoepidermoid-like carcinoma of the lung showing a crowded sheet of epithelial cells that represent the glandular component of a moderately differentiated mucoepidermoid carcinoma. The cells have delicate cytoplasm. Although many of these tumours have prominent nucleoli, this feature is not clearly demonstrated in this case (Giemsa). **C** Small tissue fragment of epithelial cells showing foamy vacuolated cytoplasm (Giemsa).

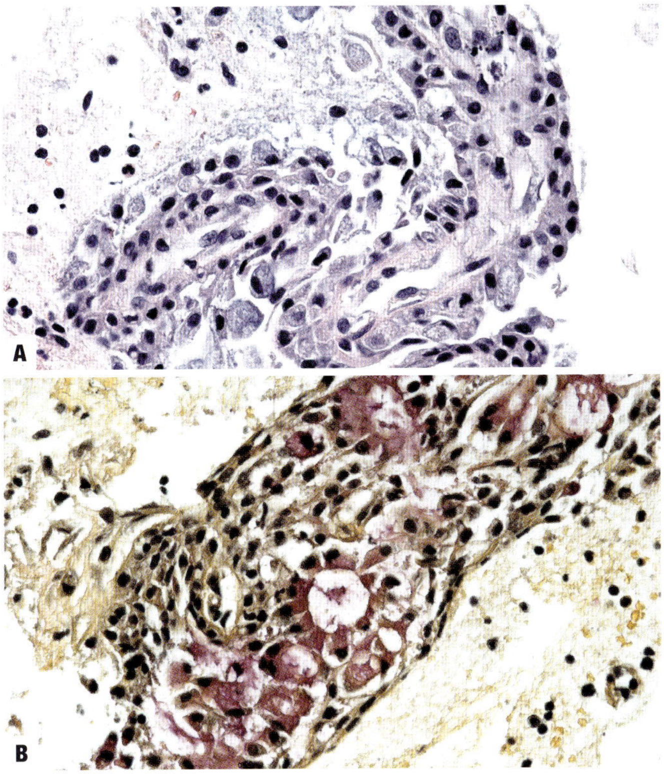

Fig. 7.27 Mucoepidermoid carcinoma. This cell block, stained with H&E (**A**) and mucicarmine (**B**) shows a large tissue fragment of epithelium composed of two distinct types of cells: cells with moderate to abundant eccentric cytoplasm, hyperchromatic nuclei, and prominent nucleoli, and cells with a low N:C ratio and eccentric cytoplasm containing microvacuolated foamy intracellular mucin. There are also occasional mucinous cells with large single mucin vacuoles.

Key diagnostic cytopathological features

Mucoepidermoid carcinoma

- Cellularity depends on the grade of tumour, with low-grade tumours producing abundant background mucin and macrophages due to cystic change, often with few epithelial tissue fragments
- Mucinous cells have goblet cell–type single large vacuoles or foamy oval regions of mucin (pink by Pap, magenta by Giemsa) and are scattered among polygonal intermediate cells in tissue fragments, as well as cohesive sheets of squamous (epidermoid) cells with denser cytoplasm and well-defined borders but lacking keratinization
- High-grade carcinomas are readily identifiable as malignant due to their atypical epidermoid cells with a lesser number of interspersed goblet-type mucinous cells, more prominent nuclear pleomorphism, larger nucleoli, necrosis, and (in some cases) mitoses

Adenoid cystic carcinoma

- Variably cellular
- Sheets with microcysts or cribriform, tubular, or complex tissue fragments and a lesser number of single cells
- Monotonous population of basaloid cells with a high N:C ratio and bland, oval to angulated nuclei with evenly dispersed dark chromatin and indistinct nucleoli
- The tumour matrix is usually sharply defined, balled up or branching, thick, and pale eosinophilic to virtually nonstaining (Pap) and magenta (Giemsa); in some cases it forms a rim surrounding basaloid tumour cells

Epithelial-myoepithelial carcinoma

- Usually highly cellular
- Two cell types, with tightly cohesive tubules or balls of basaloid epithelial cells with a high N:C ratio surrounded by larger myoepithelial cells with clear cytoplasm and oval nuclei
- Loosely cohesive tissue fragments of myoepithelial cells and stripped oval nuclei in the background
- Variable (but usually small) amount of eosinophilic (Pap) and magenta (Giemsa) matrix including stromal balls

Reference(s): {14,402,223,789}

Discussion and differential diagnosis

PSGTs are rare tumours and can mimic primary lung neoplasms owing to their growth patterns and cellular composition. They are being increasingly recognized partly because of an increasing familiarity with their counterparts in the head and neck region, and it is important to exclude the possibility of metastatic head and neck salivary gland tumours to lung before making a

Table 7.01 Salivary gland–type carcinomas: ancillary testing

Differential diagnosis	Immunocytochemistry	Molecular pathology
Mucoepidermoid carcinoma	All cell types: CK7+, TTF1– Mucous cells: MUC5AC+ Intermediate and squamous cells: CK5/6+, p40+, p63+ {757,789,356}	*CRTC1::MAML2* gene fusion (FISH or NGS) present in the majority of cases {757,356,792}
Adenoid cystic carcinoma	Myoepithelial/basal cells: p63+, S100+, SMA+, calponin+, vimentin+ Luminal cells: CK7+, EMA+, CK5/6+, KIT (CD117)+ {279,223,789}	*MYB::NFIB* or *MYBL1::NFIB* gene fusion (FISH or NGS) present in most cases (small series) {279,682}
Epithelial-myoepithelial carcinoma	Epithelial cells: CK7+, cytokeratin AE1/AE3+, MNF116+, SOX10+, EMA+ Myoepithelial cells: CK5/6+, p40+, p63+, S100+, calponin, SOX10+, SMA+ {835,684}	*PLAG1* and *HMGA2* rearrangements/amplifications (FISH) {236, 406}: *PLAG1* in 23% of cases, *HMGA2* in 26% of cases *CTNNB1* and *FGFR1* rearrangements {406} in rare cases (FISH) *HRAS* codon 61 mutations {144,931} present in ~80% of cases

NGS, next-generation sequencing; TTF1, thyroid transcription factor 1.

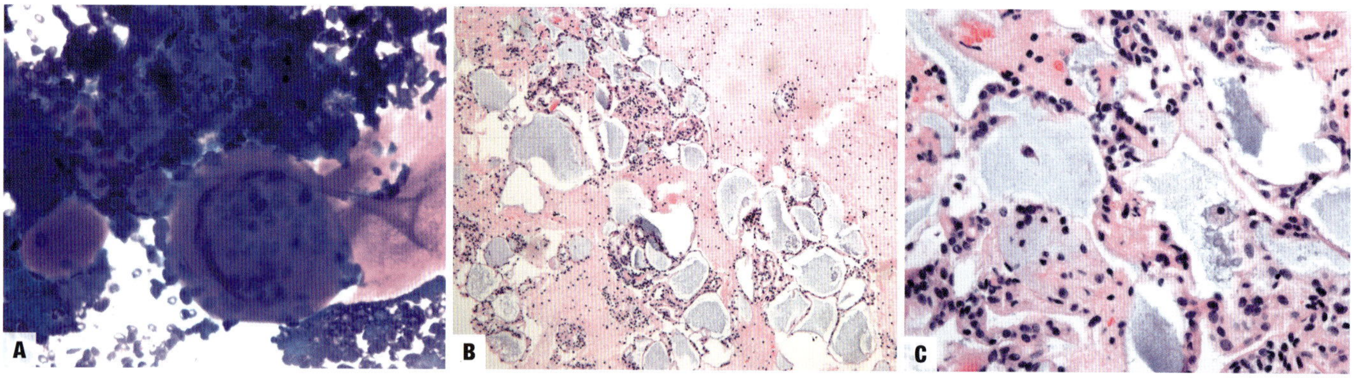

Fig. 7.28 Pulmonary adenoid cystic carcinoma. **A** FNAB showing basaloid tumour cells associated with globules of magenta stroma (Giemsa). **B** Cell block preparation showing a basaloid tumour arranged in tubular structures containing acellular stroma (H&E). **C** Higher magnification showing basaloid tumour cells arranged in cribriform architecture with acellular basement membrane material (H&E).

diagnosis of PSGT {584,446}. However, imaging features of a single mass involving the airways should favour the diagnosis of a primary lung neoplasm {575,99}.

The differential diagnosis includes primary adenocarcinoma, squamous cell carcinoma, adenosquamous carcinoma and bronchial mucous cell adenoma, other pulmonary salivary gland tumours, metastatic clear cell renal carcinoma, and perivascular epithelioid cell tumour (PEComa, clear cell tumour) {446}.

The relatively bland appearance of tumour cells with a mix of different cell types and the presence of extracellular matrix material assist in the diagnosis of PSGT.

In MEC, a mixture of mucous cells (with their eccentric goblet cell–type single vacuoles or foamy or punctate magenta [Giemsa] mucin), intermediate cells, and squamous cells is typical for this tumour, along with a lack of any keratinization {223}. In AdCC, diagnosis can be difficult in the solid-type tumour lacking cribriform foci and lacking extracellular basement membrane material. In these cases, the densely packed basaloid cells may be mistaken for small cell lung carcinoma, basaloid squamous cell carcinoma, carcinoid tumour, or even basal cell hyperplasia {789,718,14,279}.

In EMC, a dual population of small basaloid epithelial cells and larger myoepithelial cells is found, and acellular basement membrane material may by present. The differential diagnosis includes AdCC and basaloid squamous cell carcinoma {14}.

Because most PSGTs are exophytic endobronchial tumours covered by intact mucosa, these tumours may be missed by bronchial brushing or washing {223}.

Ancillary testing

An ICC panel can help to differentiate PSGT from other lung primaries such as adenocarcinoma and squamous cell carcinoma {248}. In MEC, mucous cells are positive for MUC5AC; intermediate and squamous cells are positive for CK5/6, p40, and p63; and all cells are positive for CK7 and negative for thyroid transcription factor 1 (TTF1) {757,789,356}. In AdCC, the myoepithelial cells are positive for p63, S100, SMA, calponin, and vimentin, whereas the luminal cells are positive for CK7, EMA, CK5/6, and KIT (CD117) {279,223,789}. In EMC, the epithelial cells are positive for AE1/AE3, CK7, MNF116, SOX10, and EMA, and the myoepithelial cells are positive for p63, p40, CK5/6, S100, SOX10, and SMA {835,684}.

FISH studies on cell blocks and direct smears can confirm PSGT. The *CRTC1*::*MAML2* fusion gene is specific for MEC and useful in diagnostic workups, where the FISH positive *MAML2* rearrangement should be validated by *MAML2* polymerase chain reaction or next-generation sequencing. Demonstration of *MYB* or *MYBL1* rearrangements or gene fusions by FISH or other methods can help establish a diagnosis of AdCC, and assessment of *HRAS* mutations is useful for diagnosing EMC {931,604}.

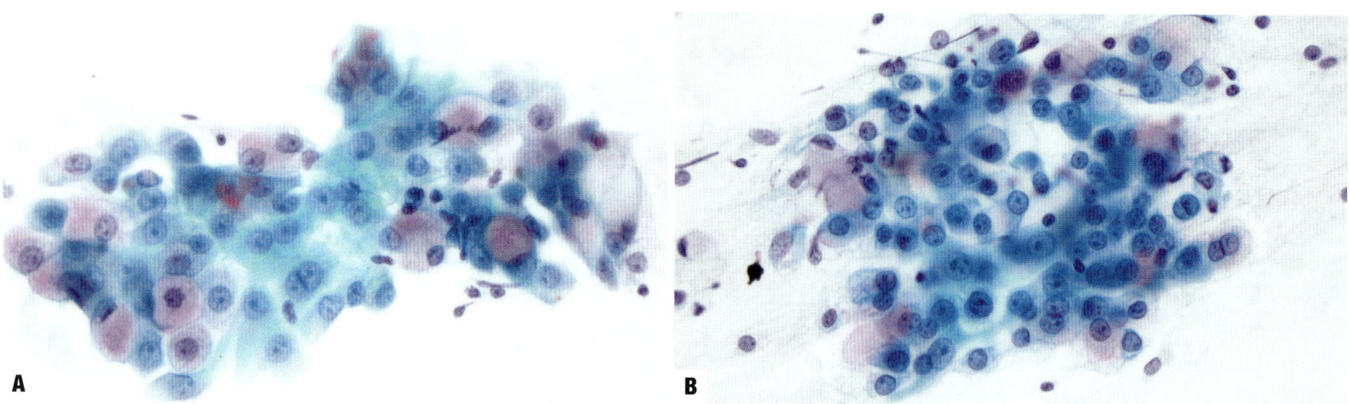

Fig. 7.29 Mucoepidermoid carcinoma. **A** Loosely cohesive tissue fragment of malignant cells characterized by their large size; their hyperchromatic nuclei with prominent single nucleoli; and their abundant, finely vacuolated, often eccentric cytoplasm, with some cells showing pale pink mucinous staining, sometimes within large single vacuoles (Pap). **B** Aspirated material displays malignant epithelial cells arranged individually or in loosely cohesive tissue fragments. The malignant cells are characterized by their large size; their hyperchromatic nuclei with prominent nucleoli; and their abundant, finely vacuolated to clear cytoplasm. The mucinous cells contain large amounts of intracytoplasmic mucin. Scattered ciliated respiratory epithelial cells and lymphocytes are seen in the background (Pap).

Adenosquamous carcinoma

Baloch ZW

Definition

Adenosquamous carcinoma is a carcinoma consisting of adenocarcinoma and squamous cell carcinoma components.

Clinical features and imaging

The relative frequency of pulmonary adenosquamous carcinoma (PASC) is reported to range from 0.4% to 5% of all lung carcinomas {485,81,946,728,1018}. Most tumours occur in patients ranging in age from 50 to 80 years (predominantly men with a strong smoking history), and < 3% of adenosquamous tumours occur in younger individuals {728,81,911}. There is a strong association with smoking history. Adenosquamous carcinoma behaves aggressively compared with other histopathological types of bronchogenic carcinoma. They usually present as large tumours at a higher clinical stage, with a frequent rate of metastases {161,1030}.

Imaging studies have shown that adenosquamous carcinoma can present in radiotherapy-related fibrosis and pneumoconiosis, and it usually occurs in the intermediate or peripheral portion of the affected lobe, but when it does occur centrally it can cause obstructive pneumonia. Adenosquamous carcinoma can show a poorly defined tumour–lung interface, pleural indentation, lobulation, spiculation, and peripheral ground-glass opacities {964,958}.

Histopathology

In surgical resection specimens, the tumours will show discrete or intermingled components of both adenocarcinoma (which tends to show acinar or solid growth with or without a lepidic pattern) and squamous cell carcinoma (either as keratinizing well-differentiated or solid poorly differentiated carcinoma). ICC for thyroid transcription factor 1 (TTF1) and p40 and a mucicarmine stain are used to highlight the adenocarcinoma component. The diagnosis of adenosquamous carcinoma can be challenging in small biopsies because it may show only one of the components, and ICC is essential to prevent the solid and non-keratinizing squamous carcinoma component being mistaken for poorly differentiated adenocarcinoma {485,81,946,728,161,64,1026,911,918}.

Key diagnostic cytopathological features

- Loosely cohesive tissue fragments and single cells showing features of adenocarcinoma and squamous cell carcinoma in a background of extensive necrosis
- Occasional keratinized cells can be seen, along with cells showing perinucleolar clearing of chromatin (Pap), prominent nucleoli, and intracytoplasmic mucin, suggesting adenocarcinoma

Reference(s): {918,877,115,834,246,905,636,549,1032}

Discussion and differential diagnosis

As in transbronchial core biopsies, the diagnosis of PASC can be challenging in FNAB samples, because of a lack of readily identifiable adenocarcinoma and squamous cell carcinoma components. It is advisable to confirm the dual differentiation by ICC before rendering a diagnosis of PASC, and most cases of PASC on FNAB have been diagnosed as poorly differentiated carcinoma with focal differentiation and a differential suggesting the possibility of PASC. The diagnosis of PASC is important in FNAB and limited tissue samples, because this tumour has the same response to treatment targeting *EGFR* mutations as adenocarcinoma, when compared with squamous cell carcinoma {485,81,946,728,161,64,1026}. The differential diagnosis of PASC includes all primary and

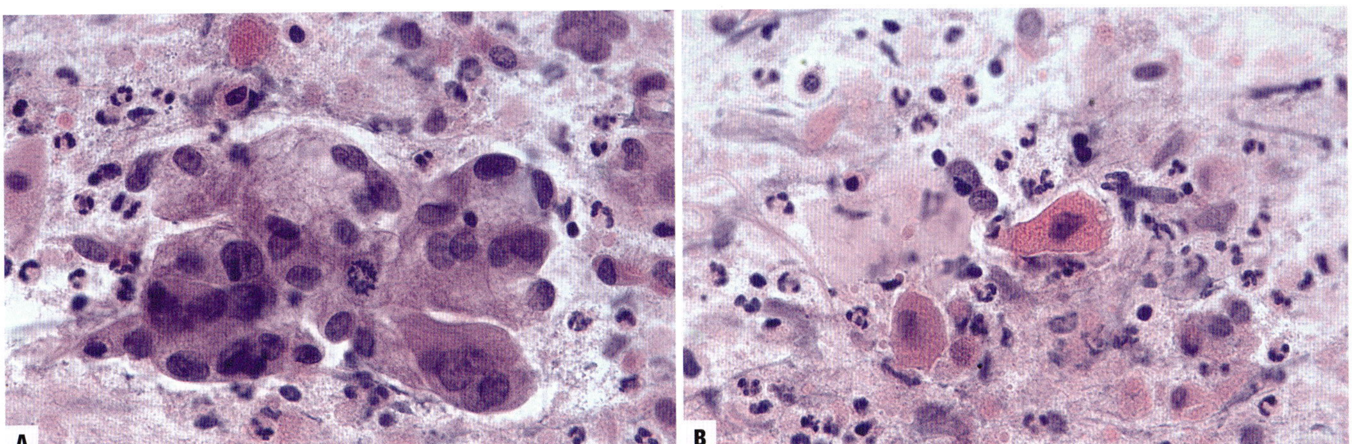

Fig. 7.30 Adenosquamous carcinoma. Pulmonary mass in left lower lobe. **A** Atypical glandular cells with enlarged, irregular nuclei and one mitosis. Adenosquamous carcinoma in concomitant histology (bronchial brushing, H&E). **B** Atypical squamous epithelium with enlarged, irregular, hyperchromatic nucleus. Adenosquamous carcinoma in concomitant histology (bronchial brushing, H&E).

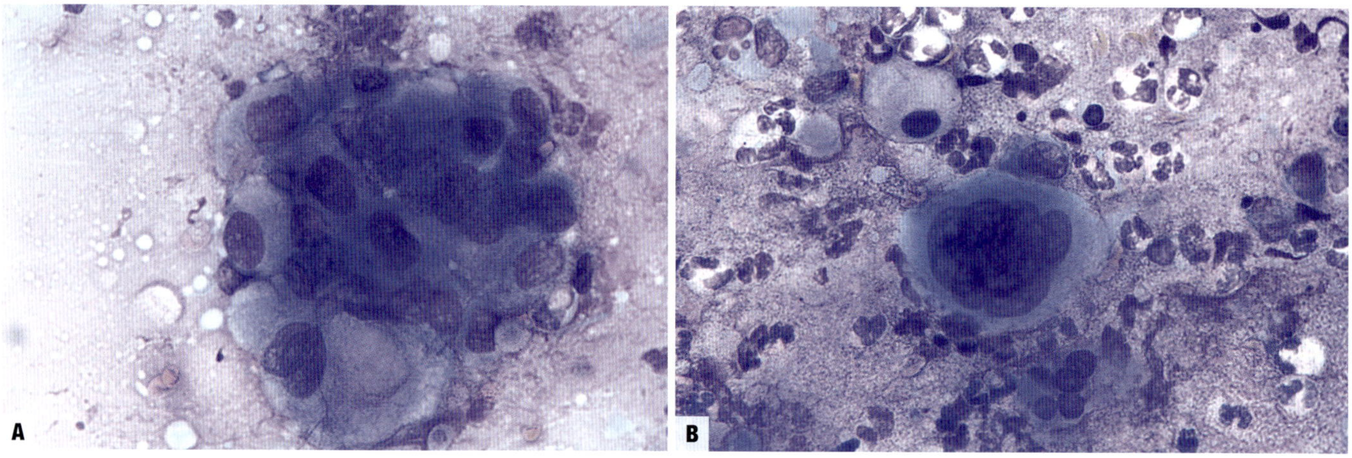

Fig. 7.31 Adenosquamous carcinoma. Pulmonary mass in left lower lobe. **A** Atypical glandular cells. Adenosquamous carcinoma in concomitant histology (bronchial brushing, Giemsa). **B** Very large atypical squamous cell with a large lobulated nucleus. Adenosquamous carcinoma in concomitant histology (bronchial brushing, Giemsa).

secondary pulmonary tumours showing varying degrees of squamous differentiation, including primary and metastatic squamous cell carcinoma, mucoepidermoid carcinoma, and metastatic endometrioid carcinoma {728}. Reactive atypia in lung parenchyma surrounding other primary tumours including squamous cell carcinoma can be mistaken for an adenocarcinoma component, leading to a misdiagnosis of adenosquamous carcinoma.

Ancillary testing

ICC with TTF1 and p40 is essential for rendering a diagnosis of PASC, especially for cases that fail to show distinct cytomorphological evidence of adenocarcinoma and squamous cell carcinoma, particularly in non-keratinizing cases. The p40 should show strong and diffuse staining to confirm the squamous component. ICC also helps in differentiating between other primary and secondary lung tumours showing squamous differentiation {485,81,946,728,161,64,1026, 582,246}. A stain for mucicarmine or PASD can be used to highlight intracytoplasmic mucin {728}. PASC may harbour gene rearrangement in *ALK*, *ROS1*, or *RET*, or gene mutation in *EGFR*, *KRAS*, *AKT1*, *ERBB2* (*HER2*), *PIK3CA*, or *STK11* {877, 140}.

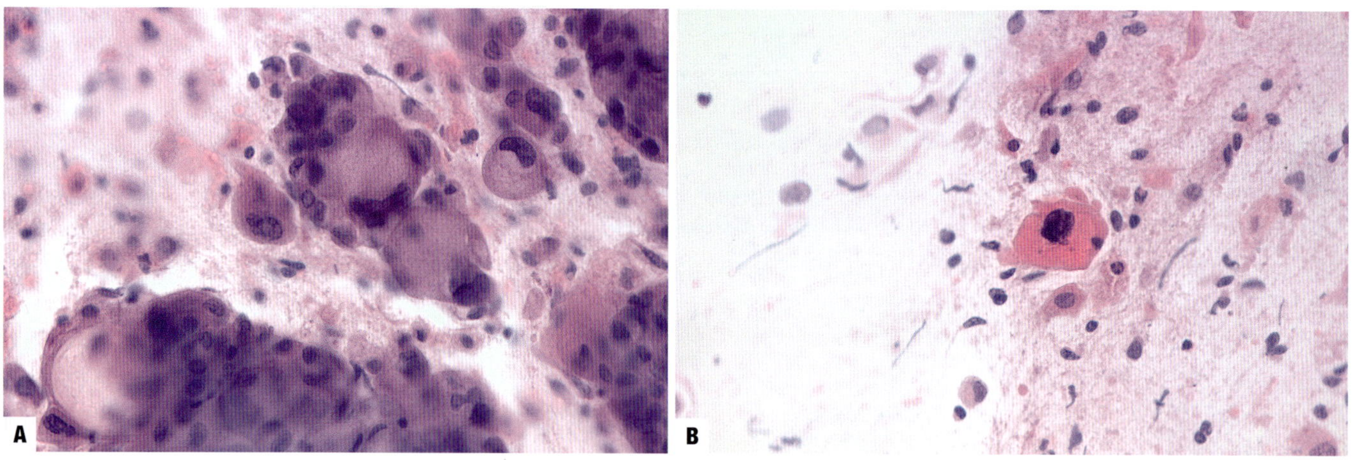

Fig. 7.32 Adenosquamous carcinoma. Pulmonary mass in left lower lobe. **A** Atypical glandular cells with enlarged, irregular nuclei and large cytoplasmic vacuoles. Adenosquamous carcinoma in concomitant histology (transbronchial FNAB, H&E). **B** Atypical squamous epithelium with enlarged, irregular, hyperchromatic nucleus. Adenosquamous carcinoma in concomitant histology (transbronchial FNAB, H&E).

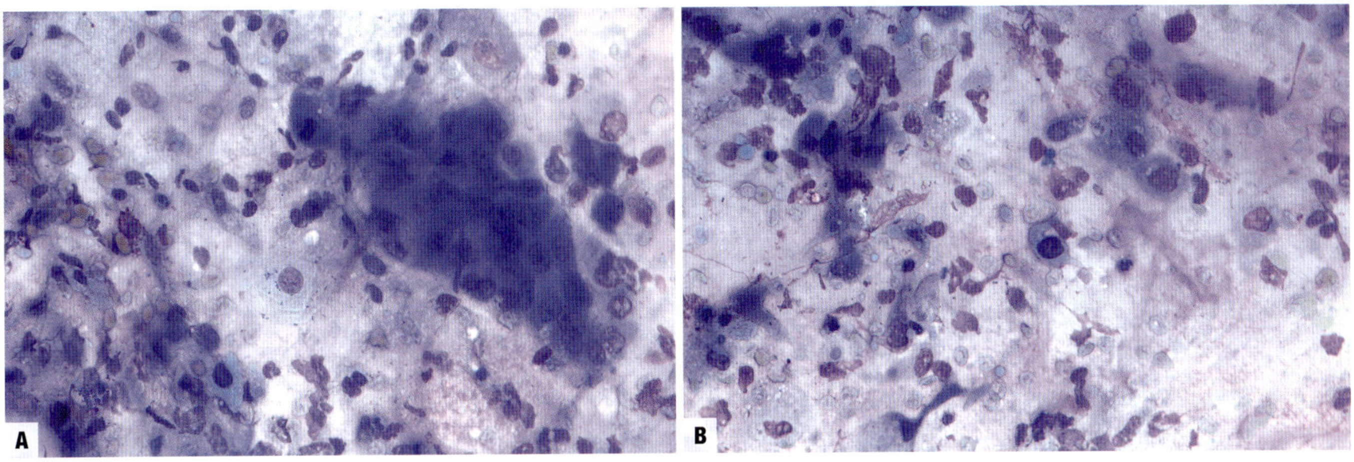

Fig. 7.33 Adenosquamous carcinoma. Pulmonary mass in left lower lobe. **A** Atypical glandular cells. Adenosquamous carcinoma in concomitant histology (transbronchial FNAB, Giemsa). **B** Atypical squamous cell with enlarged, irregular nucleus. Adenosquamous carcinoma in concomitant histology (transbronchial FNAB, Giemsa).

Pleomorphic carcinoma

Bubendorf L

Definition

Pleomorphic carcinoma is a poorly differentiated non-small cell lung carcinoma (NSCLC), including adenocarcinoma, squamous cell carcinoma, and/or large cell carcinoma containing spindle and/or giant cells, or a carcinoma that consists of spindle and/or neoplastic giant cells.

Clinical features and imaging

The signs and symptoms of pleomorphic carcinoma are similar to those of other NSCLCs. Presenting symptoms include cough, pain, haemoptysis, and dyspnoea {527,969}. Imaging shows a large central or peripheral mass, usually in the upper lobe, showing central necrosis, frequent pleural invasion, poorly defined borders with a ground-glass halo, and intense PET avidity {422,421,988,730}.

Histopathology

Pleomorphic carcinoma is composed of > 10% spindle and/or giant cells admixed with components of adenocarcinoma (in 31–72% of cases), squamous cell carcinoma (in 12–26%), or large cell carcinoma (in as many as 43%) {772,685,689}. Some tumours are composed only of spindle cells and/or tumour giant cells. The epithelial and spindle/giant cells may be intimately admixed or sharply demarcated from one another. Sometimes, osteoclast-type giant cells are scattered throughout the tumour, and these may be negative for keratin and positive for macrophage markers {689,72}. Giant cell carcinoma consists solely of highly pleomorphic giant cells with multiple irregular, sometimes multilobated nuclei and abundant eosinophilic to granular cytoplasm. Spindle cell carcinoma consists solely of neoplastic spindle cells {772,980}.

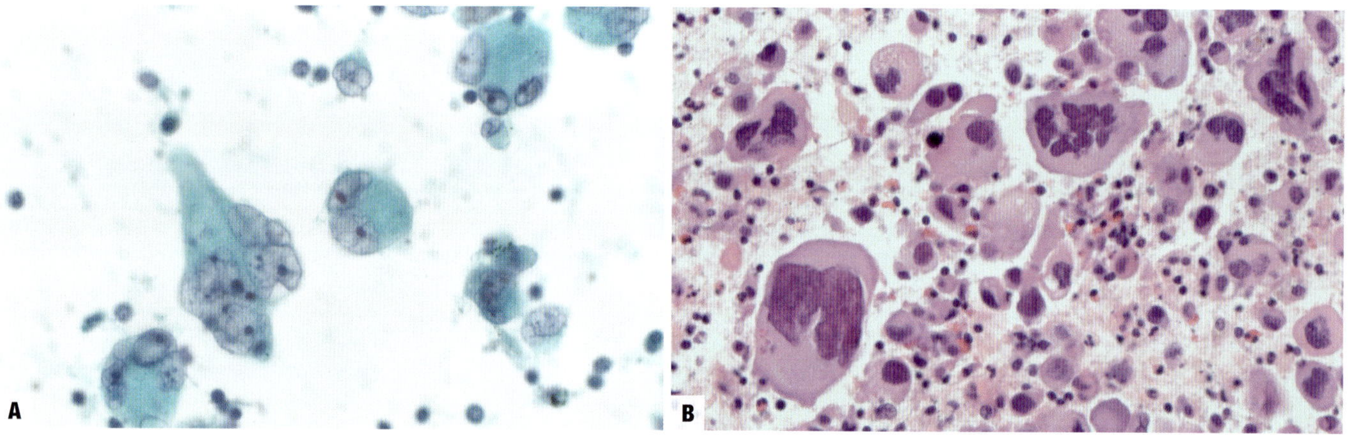

Fig. 7.34 Pleomorphic carcinoma. **A** Multinucleated tumour giant cells with highly polymorphic nuclei, positive for thyroid transcription factor 1 (TTF1) (not shown) (transbronchial FNAB from lymph node, Pap). **B** Non-small cell lung carcinoma with multinucleated giant cells showing highly pleomorphic and hyperchromatic nuclei in a background of carcinoma cells with single pleomorphic nuclei, consistent with pleomorphic carcinoma; subsequently found to be positive for TTF1, with molecular analysis showing a *KRAS* p.G12C mutation (cell block, H&E).

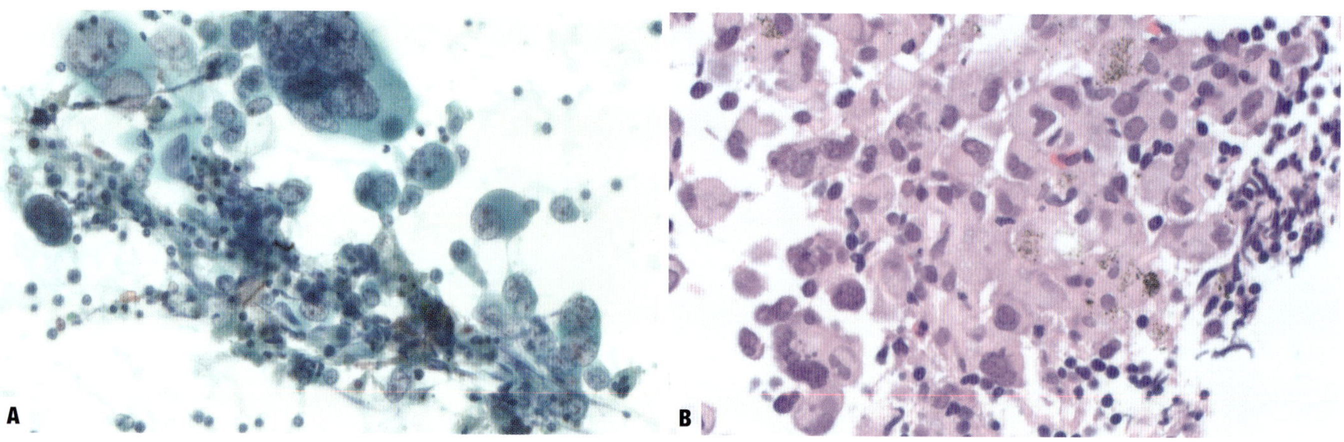

Fig. 7.35 Pleomorphic carcinoma. **A** Non-small cell lung carcinoma with multinucleated giant cells, consistent with pleomorphic carcinoma (transbronchial FNAB, Pap). Thyroid transcription factor 1 (TTF1) was positive (not shown). Molecular analysis showed a *KRAS* p.G12C mutation. **B** Same case as shown in Fig. 7.34A, showing nuclear pleomorphism (cell block, transbronchial FNAB from lymph node, H&E).

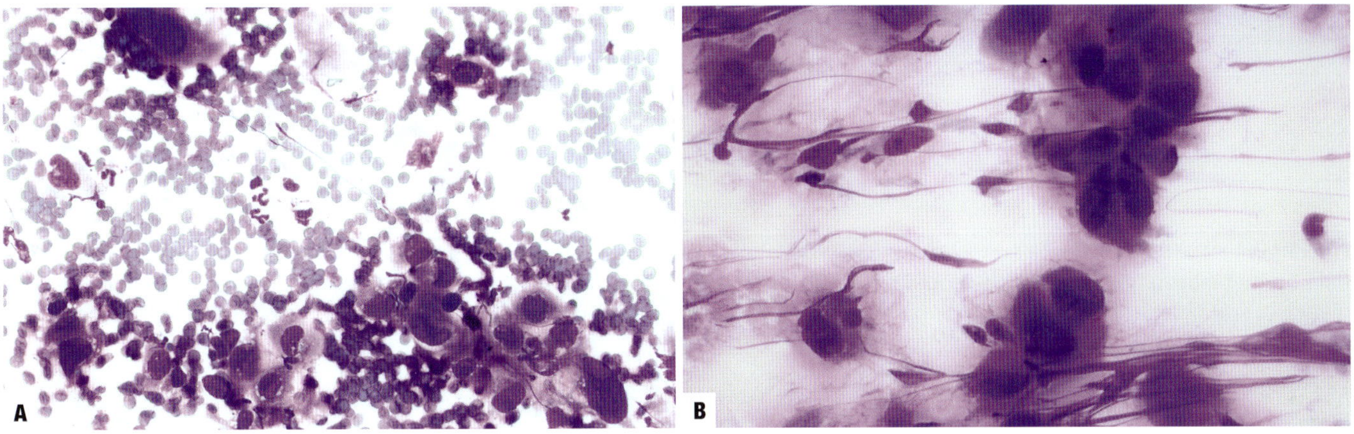

Fig. 7.36 Pleomorphic carcinoma. **A** FNAB smear showing large pleomorphic tumour cells with multinucleation and marked anisonucleosis (Giemsa). **B** FNAB smear showing large pleomorphic tumour cells with spindle to epithelioid morphology and some anisonucleosis (Giemsa).

Key diagnostic cytopathological features

- Discohesive, enlarged, and highly pleomorphic rounded or neoplastic spindle cells with prominent blue-grey (cyanophilic) (Pap) cytoplasm
- Variable number of tumour giant cells containing two or more nuclei can be present
- Large nucleoli
- Background of necrotic debris, inflammatory infiltrate, and myxoid or collagen-rich stroma often present

Reference(s): {352,147,46}

Discussion and differential diagnosis

Pleomorphic carcinoma is part of the spectrum of so-called sarcomatoid carcinomas that encompass pleomorphic carcinoma, carcinosarcoma, and pulmonary blastoma. Pleomorphic carcinoma cannot be definitively diagnosed on cytopathology, because it requires a resection specimen showing > 10% of spindle and/or giant cell components. However, if cytopathology shows NSCLC with spindle and/or giant cell carcinoma patterns, a comment should be made that their presence raises the possibility of a pleomorphic carcinoma. The differential diagnosis includes carcinosarcoma, metastatic sarcomatoid carcinoma from various sites, sarcoma, germ cell tumours, melanoma, dendritic cell sarcoma, and biphasic/sarcomatoid mesothelioma {35,689}. If adenocarcinoma or squamous cell carcinoma components are present, pleomorphic carcinoma is favoured even if keratins are completely negative in the spindle and/or giant cell component. A diagnosis of carcinosarcoma would require malignant heterologous elements such as chondrosarcoma.

Ancillary testing

Genetic events mirror those in other NSCLCs, particularly pulmonary adenocarcinoma {898,249,817}, and the frequency of *KRAS* and *EGFR* mutations is similar to that in pulmonary adenocarcinoma {898,382,502,249}. *ALK* and *ROS1* rearrangements rarely occur {898,987}. *MET* exon 14–skipping mutations are present in a subset {451,502,530}. There is a high incidence of PDL1 expression (60–90%), which is often stronger in the giant or spindle cell areas {605,419,988,503,817}.

Pulmonary blastoma

Geisinger KR

Definition

Pulmonary blastoma is a biphasic tumour composed of both a glandular carcinoma, which mirrors low-grade fetal adenocarcinoma, and a malignant stromal blastema component largely composed of primitive undifferentiated mesenchymal cells.

Clinical features and imaging

Pulmonary blastomas occur mostly in middle-aged adults with a smoking history and are only rarely seen in paediatric patients. Presenting symptoms of cough, chest pain, dyspnoea, and haemoptysis, as well as imaging of a solitary circumscribed mass in the lung periphery (frequently with a unilateral pleural effusion), are similar to those of most other non-small cell carcinomas of lung {438,726,26}.

Histopathology

Pulmonary blastoma must have both malignant epithelial and blastemal components recognizable microscopically {438,607, 35}. The epithelial component consists of a well-differentiated fetal adenocarcinoma with simple to complex glands composed of uniform epithelial cells with single, relatively bland nuclei with only small nucleoli. Within the glands, nuclear palisading is well developed, and subnuclear vacuoles are a very characteristic feature. Within some of the glandular lumina are sheets of slightly larger cells with squamoid differentiation, forming morules. Adjacent to or surrounding the glands is the blastemal sarcomatous component, comprising small, uniform malignant cells with short spindle or ovoid contours, a solitary hyperchromatic nucleus, and scant cytoplasm. Very rarely, heterologous differentiation is present.

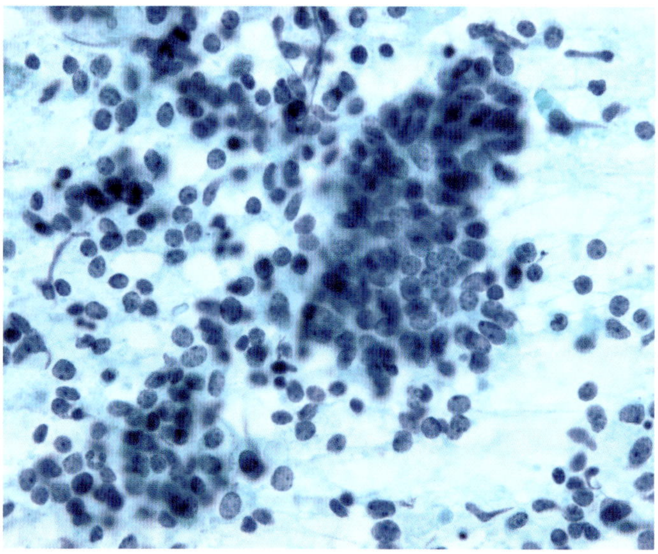

Fig. 7.37 Pulmonary blastoma. FNAB shows crowded tissue fragments of epithelial cells with regular round to oval nuclei and scattered, isolated cells with small bare nuclei, more granular cytoplasm, and small nucleoli (Pap).

Key diagnostic cytopathological features

- Moderate to highly cellular smears with two or more distinct cell populations
- Adenocarcinoma cells have relatively uniform solitary nuclei, inconspicuous nucleoli, and subnuclear vacuoles
- Squamoid cells form small sheets or morules and are larger with well-defined, denser cytoplasm, but no keratinization is seen
- Sarcomatous cells are small and homogeneous, with hyperchromatic nuclei and high N:C ratios

Reference(s): {172,519}

Discussion and differential diagnosis

If both components are recognizable, the diagnosis should be straightforward. If only the fetal carcinoma component is present, features including bland palisaded nuclei, subnuclear vacuoles, and squamoid morular elements help distinguish the tumour from adenocarcinoma. If only the blastomatous component is present, the differential diagnosis is from small cell carcinoma, which shows greater nuclear pleomorphism, nuclear moulding, and prominent crush artefact and apoptotic debris.

Ancillary testing

Both components show nuclear and cytoplasmic staining for β-catenin. The glandular component is positive for cytokeratin and often for thyroid transcription factor 1 (TTF1). Neuroendocrine markers including synaptophysin and chromogranin may be seen in the glandular and squamous and morular cells. The sarcomatous cells are positive for vimentin and SMA.
Reference(s): {1009,280,608}

Carcinosarcoma

Geisinger KR

Definition

Carcinosarcoma is a biphasic tumour usually composed of poorly differentiated non-small cell carcinomas as adenocarcinoma and/or squamous cell carcinoma and/or large cell carcinoma, and a malignant mesenchymal component, which must include heterologous differentiation.

Clinical features and imaging

As is characteristic of many poorly differentiated non-small cell carcinomas, carcinosarcoma typically arises in older adults, with a predominant male bias. The majority of patients have a strong history of cigarette smoking. The most frequent symptoms include cough and chest pain. On imaging, carcinosarcoma typically occurs in the upper lobes as a large, solitary, peripheral, well-delineated mass. The central lymph nodes may appear enlarged.

Histopathology

The diagnosis of carcinosarcoma requires both malignant components to be present: carcinomatous elements may show glandular and/or squamous differentiation or represent a large cell carcinoma, and the sarcomatous component may largely comprise nonspecific spindle tumour cells or a variable number of pleomorphic malignant giant cells, but it must also manifest chondrosarcomatous, osteosarcomatous, or rhabdomyosarcomatous differentiation by light microscopy. In both components, nuclei are large, irregular, and hyperchromatic. Nucleoli may be multiple and irregular, and macronucleoli occur.

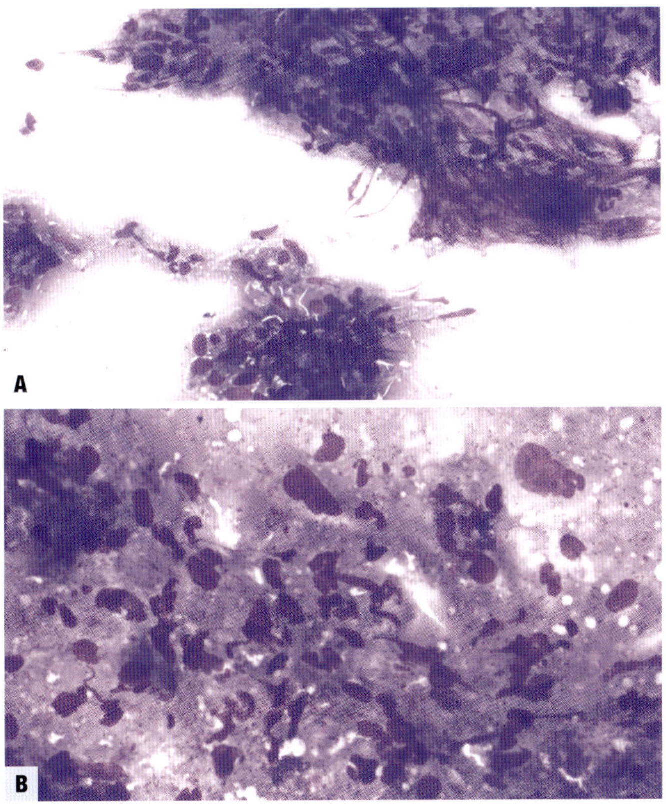

Fig. 7.38 Carcinosarcoma. **A** Relatively cohesive tissue fragments of spindle to epithelioid tumour cells with pleomorphic nuclei (Giemsa). **B** Pleomorphic large tumour cells with irregular nuclear membranes (Giemsa).

Key diagnostic cytopathological features

- High cellularity with obvious biphasic malignant components
- Adenocarcinoma, squamous, or undifferentiated carcinoma cells in loose to tightly cohesive tissue fragments and as single cells
- Malignant mesenchymal cells with spindle and/or giant cell morphology, with one or more nuclei
- Stromal heterologous differentiation consisting of primitive skeletal muscle differentiation, either as single isolated cells or in small, loosely cohesive tissue fragments, and/or malignant bone or cartilage in tissue fragments
- Large, hyperchromatic, highly pleomorphic nuclei, often with highly irregular large nucleoli
- Necrotic debris in background

Discussion and differential diagnosis

Carcinosarcoma is one of the five types of sarcomatoid carcinoma. The diagnosis of a malignancy in FNAB should be straightforward even in small samples of this tumour, but a precise diagnosis will require considerable material on direct smears and in the cell block. Only very rare isolated reports of the FNAB cytopathological findings of pulmonary carcinosarcoma have been published, and on review, most do not include descriptions of heterologous sarcomatous elements and therefore would be more accurately classified as pleomorphic carcinomas.

The differential diagnosis from a pleomorphic carcinoma, which is also in the sarcomatoid carcinoma group, is based on the identification of heterologous elements in the carcinosarcoma. The differential diagnosis from a spindle cell carcinoma is based on the recognition of a malignant glandular or squamous epithelial component in carcinosarcoma. The diagnosis of a spindle cell carcinoma should not be made in limited specimens because of the potential for sampling error where the epithelial carcinomatous elements are not present. The differential diagnosis from another biphasic neoplasm, pulmonary blastoma, can be made because its mesenchymal component is composed of primitive cells with no obvious differentiation and very high N:C ratios, and because its carcinomatous element resembles low-grade fetal adenocarcinoma. The differential diagnosis from most metastases, including those from the female genital tract, should be made on cytomorphology and the essential review of

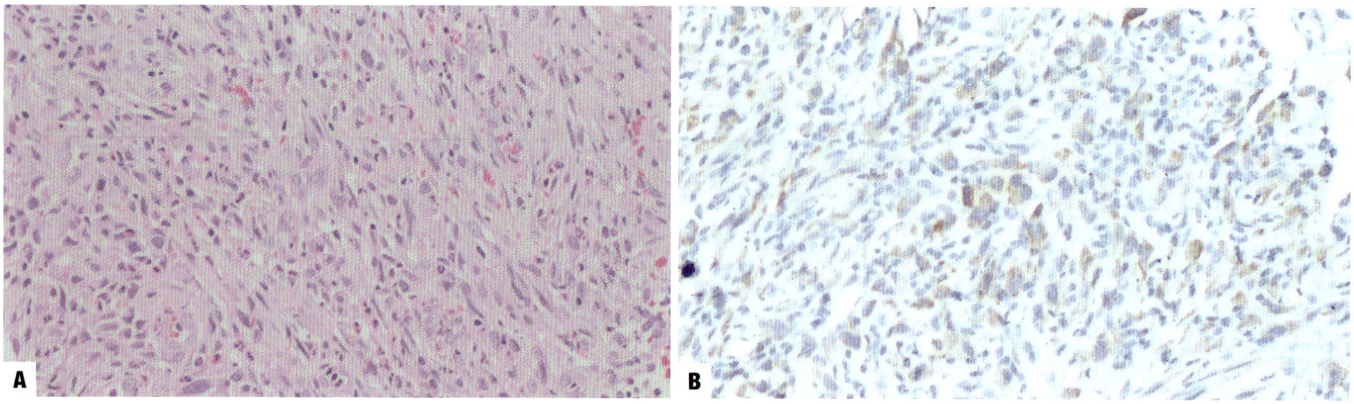

Fig. 7.39 Carcinosarcoma. **A** Biopsy shows a malignant spindle cell tumour with high-grade nuclei (H&E). **B** Corresponding biopsy shows weak positivity for pancytokeratin (ICC).

patient history, and even the great morphological mimic, melanoma, does not manifest heterologous elements.

Ancillary testing

Epithelial differentiation can be confirmed by pankeratins and CK7, with the glandular components thyroid transcription factor 1 (TTF1) and napsin A being positive, and with the squamous components being positive for p40 {772,1000}. The sarcomatous component is positive for vimentin. Desmin or myogenin may confirm muscle differentiation, and S100 supports cartilaginous differentiation.

NUT carcinoma

Jain D
Sauter JL

Definition

NUT carcinoma is a poorly differentiated carcinoma genetically defined by the presence of the nuclear protein in testis (NUT) gene (*NUTM1*) rearrangement.

Clinical features and imaging

NUT carcinoma typically presents at an advanced stage, in a wide age group of patients ranging in age from 0 to 80 years. Symptoms at presentation often include pleuritic chest pain, dyspnoea, non-productive cough, and weight loss {478,623, 897}. Local invasion, pleural invasion, and spread by lymphatic and haematogenous routes are common {47,126}. Distant metastases are common and include early metastases to bone, as well as dissemination to other distant sites, such as ovaries, liver, and brain, which occur later in the course of disease {944, 832,243,36,891,716,705}.

Features of NUT carcinoma seen on CT generally include a hypoattenuating, heterogeneously enhancing mass, often with necrosis and poorly defined infiltrative borders, with frequent invasion of adjacent structures {623,705,864,897}. NUT carcinoma on PET-CT typically shows high FDG uptake {633,820, 769}.

Histopathology

The characteristic morphology is that of an undifferentiated carcinoma. Focal abrupt keratinization is seen in approximately 33% of tumours {126}.

Key diagnostic cytopathological features

- Highly cellular smears with loosely cohesive tissue fragments and single isolated tumour cells
- Cells are round to oval and 2–3 times as large as a lymphocyte, with a high N:C ratio
- Cytoplasm is generally scant, delicate, and rarely vacuolated
- Nuclei show finely granular chromatin, discrete prominent nucleoli, and plentiful mitoses
- In cytospins, discohesive cells and tight cellular spherical tissue fragments are present and may show nuclear moulding resembling neuroendocrine tumours (NETs)
- Neutrophilic infiltrate is common
- Background shows necrosis, karyorrhectic and cellular debris, bare nuclei, and chromatinic smearing
- Rare squamous differentiation can show spindle or polygonal cells with dense cytoplasm, and keratinized cells may be seen, particularly in cell blocks
- Rarely reported in sputum samples

Reference(s): {235,56,66,447,1028}

Discussion and differential diagnosis

NUT carcinoma has nonspecific cytomorphological features and resembles the spectrum of malignant small blue round cell tumours, germ cell tumours, pure and combined small cell carcinoma with squamous cell carcinoma, basaloid squamous cell carcinoma, any undifferentiated or poorly differentiated carcinoma/adenocarcinoma, and melanoma. Because primary pulmonary squamous cell carcinomas are very rare in young nonsmokers, it is wise to consider doing NUT ICC in these cases with large mediastinal masses. Morphologically, small cell lung carcinoma demonstrates typical granular, dark and light (salt-and-pepper) chromatin and more frequent nuclear crushing and resultant chromatin smearing. Additionally, the tumour cells of small cell carcinoma do not show the prominent nucleoli seen in NUT carcinoma. Other tumours can be distinguished by a high index of suspicion for NUT carcinoma and the use of ICC and/or gene rearrangement studies.

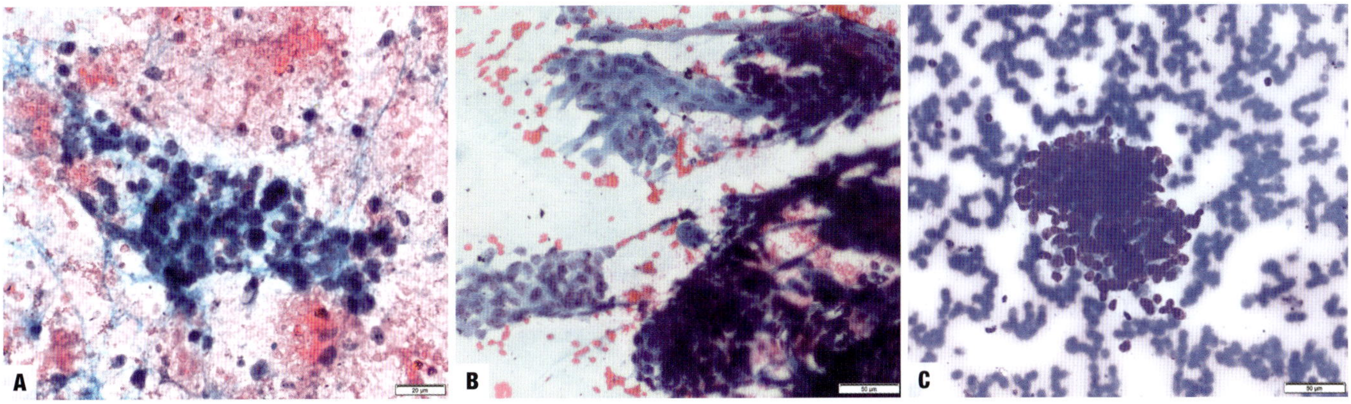

Fig. 7.40 NUT carcinoma. **A** Discohesive tissue fragment of crowded tumour cells with pleomorphic hyperchromatic nuclei (Pap). **B** Tissue fragments of polygonal tumour cells with a moderate amount of cytoplasm, indicating squamous differentiation (Pap). **C** A cohesive crowded tissue fragment of undifferentiated tumour cells with a high N:C ratio (Giemsa).

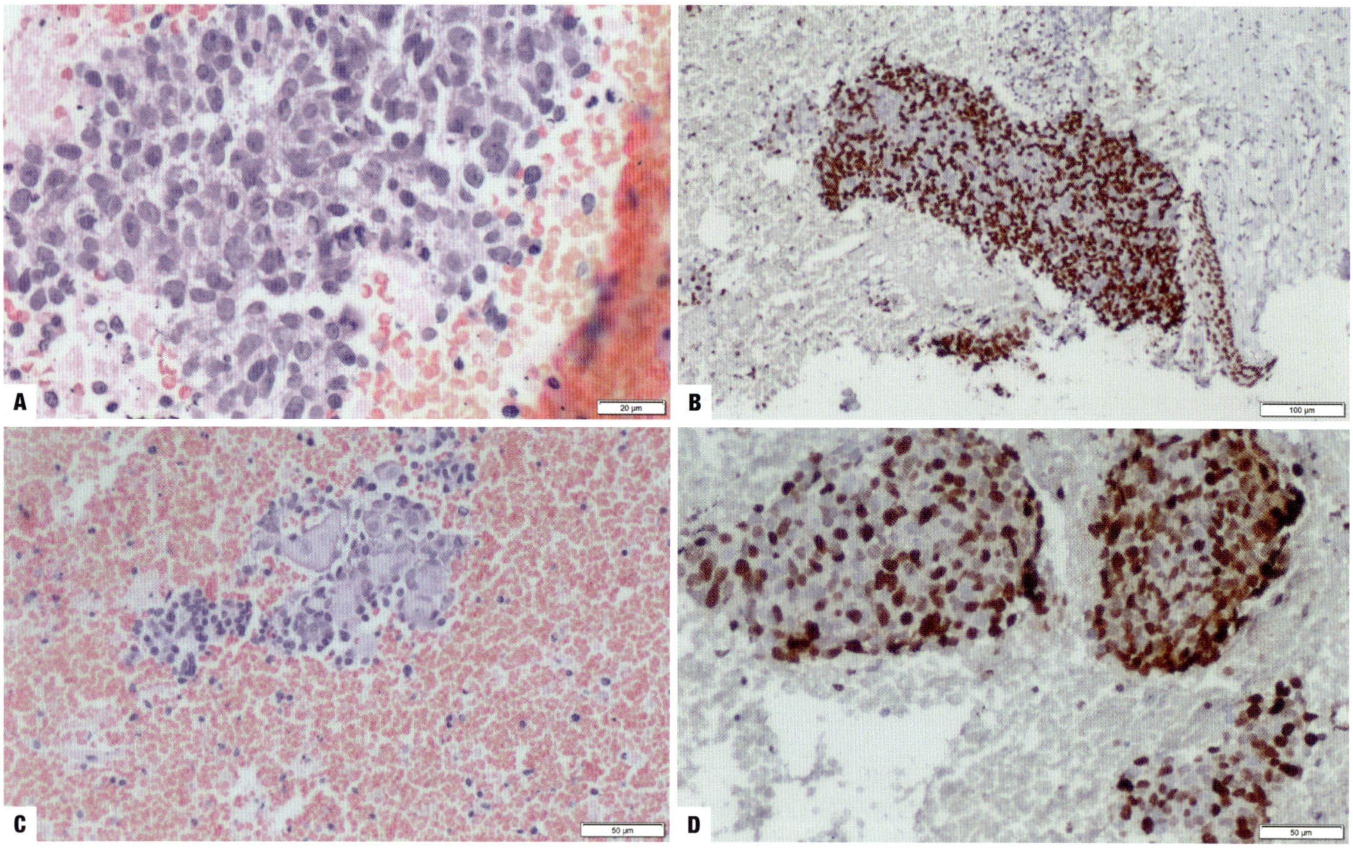

Fig. 7.41 NUT carcinoma. **A** Cell block preparation shows round tumour cells with prominent nucleoli and limited eosinophilic cytoplasm, with necrosis in the background (H&E). **B** p40 ICC shows diffuse strong nuclear positivity. **C** Cell block preparation shows squamous cells amid undifferentiated basaloid tumour cells (H&E). **D** Cell block ICC for NUT antibody (C52B1 clone) shows diffuse nuclear positivity in tumour cells.

Ancillary testing

NUT carcinomas are commonly (but not always) positive for pankeratins and for p63 (which is more often positive than p40) {544,694,354,146}. They are usually negative for neuroendocrine markers and thyroid transcription factor 1 (TTF1), with few exceptions {694,846,354,891}. Cell blocks are invaluable for the demonstration of the *NUTM1* rearrangement, either by FISH or ICC {342}. Speckled nuclear expression in > 50% of tumour nuclei in ICC using clone C52B1 is required for establishing the diagnosis. The ICC has 100% specificity and 87% sensitivity {310}. Alternatively, demonstrating *NUTM1* rearrangement can be done by molecular methods such as karyotyping, FISH, PCR, or next-generation sequencing–based methods {830, 902,867}.

Thoracic SMARCA4-deficient undifferentiated tumour

Sauter JL
Jain D

Definition

Thoracic SMARCA4-deficient undifferentiated tumour (SMARCA4-UT) is a high-grade undifferentiated malignant epithelial neoplasm that occurs in adults and has significant thoracic involvement. Deficiency of SMARCA4 (BRG1) must be confirmed by ICC or molecular methods.

Clinical features and imaging

SMARCA4 (BRG1) is a central component of the SWI/SNF chromatin-remodelling complex. Thoracic SMARCA4-UTs occur in adults (age range: 27–90 years) and have a male predilection. They often occur in patients with a significant smoking history {475,1004,803,738,690}. Symptoms at presentation include dyspnoea, chest pain, weight loss, and symptoms related to metastases, such as seizures and bone pain {803}. SMARCA4-UTs often present at an advanced stage, and they have an aggressive course and a poor prognosis. The reported median overall survival time is 4–7 months {475,1004,803,738,690,180}. Metastatic sites include lymph nodes, bone, adrenal glands, brain, and abdomen/pelvis {1004,803,180,738}. SMARCA4-UTs behave more aggressively than SMARCA4-deficient conventional non-small cell lung carcinoma (NSCLC) {475,738}.

Imaging features include large, poorly defined, compressive, PET-avid masses involving the mediastinum, pulmonary hilum, lung, and/or pleura. Focal lung involvement occurs in most cases {475,1004,803,738,690,180}.

Histopathology

SMARCA4-UTs typically show undifferentiated morphology characterized by diffuse sheets of discohesive round to epithelioid cells, which are relatively monotonous, but mild to moderate cellular pleomorphism can be seen. Rhabdoid features may be

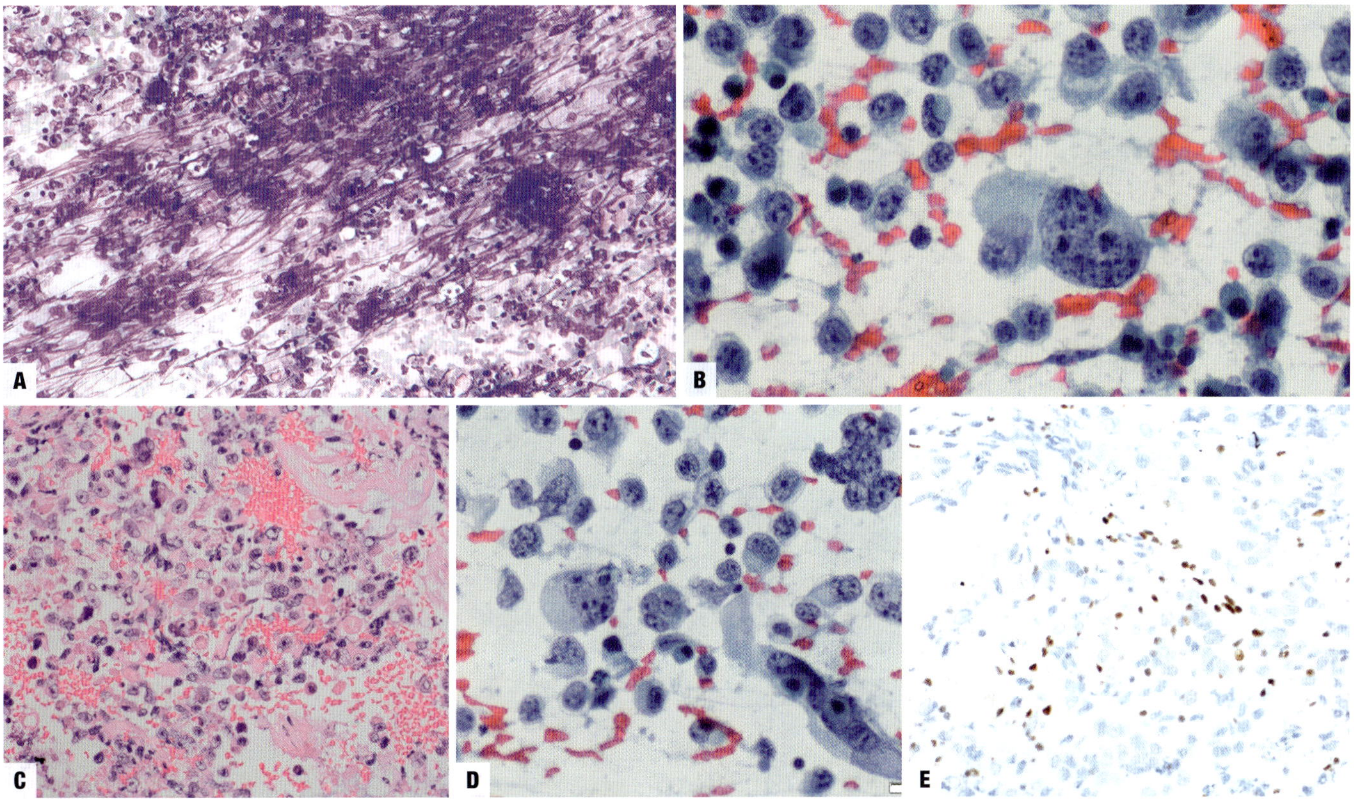

Fig. 7.42 Thoracic SMARCA4-deficient undifferentiated tumour. **A** Rare small tissue fragments are present, with abundant chromatinic streaking artefact and some single rounded intact tumour cells with fragile cytoplasm (Giemsa). **B** Highly pleomorphic dispersed tumour cells with eccentric cytoplasm in most cells, with cytoplasmic densities pushing into the curved nucleus of some cells, and hyperchromatic coarse chromatin with perinucleolar clearing and large nucleoli; occasional giant cells with large highly pleomorphic nuclei are seen (Pap). **C** High-power magnification of cell block, highlighting discohesive tumour cells with round to oval, moderately pleomorphic nuclei with nuclear irregularities, vesicular chromatin, and prominent nucleoli. Many tumour cells display eccentric dense eosinophilic cytoplasm, but classic rhabdoid morphology is not seen (H&E). **D** Highly pleomorphic tumour cells with eccentric cytoplasm (in most cells) and highly pleomorphic nuclei with coarse chromatin and prominent nucleoli (Pap). **E** Cell block ICC for SMARCA4 (BRG1) shows complete loss of expression of SMARCA4 in tumour cells, in the presence of a positive internal control demonstrated by nuclear positivity in benign cells.

present, albeit focally, in some tumours. Nuclei show perinucleolar clearing of the chromatin and prominent nucleoli. Plentiful mitoses and tumour necrosis are common. Spindle cells, clear cells, myxoid change, sclerosis, and an alveolar pattern are rare but have been reported {1004,690,738}. Gland formation or keratinization is generally absent, but 5% of reported cases show undifferentiated morphology adjacent to areas of conventional NSCLC {738}.

Key diagnostic cytopathological features

- Hypercellular smears with dispersed single cells or loosely cohesive sheets
- Cells are round to ovoid or polygonal, intermediate in size, and often relatively monotonous, but pleomorphism does occur
- Cell borders may be prominent or poorly defined with fragile cytoplasm
- Rhabdoid morphology characterized by globular eosinophilic (Pap) perinuclear inclusions or cytoplasmic condensation may be seen but is not required for diagnosis and may not be well demonstrated in smears
- Nuclei are enlarged and round to oval but can show irregularities, with prominent nucleoli and perinucleolar clearing (Pap) in cells with eccentric cytoplasm
- Mitoses are frequent and apoptotic nuclei may be seen with rare streaking artefact
- Background is often necrotic and/or inflammatory, and multinucleation, giant cells, and bare nuclei in the background have been reported

Reference(s): {888,557,547,609}

Discussion and differential diagnosis

The differential diagnosis is broad and includes any poorly differentiated or undifferentiated malignant epithelioid neoplasm, including neuroendocrine carcinomas, germ cell tumours, NUT carcinoma, lymphoma, melanoma, mesothelioma, and sarcoma (including rhabdomyosarcoma, *CIC*-rearranged sarcoma, malignant rhabdoid tumour, and epithelioid sarcoma). Appropriate ICC panels can aid in this differential diagnosis. NSCLC can usually be distinguished by the degree of glandular or squamous differentiation and ICC.

Ancillary testing

The typical immunophenotype of SMARCA4-UT is loss of SMARCA4 (BRG1) and SMARCA2 (BRM); expression of CD34, SOX10, and/or SALL4; and absent or focally weak claudin-4 and keratin expression {1004,803,690,738}. Some cases show a severe reduction of SMARCA4 (BRG1) expression rather than a complete loss {1004,738,547}. SMARCB1 (INI1) expression is retained. Synaptophysin expression is common {180,738}, and expression of thyroid transcription factor 1 (TTF1), p63, p40, or WT1 has been reported in rare cases {475,1004,738}. As many as 5% of conventional NSCLC are deficient in SMARCA4 {542,646,1005,331,187,613} but may be distinguished by the presence of gland formation or keratinization, indicating adenocarcinoma or squamous cell carcinoma. Keratins and claudin-4 may be helpful, because expression of these markers is absent or only focally weak in SMARCA4-UT. Expression of SMARCA2 (BRM) is also typically lost in SMARCA4-UT but retained in carcinomas. Because none of these morphological or ICC features are entirely sensitive or specific, rare cases with features of both SMARCA4-UT and carcinoma remain difficult to classify.

Sequencing can confirm the presence of *SMARCA4* mutation, but loss of SMARCA4 (BRG1) expression by ICC is sufficient for diagnosis. *SMARCA4* FISH has limited utility {738}.

Carcinoid/neuroendocrine tumours of the lung

Michael CW
Dalurzo ML
Papotti M
Rekhtman N
Vivero M

Definition

Carcinoid/neuroendocrine tumours are well-differentiated neuroendocrine malignancies showing pure neuroendocrine differentiation.

Clinical features and imaging

Pulmonary neuroendocrine tumours (NETs) are also known as carcinoid tumours and account for approximately 2% of all lung malignancies; they can be subtyped as typical carcinoid tumours (TCs), accounting for 80–90% of cases, and atypical carcinoid tumours (ACs), accounting for only a minority of cases {734,109,910}. NETs are not related to smoking, have a median patient age of 55 years {693,734,551}, and can arise in adolescents {1010,487}.

Approximately 80% of lung NETs are central and present on imaging as a well-defined, round or ovoid endobronchial or peribronchial nodule, whereas 20% are peripheral and present as sharply circumscribed intraparenchymal nodules {379,558, 1033}. Clinically, central NETs may present with symptoms related to bronchial obstruction, whereas peripheral NETs are generally asymptomatic. Symptoms related to hormone secretion are rare {313,551}. NETs typically show milder FDG uptake on PET scans {442,1033}, although FDG avidity is increased in ACs.

Regional lymph node metastases occur in < 5% of TCs and 30–50% of ACs. Distant metastases are rare for TCs but occur in 20–30% of ACs {734,507,551}. Metastasis can occur to a variety of sites but most commonly involves the liver, bone, and brain {150,737,328}.

Histopathology

Neuroendocrine architecture is present, characterized by an organoid, nested, or nodular arrangement; trabecular patterns; cell cords; and frequent rosettes. Cells are polygonal or plasmacytoid, with round nuclei showing uniform smooth nuclear membranes and granular salt-and-pepper chromatin. Histopathological variants include the spindle or fusiform cell pattern (which is most commonly peripherally located {677}), as well as glandular, oncocytic, papillary, and pigmented NET {734,910}. NETs are subtyped as TC (> 2 mitoses/2 mm^2 and lacking necrosis) or AC (2–10 mitoses/2 mm^2 and/or featuring necrosis, which is usually focal, punctate, and comedo-like). NETs with mitotic counts exceeding 10 mitoses/2 mm^2 are increasingly recognized {737,741,719,781,329}.

Key diagnostic cytopathological features

- High cellularity
- Small, discohesive sheets; larger tissue fragments consisting of plexiform, branching, thin fibrovascular strands surrounding and attached to sheets of neoplastic cells; trabeculae, cords, and single intact cells; a papillary or acinar-like architecture can be seen
- Pseudorosettes are observed in half of the cases
- Stripped branching and anastomosing fibrovascular strands without attached neoplastic cells may be present
- Cells are uniform, round to oval, and occasionally spindle, with well-defined margins
- Eccentric cytoplasm produces a plasmacytoid appearance, or the nuclei can be central (Giemsa)
- Nuclei are monotonous, are round or ovoid with smooth contours, and show salt-and-pepper finely granular chromatin (Pap)
- Nucleoli are small or inconspicuous
- Binucleation, intranuclear pseudoinclusions, and nuclear grooves may be seen
- Cytoplasm is moderate in amount and finely granular, with eosinophilic (H&E), greyish-blue (Pap), or red to magenta granules (Giemsa)

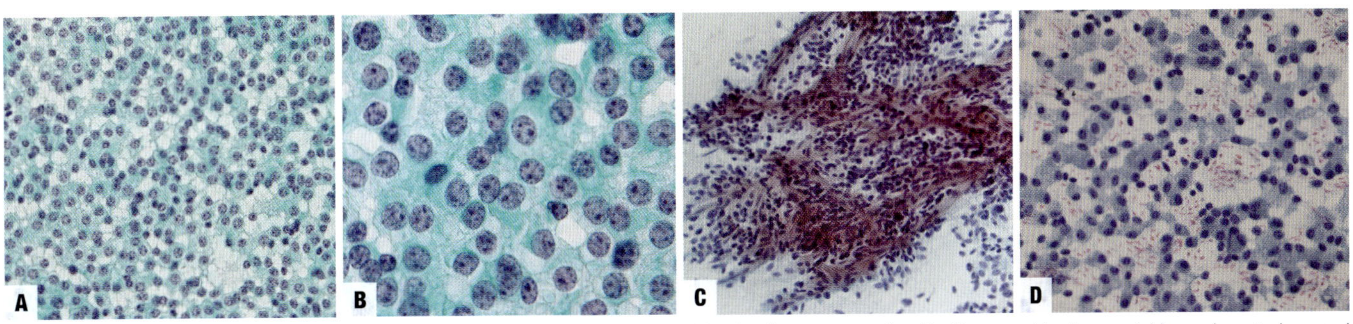

Fig. 7.43 Neuroendocrine tumour (NET). **A** Lower-power view shows many round or ovoid and uniform tumour cells with often eccentric plasmacytoid granular cytoplasm and minimally pleomorphic round nuclei with finely granular, uniform, salt-and-pepper chromatin (Pap). **B** High-power view shows typical finely granular salt-and-pepper chromatin in the round nuclei of the tumour cells, with many cells showing plasmacytoid eccentric granular cytoplasm (Pap). **C** Branching, anastomosing capillaries enclosing nests of cells and with attached small sheets of round to oval tumour cells with scant eccentric cytoplasm and uniformly granular salt-and-pepper chromatin in round nuclei (Pap). **D** Loosely cohesive population of round cells with moderate to abundant eccentric cytoplasm, giving a plasmacytoid appearance, and with bland nuclei with uniformly granular salt-and-pepper chromatin and inconspicuous or small nucleoli (Pap).

- Numerous naked nuclei are present in a finely granular background related to the release of granules from fragmented cytoplasm
- Oncocytic variant shows more granularity and deep eosinophilia in the cytoplasm
- Pigmented variant shows small melanin pigment granules

Reference(s): {345, 683, 879, 788, 870, 165, 576, 785, 360, 994, 579}

Discussion and differential diagnosis

The diagnosis can be established by FNAB or by exfoliative samples if the tumour erodes the overlying mucosa {511}. NET is rarely seen in sputum samples, where neoplastic cells are usually discohesive, although expectorated tissue fragments and large tissue fragments have been reported in patients with haemoptysis {171}. In cell blocks, solid or organoid fragments of uniform cells with no crush artefact suggest NET. In the spindle cell variant, the cells present as loosely cohesive

Table 7.02 Cytopathological features of neuroendocrine tumours (NETs)

Feature	NET / typical carcinoid	NET / atypical carcinoid	LCNEC	SCNEC
Pattern at low magnification	Trabeculae; branching fibrovascular strands with attached tumour sheets, cords, and loosely cohesive sheets; and plentiful dispersed single cells and stripped nuclei		Irregular tissue fragments and sheets, with some dispersed cells in a necrotic background	Irregular tissue fragments and sheets, with chromatinic smearing and apoptotic debris
Necrosis	Absent	Rare single cell	Extensive	Extensive
Complex branching fibrovascular strands	Present in ~50%	Present in ~50%	May be present	Absent
Cellular features				
Disorganization	Absent	May be focal	Present	Present
Pleomorphism	Minimal	Mild and focal	Marked	Moderate
Size	Small to medium	Small to medium	Large, at least focally	Intermediate
Plasmacytoid cells	Present	Present	Absent	Absent
Spindle cells	Present, may dominate	Present, may dominate	Absent	Absent
Nuclear features				
Size	Small	Small	Large	Intermediate (> 3× lymphocyte diameter)
Atypia	Absent	May be focal	Marked	Marked
Nucleoli	Small	Small or focally prominent	Very prominent, at least focally	Few
Chromatin	SAPC+	SAPC+/coarse	SAPC+/coarse	SAPC+
Moulding	Focal, mild	Focal, moderate	Focal, moderate	Prominent
Palisading	Absent	Absent	Frequent	Less frequent
Mitosis	Very rare	Rare	High	High
Crush artefact	Absent	Focal	May be present	Significant
Cytoplasmic features				
Amount	Moderate to abundant	Scant to moderate	Moderate to abundant	Scant
Granularity	Present	Present	Absent	Absent
Melanin pigment	May be present	May be present	Absent	Absent
NE markers	React with most markers	React with most markers	React with ≥ 2 markers	React with ≥ 2 markers; some cases may not react with any markers
Chromogranin	Diffuse (97%)	Diffuse (79%)	Focal (41%)	Focal (47%)
Synaptophysin	Diffuse (97%)	Diffuse (79%)	Focal (69%)	Focal (67%)
CD56	83%	57%	53%	97%
TTF1	~50%	~50%	~50%	90%
Ki-67	< 5%	5–10%[a]	> 40%	> 40%

LCNEC, large cell neuroendocrine carcinoma; NE, neuroendocrine; SAPC, salt-and-pepper chromatin; SCNEC, small cell neuroendocrine carcinoma; TTF1, thyroid transcription factor 1.

[a]Cases with higher mitotic rate and Ki-67 proliferation index may occur and are currently classified as LCNEC.

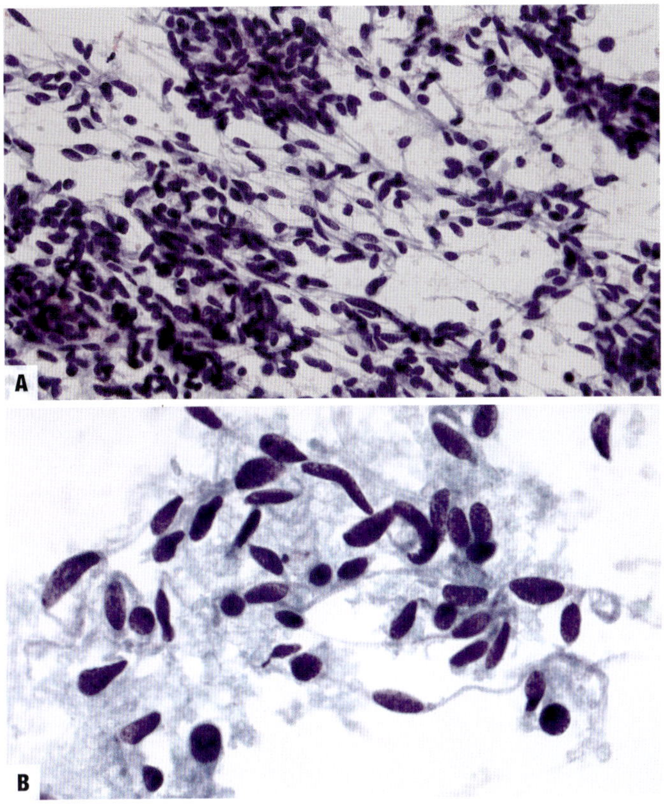

Fig. 7.44 Neuroendocrine tumour (NET). **A** Spindle cells haphazardly arranged as small discohesive tissue fragments and dispersed single cells, with elongated nuclei with fine chromatin and inconspicuous nucleoli (Pap). **B** Long, slender cytoplasm and elongated curved nuclei of the spindle cell NET (Pap).

and haphazardly arranged curved spindle cells with pulled-out slender cytoplasm {627}.

Because of the lower cellularity of cytopathology samples compared with resections, mitotic counts may be difficult to assess accurately {751,919,178,586}. Although the presence of mitotic figures, disorganized architecture, cellular atypia, and single cell necrosis are features that were reported to favour AC in cytopathology, distinction between TC and AC is not possible in the majority of cases and is best deferred to surgical resection {345,627}. In cytopathology, well-differentiated NET should be reported as "well-differentiated neuroendocrine tumour NOS" because these tumours cannot be graded {737}.

Technically adequate sample processing, good cellular preservation, and ICC are necessary to distinguish NET from its potential mimics {743,870}. The differential diagnosis includes small cell neuroendocrine carcinoma (SCNEC) and large cell neuroendocrine carcinoma (LCNEC) (see Table 7.02), low-grade adenocarcinoma, lymphoma, and other rare malignancies including adenoid cystic carcinoma and paraganglioma {870,14,265,718,994}. NET, especially the spindle pattern, may be confused with bronchial cells on bronchial brush {345,19}. Other differential diagnoses include metastatic breast lobular carcinoma and plasmacytoma {353}, melanoma for the pigmented variant {545}, metastatic oncocytic tumours for the oncocytic variant, and low-grade mesenchymal tumours for the spindle cell pattern {643,27,184,352} (see Table 7.03).

Metastatic extrapulmonary NETs are morphologically and immunocytochemically similar to primary lung NET and may require organ-specific ICC and clinical context for diagnosis {353}.

Ancillary testing

Between 90% and 100% of NETs diffusely express neuroendocrine markers including INSM1, chromogranin, synaptophysin, and CD56 {1000,950,222,317,860}. Thyroid transcription factor 1 (TTF1) expression in pulmonary NET varies from 0% to 69%, with higher rates in spindle cell NET and AC {317,1019,677,923}. The Ki-67 proliferation index is low in TC (1–5%) and higher in AC (3–10%) {562,687}. Although this is not included in the diagnostic criteria, it may assist in differentiating NET from high-grade pulmonary neuroendocrine neoplasms in small specimens {1000, 562,687,492,734,95}, but some NETs, particularly metastatic tumours, may have an elevated Ki-67 index {737} and definitive classification should be deferred to a surgical specimen. The Ki-67 proliferation index may predict response to therapy in advanced-stage NET {686,109}, but it is not widely used for clinical management. There is currently no clinical role for cytogenetic or molecular testing in pulmonary NETs, because they have not been shown to harbour actionable targets of therapy {737,13}. PDL1 is expressed in a subset of pulmonary NETs, and immunotherapy may improve outcomes in advanced disease but is not currently the standard of care {554,431}.

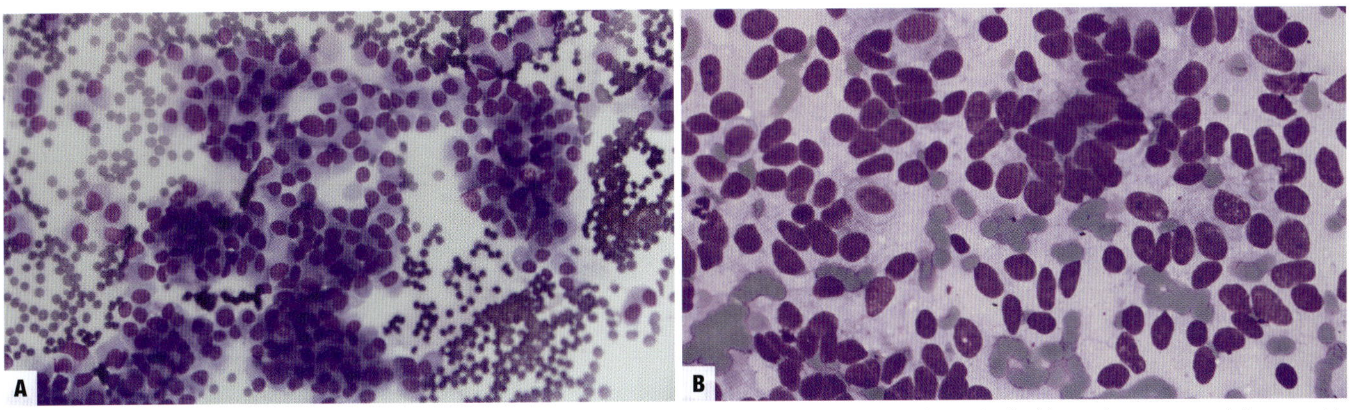

Fig. 7.45 Neuroendocrine tumour (NET). **A** Small, loosely cohesive sheets and more 3D small tissue fragments of round to oval cells with a moderate amount of often eccentric cytoplasm (Giemsa). **B** Round to oval nuclei with very focal subtle moulding in mildly crowded tissue fragments showing pseudorosettes. The cells are slightly larger, and the nuclei exhibit some variation in size and shape with occasional conspicuous nucleoli, raising the possibility of an atypical carcinoid (Giemsa).

Table 7.03 Differential diagnosis of spindle cell carcinoid

Differential diagnosis	Cytopathological features	Immunostains
Spindle cell carcinoid	Loosely cohesive or single spindle cells with slender, elongated cytoplasm Haphazardly arranged cells Frequently curved or form arches Plexiform vessels present in 50% of cases No cytopathological atypia, mitoses, or necrosis in typical carcinoid Mild atypia, focal necrosis, or mitoses in atypical carcinoid	Positive for NE markers (CD56, chromogranin, synaptophysin, and INSM1) Positive for pancytokeratin
Bronchial cells	Ciliated columnar cells Mostly single cells Lack of cellular curves and arches Nucleus slightly smaller Plexiform vessels absent	Negative for NE markers
Melanoma	Loosely cohesive or single cells Larger nuclei with more atypia Lack of cellular curves and arches Plexiform vessels absent	Negative for NE markers and cytokeratins Positive for S100, HMB45, melan-A (MART1), and SOX10
Solitary fibrous tumour	Poorly cellular smears Thick fragments of spindle cells Occasional collagen fragments Plexiform vessels absent Primarily pleural-based	Negative for NE markers Positive for STAT6, BCL2, CD34, CD99, EMA, and actin
Metastatic sarcomas	Aggregates of spindle cells with various atypia Plexiform vessels absent	Negative for NE markers Positive for vimentin and other stains, depending on original sarcoma
Sarcomatoid carcinoma	More prominent atypia, mitoses, and necrosis Plexiform vessels absent	Negative for NE markers Positive for cytokeratins; TTF1 or p40 may be positive
Sarcomatoid mesothelioma	Less cellular smears with few cohesive groups of atypical spindle cells Collagenous stroma +/– Primarily pleural-based	Negative for NE markers Positive for cytokeratins and mesothelial markers

NE, neuroendocrine; TTF1, thyroid transcription factor 1.

Small cell lung carcinoma

Michael CW
Papotti M
Rekhtman N
Vivero M

Definition

Small cell lung carcinoma (SCLC) is a malignant epithelial tumour composed of small cells with scant cytoplasm, finely granular nuclear chromatin, absent or inconspicuous nucleoli, a high mitotic count, and frequent necrosis, and in most cases it expresses neuroendocrine markers. SCLC can be combined with non-small cell carcinoma.

Clinical features and imaging

SCLC accounts for approximately 15% of all lung carcinomas and has a strong association with smoking {914,734,782}. SCLC may also occur when non-small cell lung carcinoma acquires resistance to tyrosine kinase inhibitor therapy {827,1011,720}.

Most SCLCs are at an advanced stage and metastatic on presentation. Common sites of metastasis include the brain, liver, bone, and adrenal glands {782}. Malignant pleural and pericardial effusions may occur. Patients may present with respiratory symptoms including cough, dyspnoea, or haemoptysis, and paraneoplastic syndromes are common, whereas distant metastases are associated with fatigue, weight loss, and neurological symptoms {943,782}. Despite initial chemosensitivity, stage IV SCLC has a poor prognosis, with a median survival time of < 1 year {782}.

Histopathology

SCLC is characterized by small cells with nested or sheet-like growth {632}. Pseudorosettes can be present, usually focally. Cells are ovoid or elongated, with scant cytoplasm, nuclear moulding, and finely granular chromatin. Large areas of necrosis or smaller areas of pinpoint necrosis are common. The mitotic count is > 10 mitoses/2 mm^2 (median: 80 mitoses/2 mm^2). Crush artefact may be prominent in small biopsies, obscuring tumour morphology and mitotic figures.

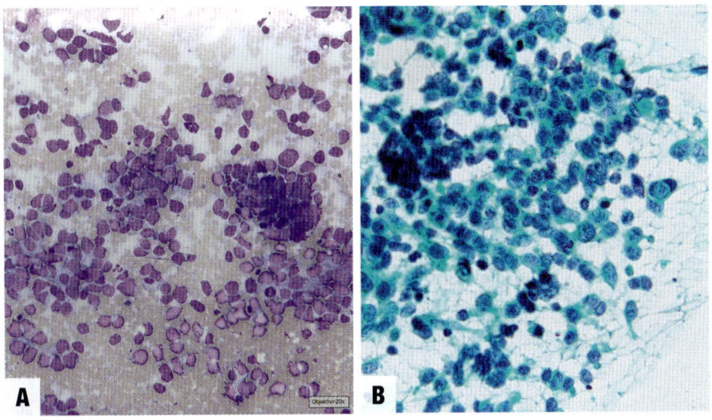

Fig. 7.47 Small cell lung carcinoma. **A** Discohesive tissue fragments of atypical cells with a high N:C ratio, nuclear moulding, and hyperchromasia. There is minimal apoptosis. At the lower right is one mitosis (transbronchial FNAB, Giemsa). **B** Many loosely cohesive small and atypical cells show a high N:C ratio. The nuclei show fine granular chromatin and cytoplasm is scant. Some cells in the right of the field show close cell-to-cell contact.

Key diagnostic cytopathological features

- Crowded irregular tissue fragments in a background of discohesive cells forming doublets, triplets, and cell cords, as well as many single intact cells
- Pseudorosettes may occasionally be present
- Cell size < 3 times that of a small lymphocyte; occasionally larger cells
- Scant cytoplasm, although a moderate amount of pale eosinophilic (Pap) cytoplasm can be seen in a subset of cases
- Nuclei are angulated, and nuclear moulding is best appreciated on Giemsa-stained smears
- Finely granular chromatin pattern, best appreciated on Pap-stained smears

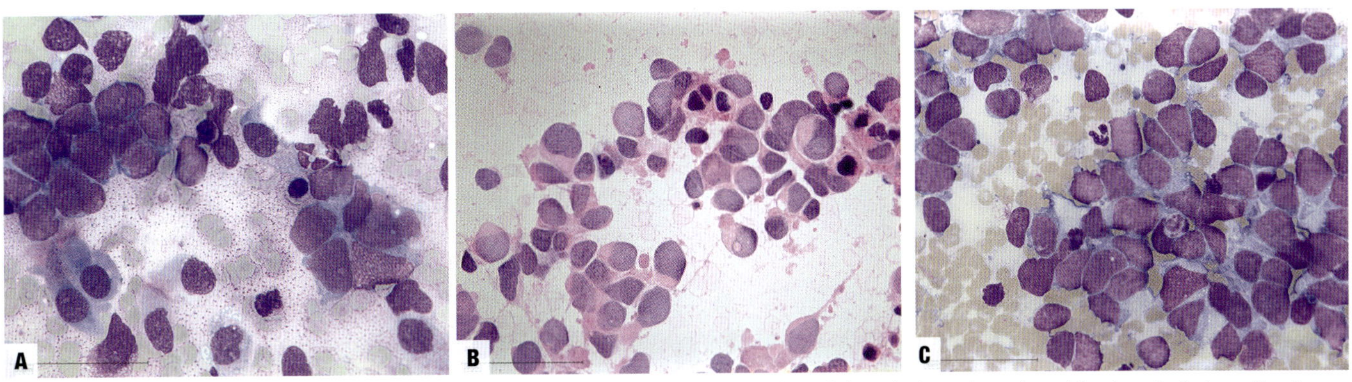

Fig. 7.46 Small cell lung carcinoma. **A** Small tissue fragments of atypical cells showing nuclear moulding, with irregular, hyperchromatic nuclei and scant cytoplasm. The chromatin is dense and finely granular without prominent nucleoli. Stripped nuclei are present in the background, and in the lower left of the smear, two normal ciliated bronchial cells are present for size comparison (bronchial brushing, Giemsa). **B** Loosely cohesive small sheets of atypical cells showing nuclear moulding, limited (often eccentric) cytoplasm in most cells, and hyperchromatic moderately pleomorphic nuclei with fine uniform chromatin and no discernible nucleoli. Some very dark nuclei of degenerating tumour cells are also present (transbronchial FNAB, H&E). **C** Tissue fragments of cells with a high N:C ratio, minimal but usually eccentric cytoplasm, focal pseudorosette architecture, and moulding of tumour cells. Nuclei show a fine chromatin pattern. Two blue bodies indenting the nuclei are seen at 4 o'clock (transbronchial FNAB, Giemsa).

- Occasional small nucleoli may be seen, but no large or frequent nucleoli
- Chromatin smearing representing nuclear crush artefact may limit cytomorphological assessment
- Mitoses are usually plentiful but may be difficult to appreciate
- Blue bodies, which are small, round, and blue (Giemsa), impinge the nuclear margin but are not entirely specific
- Background of necrotic and apoptotic debris
- In sputum samples, the neoplastic cells are usually degenerated with small dark nuclei and tend to be found along mucous strands
- In liquid-based cytopathology, the neoplastic cells are more discohesive, with more conspicuous nucleoli and subtle moulding, and exhibit dark, even chromatin that stands out against the lighter chromatin of benign background cells; chromatin smearing (an artefact induced by manual spreading) is more subtle and appears as slightly elongated nuclei or tangles of thread-like material

Reference(s): {732,345,997,523,336,632,875,49,567}

Discussion and differential diagnosis

Cytopathology has a sensitivity of 79% and an accuracy of 94% in the diagnosis and staging of SCLC {732}. The differential diagnosis includes other neuroendocrine neoplasms, carcinomas, and small blue cell tumours (see Table 7.04). It should be noted that although the cells are small in relation to non-small cell lung carcinoma, the nuclei are larger than those seen in most lymphoid cells and larger than those seen in bronchial cells.

Basaloid squamous cell carcinoma is characterized by nests of small to medium-sized cells with high N:C ratios, often with peripheral palisading, and by a high mitotic count. There may be stromal wrapping of tissue fragments.

Small round cell sarcoma, i.e. Ewing sarcoma / primitive neuroectodermal tumour, shares some features with SCLC including rosette or pseudorosette formation, a high N:C ratio, and a necrotic background, with poorer cellular cohesion and less crush artefact.

NUT carcinoma and SMARCA4-deficient thoracic tumours can have a high N:C ratio and mimic SCLC, although some will show focal abrupt keratinization in tissue fragments or in the background.

Extrapulmonary small cell carcinoma is cytopathologically and immunocytochemically indistinguishable from pulmonary SCLC, including a shared thyroid transcription factor 1 (TTF1) reactivity. Only the clinical history can assist in the correct diagnosis {141}.

Merkel cell carcinoma is indistinguishable from SCLC on cytopathology. Clinical history and ICC are required.

Pulmonary or mediastinal lymphomas, including diffuse large B-cell, mantle cell, follicular, MALT, Burkitt, and T-cell lymphomas, share many features with SCLC, including varying degrees of crush artefact. Lymphoma cells are usually very discohesive and predominantly present as single cells, with characteristic nuclear features in many cases.

Reserve/basal cell hyperplasia appears in exfoliated samples as tightly cohesive tissue fragments with rare isolated cells in a background of other reactive changes. The cells lack nuclear atypia and necrosis and are non-reactive to neuroendocrine markers {879,785}.

Ancillary testing

ICC is routinely utilized to confirm the diagnosis of SCLC and exclude the possibility of mimics, particularly the basal cell variant of squamous cell carcinoma {903,914}. The majority of SCLCs express neuroendocrine markers, including chromogranin A, synaptophysin, CD56 (NCAM), and INSM1 {914,734,764,593}. Staining for chromogranin A is typically weak. Approximately 20% of SCLCs are negative for both synaptophysin and chromogranin A, although they are typically positive for CD56 and/or INSM1 {734,764,593}. Importantly, CD56 is the least specific of the neuroendocrine markers and can be expressed in a variety of non-neuroendocrine tumours. Occasional SCLCs with minimal or no expression of standard neuroendocrine markers do occur, and they can be diagnosed in the context of appropriate cytomorphology and exclusion of mimics {914,734}. SCLC is usually positive for pancytokeratins, with a characteristic dot-like cytoplasmic staining, but it is negative in high-molecular-weight keratins such as CK5/6. TTF1 is positive in 90% of SCLCs, but it is not specific for lung origin {914,734}. Napsin A is consistently negative in SCLC {740}. Diffuse expression of the squamous markers p63, p40, and CK5/6 excludes the diagnosis of SCLC, but a patchy expression or labelling of scattered cells may occur in SCLC {914,734}. Nearly all SCLCs harbour inactivating *RB1* and *TP53* mutations, associated with the loss of RB1 and aberrant p53 expression by ICC {782}. The Ki-67 proliferative index is 65–100%.

ICC is required for the distinction of the following specific tumours:

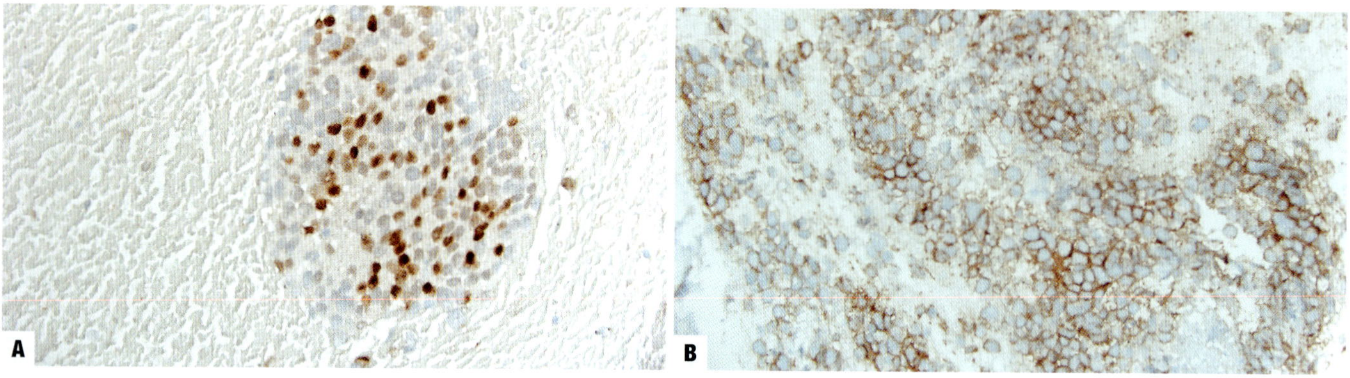

Fig. 7.48 Small cell lung carcinoma. **A** INSM1 shows strong nuclear expression in carcinoma cells (cell block, ICC). **B** CD56 shows diffuse strong membranous expression (cell block, ICC).

- Basaloid squamous cell carcinoma, which is non-reactive to neuroendocrine markers and strongly reactive to p40, p63, and high-molecular-weight cytokeratins such as CK5/6 {876,879}
- Ewing sarcoma / primitive neuroectodermal tumour, which is positive for synaptophysin, CD99, and FLI1 and negative for cytokeratin, and which has the *EWSR1::FLI1* fusion {879, 23,535,578,793}
- SMARCA4-deficient thoracic tumours, which show a loss of SMARCA4 protein expression, and NUT carcinoma, which shows nuclear localization of NUT protein in tumour cells {124,609,738}
- Merkel cell carcinoma, which shows CK20 perinuclear dot positivity; Merkel cell polyomavirus ICC confirms the diagnosis {141,52}

ICC and flow cytometry assist the diagnosis of SCLC and lymphoma, respectively. Lymphomas express clonal lymphoid markers and are negative in neuroendocrine markers and cytokeratin {879,136,386}.

Table 7.04 Differential diagnosis of neuroendocrine carcinomas

Differential diagnosis	Characteristic features	Immunocytochemistry
Singly scattered bronchial cells	Nucleus slightly smaller, with fine chromatin Columnar ciliated cells Adjacent goblet cells	Negative for NE markers
Small cell carcinoma and large cell carcinoma	More atypia and necrosis, plentiful mitoses and nuclear moulding Plexiform capillaries absent in SCNEC More cohesive tissue fragments	Ki-67 > 40%
Merkel cell carcinoma	Small cohesive tissue fragments or single cells Scant cytoplasm, moulding, and crush artefact Atypia at least focally	Positive for NE markers Positive CK20 (dot-like) Positive for MCPyV large T antigen
Adenocarcinoma of lung	3D tissue fragments, coarse chromatin, prominent nuclei SAPC absent Vacuolated cytoplasm	TTF1 is not helpful Negative for NE markers and positive for napsin A and CK7
Adenoid cystic carcinoma	Tight small blue cell tissue fragments Scant cytoplasm Metachromatic material +/− Demonstrates dual luminal epithelial and subluminal myoepithelial cells	Negative for NE markers and TTF1 Luminal epithelium positive for low-molecular-weight keratin and KIT Abluminal myoepithelial cells positive for p63/p40, SMA, S100, and SOX10 MYB positive in most cases
Lobular carcinoma of breast	Plasmacytoid cells with high N:C ratio Variable nuclear atypia SAPC absent Intracytoplasmic lumina	Negative for NE markers Positive for GATA3, ER, and PR Variable reaction with GCDFP and mammaglobin
Lymphoma	Small discohesive cells Scant cytoplasm SAPC absent Numerous fragments of lymphoid cell cytoplasm	Positive for lymphoid markers Negative for keratins and NE markers
Oncocytic neoplasms	Sheets, tissue fragments, or single cells Large cells with abundant granular cytoplasm Prominent nuclei	Negative for NE markers Additional stains depending on primary origin
Melanoma	Plasmacytoid, round to oval to spindle cells Moderate dusty cytoplasm Large nuclei with prominent cherry-red nucleoli Background melanin pigment +/−	Negative for NE markers and keratins Positive for S100, HMB45, melan-A (MART1), and SOX10
Paraganglioma	Small tissue fragments or single cells Fine chromatin Moderate to abundant pale cytoplasm	Positive for NE markers Negative for cytokeratins S100 highlights sustentacular cells

NE, neuroendocrine; MCPyV, Merkel cell polyomavirus; SAPC, salt-and-pepper chromatin; SCNEC, small cell neuroendocrine carcinoma; TTF1, thyroid transcription factor 1.

Large cell neuroendocrine carcinoma

Michael CW
Papotti M
Rekhtman N
Vivero M

Definition

Large cell neuroendocrine carcinoma (LCNEC) is a high-grade non-small cell carcinoma with neuroendocrine morphology that expresses neuroendocrine immunocytochemical markers.

Clinical features and imaging

LCNEC has a peripheral location in > 75% of cases and rarely involves the main airways {480}. It has a strong association with smoking, and the clinical presentation is similar to that of other non-small cell lung carcinomas (NSCLCs). Half of the cases are inoperable at diagnosis, with distant metastases mostly to brain, liver, and bone {428,600}.

The imaging features are similar to those of other NSCLCs: irregular tumour borders and expansive growth in peripheral lung fields by CT. Mediastinal lymphadenopathy is common, whereas obstructive pneumonia is rare {655,480,9}.

Histopathology

LCNECs vary in size from 10 to 100 mm and are tan-red and necrotic. Microscopically, an organoid growth pattern with nests, trabeculae, rosettes, and palisading is observed, with a variable desmoplastic reaction and generally extensive necrosis. Tumour cells are large (usually more than the diameter of three small lymphocytes), with nuclear atypia, coarsely granular chromatin, prominent nucleoli, and abundant weakly eosinophilic (Pap) cytoplasm. The diagnosis is confirmed by a mitotic count exceeding 10 mitoses/2 mm^2, with a wide variation (median: 70 mitoses/2 mm^2) {917,910,734,748}. In some cases, combined tumours occur, with LCNEC components and small cell lung carcinoma, squamous cell carcinoma, or adenocarcinoma components {910,915,917}.

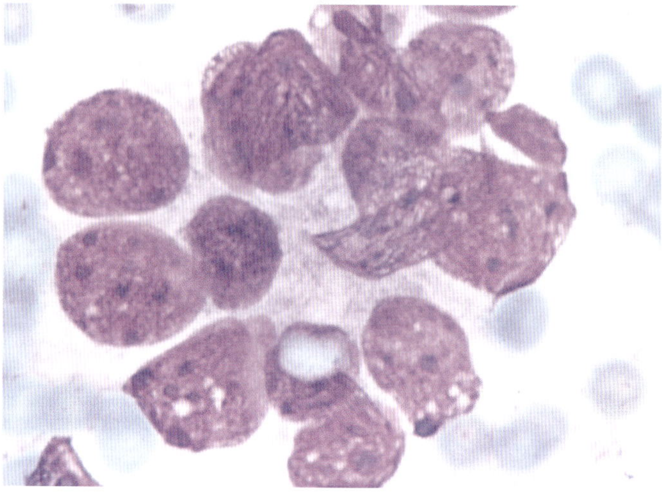

Fig. 7.50 Large cell neuroendocrine carcinoma (LCNEC). Large cells with a high N:C ratio, indistinct pale cytoplasm, and enlarged pleomorphic nuclei with granular chromatin and conspicuous nucleoli (Giemsa).

Key diagnostic cytopathological features

- Moderately to highly cellular
- Small, cohesive or loosely cohesive tissue fragments in a background of single cells and necrosis; rare cases present as predominantly single intact cells, mimicking lymphoma
- Thin fibrovascular strands may traverse the tissue fragments
- Cells are intermediate to large in size, i.e. usually greater than the diameter of three lymphocytes, with moderate to abundant cytoplasm
- Nuclear moulding may be present but is subtler than in small cell lung carcinoma, and the chromatin is typically

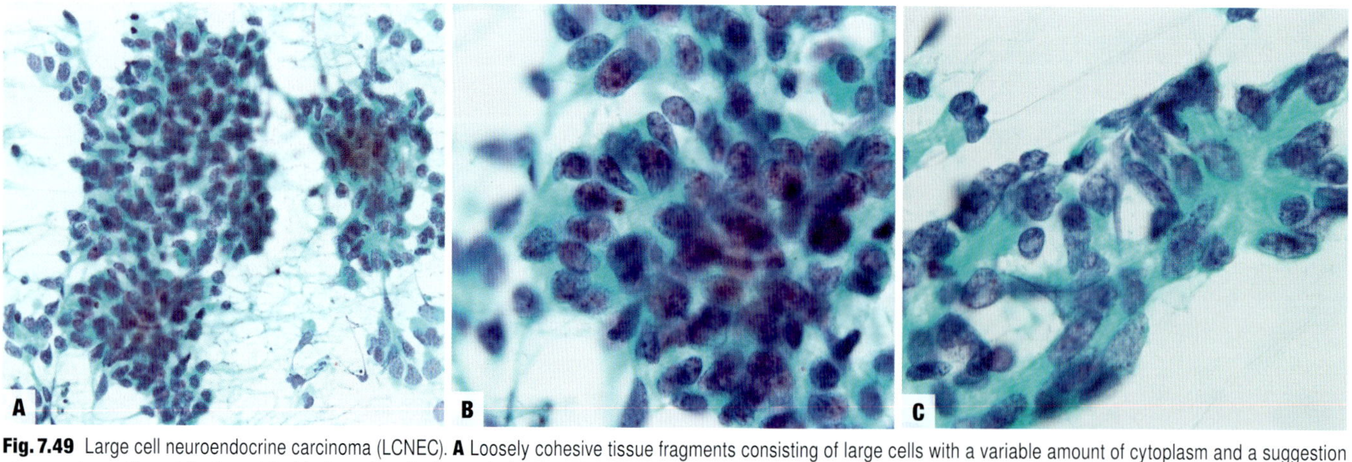

Fig. 7.49 Large cell neuroendocrine carcinoma (LCNEC). **A** Loosely cohesive tissue fragments consisting of large cells with a variable amount of cytoplasm and a suggestion of a pseudorosette architecture at 3 o'clock, and markedly atypical enlarged and hyperchromatic nuclei (Pap). **B** Higher-power view showing a pseudorosette architecture and pleomorphic nuclei in large cells (Pap). **C** Tissue fragment showing a rosette-like architecture, with large cells with eccentric cytoplasm and enlarged pleomorphic nuclei with granular chromatin (Pap).

Table 7.05 Differential diagnosis of large cell neuroendocrine carcinoma (LCNEC)

Feature	LCNEC	SCLC	NSCLC	Lymphoma
Tissue fragments	++	++	+++	–
Single intact cells	++	++	++	+++
Pseudorosettes	+/–[a]	+/–	–	–
Doublets and triplets	+/–	+++	–	–
Spindle cells	+	––/+	–	–
Nuclei				
Pseudorosette	++	+	–	–
Moulding	++	+++	–	–
Irregular membrane	++	+	+++	Varies by type
Chromatin				
Fine granular	+/–	+++	–	–
Coarse	+/–	–	++	++
Smearing	+/++	+++	–	+/–
Nucleoli				Vary by type
Inconspicuous	+/++	+++	–	
Prominent	++/+	–	++/+++	
Traversing vessels	+/++	–	+/–	–
Neuroendocrine markers	+++	+++	–/+	–

NSCLC, non-small cell lung carcinoma; SCLC, small cell lung carcinoma; +, occasionally present; ++, commonly present; +++, main feature; –, absent; –– predominantly absent.
[a]Best seen on cell blocks.

granular and fine but can be coarse or show perinucleolar clearing in the Pap-stained specimen
- Nucleoli range from inconspicuous to large
- Chromatinic smearing is common
- Necrosis is prominent in most cases
- Mitoses are frequent

Reference(s): {977,997,537,384,345,365}

Discussion and differential diagnosis

The definitive diagnosis of LCNEC is difficult in cytopathology because of morphological overlap with small cell lung carcinoma, NSCLC, and (rarely) lymphoma, which have to be considered in the differential diagnosis, along with neuroendocrine tumour (NET) (atypical carcinoid) (see Table 7.05). However, the diagnosis may be suggested in cases with cellular cell blocks that allow for the assessment of neuroendocrine morphology (including nesting, palisading, and rosettes) and ICC.

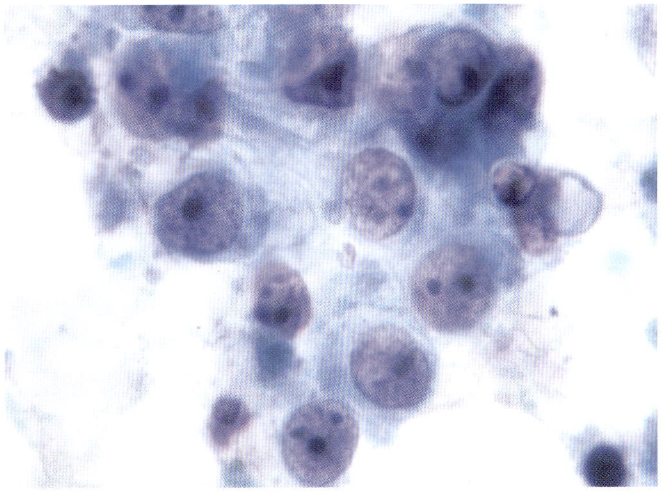

Fig. 7.51 Large cell neuroendocrine carcinoma (LCNEC). Small tissue fragment consisting of large cells with a moderate amount of often eccentric cytoplasm, large pleomorphic nuclei, a mix of fine and coarser chromatin, and prominent nucleoli (Pap).

Ancillary testing

LCNECs are positive for thyroid transcription factor 1 (TTF1), synaptophysin, chromogranin, CD56, and INSM1 in 75% of cases {523,950,1025}. Neuroendocrine markers must be interpreted in the context of neuroendocrine cytomorphology and appropriate clinical history, because NSCLC and metastatic disease can be positive for these markers {950,396,1000}. The Ki-67 proliferation index is primarily used to separate high-grade from low-grade neuroendocrine neoplasms. LCNEC typically demonstrates a Ki-67 proliferation index > 40% {562, 687}, and although it is not included in the diagnostic criteria, Ki-67 can be useful in cytopathology specimens and small biopsies to differentiate high-grade neuroendocrine carcinoma from NET (atypical carcinoid tumour) {562,687}. A subset of LCNECs harbour canonical and non-canonical non-small cell carcinoma mutations {562,741}, including established and potential targets of therapy {577,477,555}. Some LCNECs may also express PDL1, providing a different therapeutic approach, if clinically appropriate {330}. Predictive ICC for ALK, ROS1, and PDL1, as well as single-gene or next-generation sequencing, may inform clinical management.

Lymphomas

Monaco SE
Lin O

Definition

Primary pulmonary extranodal marginal zone lymphoma (EMZL) is a low-grade B-cell lymphoma that is believed to arise from the marginal zone B cells of the bronchial mucosa-associated lymphoid tissue.

Primary pulmonary diffuse large B-cell lymphoma (DLBCL) is a B-cell lymphoma with the same morphological, immunophenotypic, and molecular features as systemic or nodal DLBCL.

Clinical features and imaging

EMZL is a mucosa-associated lymphoma (a MALT lymphoma) and the most common type of primary pulmonary lymphoma, representing 70–90% of all primary lymphomas involving the lung {794,83,696}. There is a slight female patient predominance, and it is associated with cigarette smoking and autoimmune diseases. A monoclonal gammopathy is detected in approximately 60% of patients {448}. The most common imaging finding is the presence of solitary or multiple nodules of < 50 mm in one lung, although other patterns, including poorly defined infiltrates with CT attenuation containing air bronchograms and a peripheral mass with pleural thickening, have also been described.

Primary pulmonary DLBCL represents approximately 10% of all primary lymphomas arising in the lung {794,411}. The median age at presentation is approximately 60 years; however, paediatric cases have been described, particularly in immunodeficient patients. There is no sex preference. There is a spectrum of imaging findings, including areas of consolidation, solitary or multiple nodules, and an interstitial infiltrate or ground-glass appearance with or without mediastinal lymphadenopathy. Most lesions are bilateral. Cavitation or central necrosis is a common feature {843}.

Histopathology

EMZL presents in resected lung specimens as a tan-white, light-grey homogeneous unencapsulated mass with relatively well-defined borders and peripheral areas of consolidation.

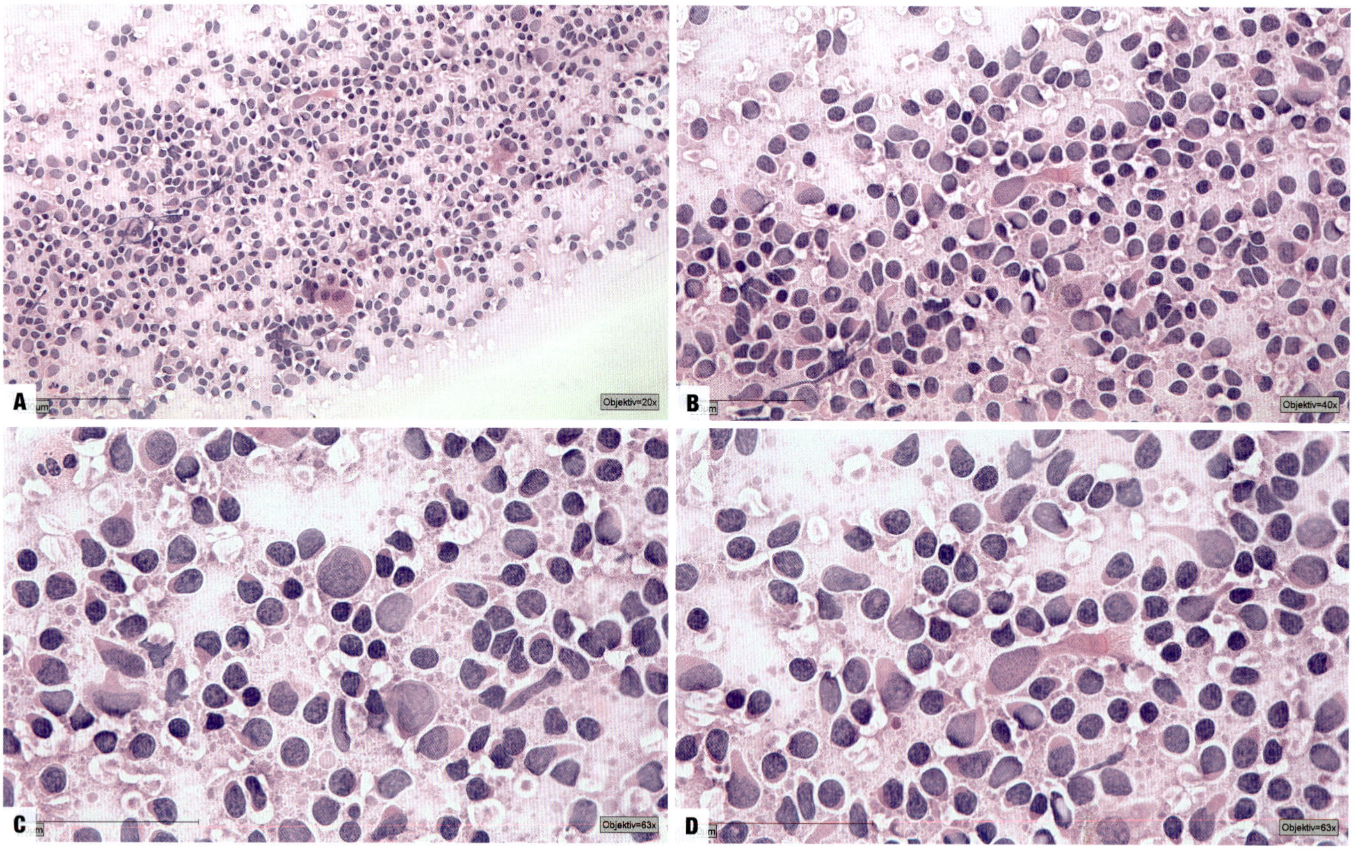

Fig. 7.52 MALT lymphoma. Chronic cough, persistent infiltrates, and atelectasis in the right upper lobe. Concomitant histology: MALT lymphoma in the right upper lobe. **A,B** Cellular smear with numerous lymphoid cells of varying size. Only a few respiratory epithelial cells are present (bronchial brushing, H&E). **C** Cellular smear with numerous lymphoid cells of varying size, some with a large nucleus and dense cytoplasm. Many cytoplasmic fragments in the background (bronchial brushing, H&E). **D** Cellular smear with numerous lymphoid cells of varying size. Many cytoplasmic fragments in the background, with one ciliated respiratory epithelial cell (bronchial brushing, H&E).

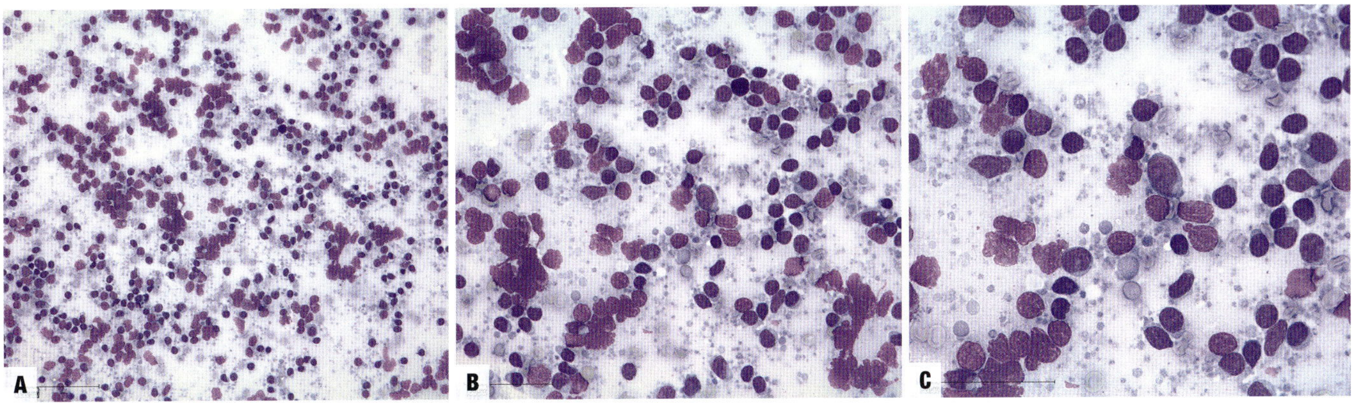

Fig. 7.53 MALT lymphoma. Chronic cough, persistent infiltrates, and atelectasis in the right upper lobe. Concomitant histology: MALT lymphoma in the right upper lobe. **A–C** Numerous lymphoid cells of varying size. In the centre there is a blastic cell with a large nucleolus. Many degenerated nuclei are present and there are many cytoplasmic fragments in the background (bronchial brushing, Giemsa).

Microscopically, dense lymphoid infiltrates disrupt the lung parenchyma as discrete nodular lesions or as a lymphangitic distribution along the pleura or around bronchovascular bundles. Reactive lymphoid follicles and lymphoepithelial lesions are frequently seen {696}.

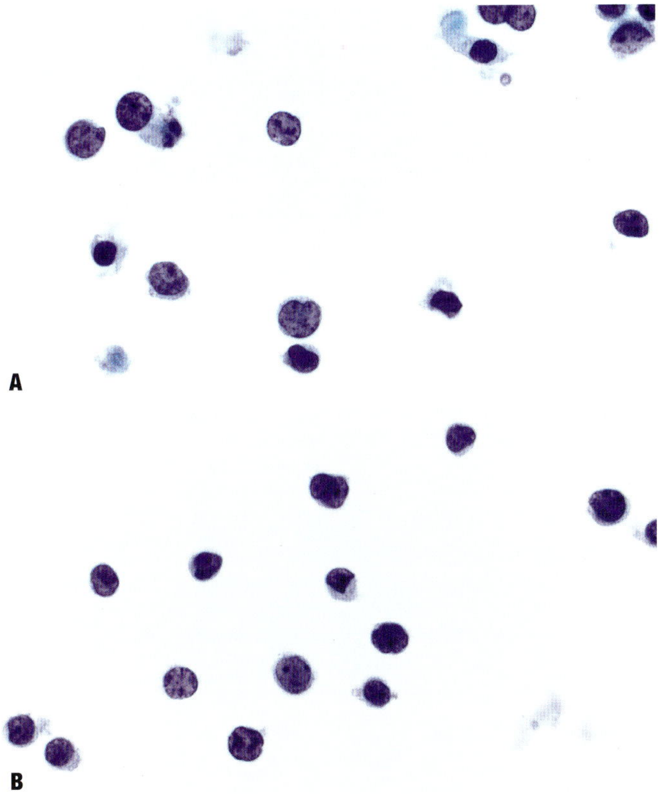

Fig. 7.54 Diffuse large B-cell lymphoma. **A** Pulmonary diffuse large B-cell lymphoma consisting of medium-sized to large atypical lymphoid cells with a high N:C ratio, mildly irregular nuclear contours, fine even chromatin, and inconspicuous nucleoli, from an endobronchial ultrasound–guided transbronchial FNAB of a lower lobe lung mass (liquid-based preparation, Pap). **B** Pulmonary diffuse large B-cell lymphoma consisting of atypical medium-sized to large atypical lymphoid cells (note the comparison with a bronchial epithelial cell in the upper-right corner), from an endobronchial ultrasound–guided transbronchial FNAB of a large right lower lobe lung mass. Immunostaining showed the atypical lymphoid cells to be positive for CD20, with a Ki-67 proliferation index of approximately 80% (not shown) (liquid-based preparation, Pap).

Pulmonary DLBCL shows a dense lymphoid infiltrate composed of medium-sized to large lymphoid cells with perinucleolar clearing of the chromatin and often single or multiple nucleoli. Mitotic figures and apoptotic cells are frequently seen, as well as infiltration of bronchial walls.

Key diagnostic cytopathological features

Extranodal marginal zone lymphoma

- Relatively cellular smears
- Mix of small lymphocytes, centrocytes, and monocytoid cells with clear cytoplasm, as well as a relative abundance of plasma cells or plasmacytoid cells, which are best observed with Giemsa staining
- Lymphoid cell cytoplasmic fragments (lymphoglandular bodies) are seen in the background with Giemsa staining
- Amyloid can be present

Reference(s): {434,391}

Diffuse large B-cell lymphoma

- Variable cellularity
- Relatively monotonous intermediate and (predominantly) large lymphoid cells, mostly arranged as single cells, although pseudoaggregation may occur
- Nuclei may show a prominent central single nucleolus and eccentric cytoplasm in the immunoblastic subtype, or one to three marginal nucleoli in the centroblastic subtype, with scant amphophilic to basophilic cytoplasm; pleomorphic variants can also occur
- Cytoplasm can be eccentric or more circumferential and is well defined
- Mitoses and apoptotic bodies are frequent
- Lymphoid cell cytoplasmic fragments (lymphoglandular bodies) are seen in the background with Giemsa staining

Reference(s): {794}

Discussion and differential diagnosis

The diagnosis of EMZL of the lung on FNAB, bronchial wash, or sputum samples can be difficult, and the differential diagnosis includes reactive lymphoid processes and other types of low-grade B-cell lymphomas, such as small lymphocytic lymphoma, mantle cell lymphoma, low-grade follicular lymphoma, and lymphoplasmacytic lymphoma. Flow cytometry is required.

Pulmonary DLBCL is thought to arise from a transformation from previous marginal zone lymphoma or to represent de novo disease. The differential diagnosis includes poorly differentiated non-small cell carcinomas of the lung and metastatic carcinomas to the lung, metastatic melanoma, and other metastatic diseases to the lung. The neoplastic cells in DLBCL can show pseudoaggregation, whereas some carcinomas and melanomas can present predominantly as single cells.

Ancillary testing

EMZL has admixed CD3+ and CD5+ T cells among the CD20+, CD79a+, and PAX5+ B cells, and it lacks a characteristic ICC phenotype marker, which makes ICC of limited use. Flow cytometry studies are critical in detecting the presence of a CD20 clonal B-cell population and demonstrate CD5− and CD10− B cells. Coexpression of CD43 is seen in 30–80% of cases. Molecular studies demonstrate the presence of a clonal B-cell population. FISH studies may demonstrate the presence of *MALT1* rearrangement or trisomy 3 {434}.

DLBCL often requires ICC to exclude poorly differentiated carcinomas and melanoma and to demonstrate a lymphoid origin. Flow cytometry can demonstrate B-cell monoclonality and exclude other lymphomas to make a precise classification: the cells are typically positive for CD20, PAX5, and CD79a and negative for CD5, CD10, BCL2, BCL6, cyclin D1, and CD3. Flow cytometry, however, has a lower sensitivity for DLBCL (owing to cell fragility, which can yield false negative results) and should be interpreted with care. FISH studies for *BCL2*, *BCL6*, and *MYC* are used to rule out double-hit high-grade B-cell lymphomas, which have a similar cytomorphology.

Pulmonary Langerhans cell histiocytosis

Maleki Z

Definition

Langerhans cell histiocytosis (LCH) is a clonal neoplasm of myeloid dendritic cells expressing a Langerhans cell phenotype (positive for CD1a and CD207) occurring in the lung interstitium.

Clinical features and imaging

LCH affects both sexes equally, presenting in patients aged 18–70 years (mean: 40 years). LCH is mostly seen in smokers {722}. If it presents in the lungs in adults, only 15% of cases are associated with extrapulmonary involvement, whereas the disseminated type of LCH can involve the lungs in paediatric cases. Patients may present with pulmonary symptoms including cough, shortness of breath, or chest pain, or with systemic symptoms including fever, weight loss, and malaise.

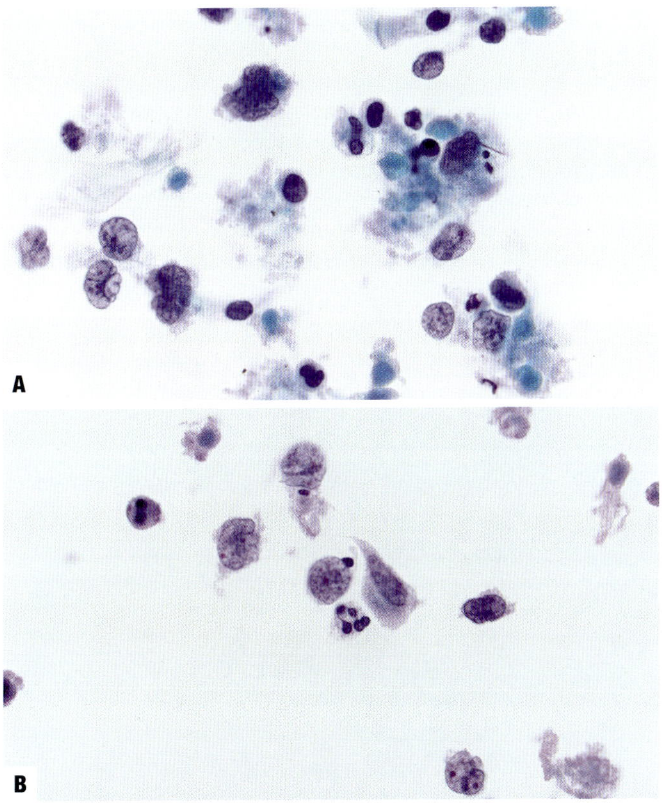

Fig. 7.55 Pulmonary Langerhans cell histiocytosis. **A** Langerhans cells with enlarged, deeply indented and convoluted nuclei with fine chromatin and indistinct nucleoli, from endobronchial ultrasound–guided transbronchial FNAB of an upper lobe lung nodule. Note the occasional eosinophils in the background. This case was *BRAF* p.V600E–mutant (liquid-based cytopathology, Pap). **B** Langerhans cells with markedly indented and convoluted nuclei and fine chromatin (note size comparison to the benign bronchial epithelial cell in the upper-right corner), from an endobronchial ultrasound–guided transbronchial FNAB of an upper lobe lung nodule. These cells were positive for CD1a (not shown), and molecular testing demonstrated the characteristic *BRAF* p.V600E mutation (liquid-based cytopathology, Pap).

Occasionally patients develop pleural effusions. Pulmonary function tests are abnormal in 85% of cases, with evidence of restrictive deficits, obstructive deficits, mixed restrictive/obstructive deficits, and isolated decreased diffusing capacity.

CXR show interstitial lung disease. CT scans show bilateral nodules, or nodules with cystic changes with a predilection for the mid and upper lung zones {1}.

The prognosis is generally good, but a subset of patients develop pulmonary insufficiency due to subsequent fibrosis and cystic change.

Histopathology

LCH nodules show a highly cellular proliferation of Langerhans cells around small airways, primarily bronchioles and alveolar ducts. Langerhans cells are large, with pale eosinophilic cytoplasm and with nuclei that show prominent folding of the nuclear membrane. Interspersed eosinophils and pigmented alveolar macrophages are common.

Key diagnostic cytopathological features

- Moderate to high cellularity
- Dispersed Langerhans cells characterized by their large size; abundant finely granular, delicate cytoplasm; and elongated pale nuclei with plentiful nuclear grooves and folded nuclear membrane
- Langerhans cells may be variable in size, with anisonucleosis, binucleation, and multinucleation
- Plentiful eosinophils admixed with other inflammatory cells, including lymphocytes, in the background
- No evidence of phagocytosis
- Charcot–Leyden crystals may occasionally be seen

Discussion and differential diagnosis

Hodgkin lymphoma is the most important differential diagnosis from LCH, because both have large cells in a mixed inflammatory cell background. However, Langerhans cells are large, with abundant clear to finely granular cytoplasm, nuclear grooves, and folded nuclear membrane. Reed–Sternberg cells in Hodgkin lymphoma are characterized by abundant cytoplasm, large twin nuclei, fine chromatin, and prominent large single nucleoli in each nucleus. Eosinophils in LCH are more abundant than in Hodgkin disease, which usually shows more abundant lymphocytes {831}.

Ancillary testing

Langerhans cells are characterized by the expression of CD1a, CD207, and S100 by ICC and Birbeck granules by electron microscopy. Hodgkin and Reed–Sternberg cells are positive for CD30 and (in most cases) CD15. In bronchoalveolar lavage (BAL), > 5% of cells must be positive for CD1a to make the diagnosis.

Erdheim–Chester disease

Monaco SE

Definition

Erdheim–Chester disease (ECD) is a rare histiocytic neoplasm characterized by a clonal systemic proliferation of histiocytes with foamy cytoplasm and Touton giant cells.

Clinical features and imaging

ECD typically presents in adults, with involvement of the long bones of the lower extremity, but it can also be seen in extraskeletal sites, such as the retroperitoneum, brain, skin, and thoracic cavity. Approximately half of all cases will have pulmonary or pleural involvement, and patients may be symptomatic with dyspnoea or cough or they may simply present with manifestations from involvement of other areas, such as bone pain, given that skeletal involvement is almost always seen. Unlike with pulmonary Langerhans cell histiocytosis (LCH), ECD has no known association with smoking. However, extraskeletal involvement, such as lung involvement, is associated with a worse prognosis in ECD. Bone scans in these patients will show bilateral, symmetrical labelling. Chest CT may show subtle inflammatory-type findings, with micronodules, ground-glass opacities, and thickening of the fissures.

Histopathology

The lesions appear fibrotic with a xanthogranulomatous infiltrate or just as non-diagnostic fibrotic tissue. The histiocytes can be challenging to identify, given the low N:C ratio of the cells and the bland nuclear features. Multinucleated and Touton giant cells are also seen, with a variably prominent lymphoplasmacytic infiltrate.

Key diagnostic cytopathological features

- Loosely cohesive and discohesive histiocytes with abundant foamy cytoplasm
- Multinucleated or Touton-type giant cells may be seen
- Histiocytes have oval or kidney-shaped nuclei without grooves and without prominent nucleoli
- Nuclei may appear as stripped oval nuclei
- Background may show metachromatic fibrotic material or inflammatory cells, particularly lymphocytes and plasma cells

Discussion and differential diagnosis

ECD is a rare non–Langerhans cell histiocytosis that is unique in that it has the same BRAF p.V600E mutations as are seen in LCH but is a distinct entity with a different immunophenotype {321}. The *BRAF* mutations are important because they allow the BRAF VE1 immunostain to be utilized for diagnosis and BRAF inhibitors to be used for treatment. Other targetable MAPK/ERK pathway mutations can also be identified, and so the main reason for biopsy in these patients is to obtain material for mutation testing in order to select the appropriate treatment {298}. The differential

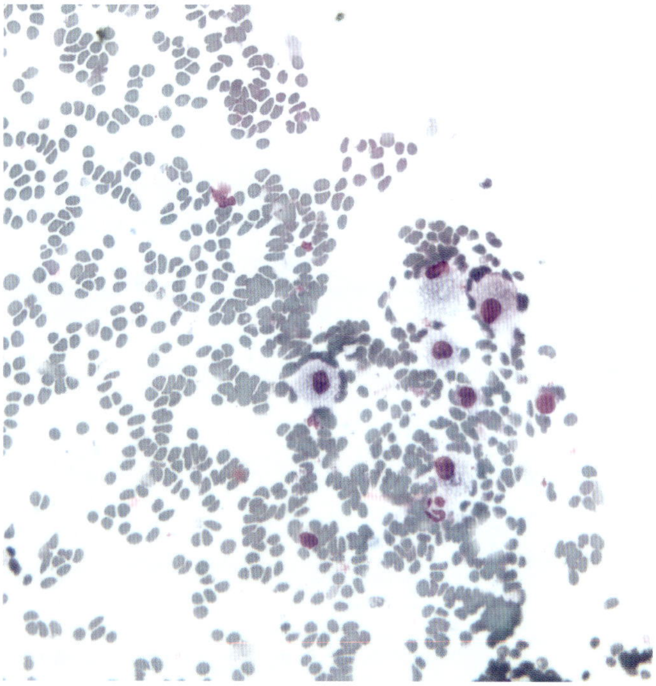

Fig. 7.56 Erdheim–Chester disease. Dispersed large histiocytes with rounded, mildly pleomorphic nuclei and abundant finely granular, often eccentric cytoplasm (Giemsa).

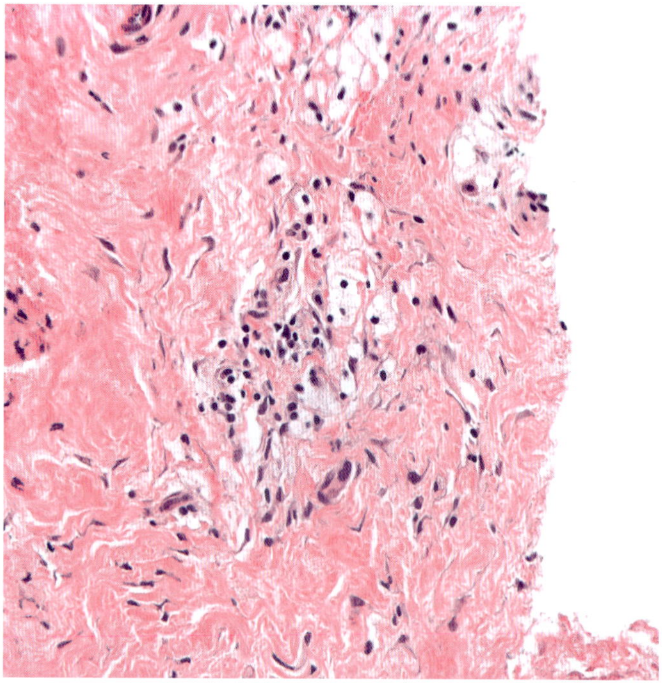

Fig. 7.57 Erdheim–Chester disease. Surgical resection showing scattered large histiocytes with round, minimally irregular nuclei and abundant finely granular, often eccentric cytoplasm with occasional lymphocytes and plasma cells in a dense fibrotic stroma (H&E).

diagnosis is broad because the cytopathological features are relatively nonspecific and rely on correlation with clinical history and imaging findings and the ICC. The differential diagnosis includes LCH, reactive histiocytic proliferations, and mesenchymal tumours. The reactive diagnoses include xanthogranulomatous infiltrates that can occur after treatment or with infection, and the foamy granulomatous inflammation seen with atypical mycobacterial infections. Cases may appear non-diagnostic because the fibrotic tissue yields fragments that are acellular, and these cases will typically undergo core needle biopsy. Low-grade sarcomas and well-differentiated liposarcomas are also a consideration for pulmonary metastases.

Ancillary testing

The ECD histiocytes stain positively for CD68, CD163, factor XIIIa, and fascin, and negative for CD1a and CD207 (langerin) and are usually negative for S100, although weak S100 staining can be seen in about 20–30% of cases {298}. The BRAF VE1 stain also shows cytoplasmic positivity, reflecting the presence of the BRAF p.V600E mutations in over half of these cases.

Chapter 7

Spindle cell tumours

Hiroshima K
Engels M
Michael CW
Önal BÜ

Definition

Malignant spindle cell tumours encompass a wide range of malignant neoplasms composed almost exclusively of spindle cells or those in which spindle cells are a major component of the lesion.

Clinical features and imaging

The wide range of spindle cell tumours has no distinctive clinical presentations or imaging.

Histopathology

Spindle cell carcinoma is a subtype of pleomorphic carcinoma consisting solely of neoplastic spindle cells, with markedly atypical or deceptively bland nuclei {772,980,264}.

Spindle cell neuroendocrine (carcinoid) tumour (spindle cell NET) consists of small to intermediate-sized spindle cells with finely granular or pale cytoplasm and uniform round to elongated nuclei with fine to coarsely granular, evenly dispersed chromatin and inconspicuous to single round nucleoli. There may be a mix with other variants.

Pulmonary blastoma shows a biphasic pattern of primitive mesenchymal cells that are closely packed, primitive, oval to spindle, small blastema-like cells, which focally show bizarre nuclei, mixed with fibroblast-like cells, glandular structures resembling endometrioid carcinoma, and morules {438,1009}.

Pulmonary artery intimal sarcoma is a poorly differentiated mesenchymal tumour with fibroblastic and myofibroblastic differentiation, which occasionally shows leiomyosarcomatous, rhabdomyosarcomatous, or angiosarcomatous components {896,355}.

Leiomyosarcomas are high-grade and hypercellular and consist of long, intersecting fascicles that are parallel and perpendicular to the plane of section and consist of spindle cells with moderate to abundant pale to eosinophilic cytoplasm and moderately pleomorphic plump nuclei with blunt ends (cigar-shaped). Mitoses (including atypical mitoses) are frequent {981}. Necrosis is found in larger tumours.

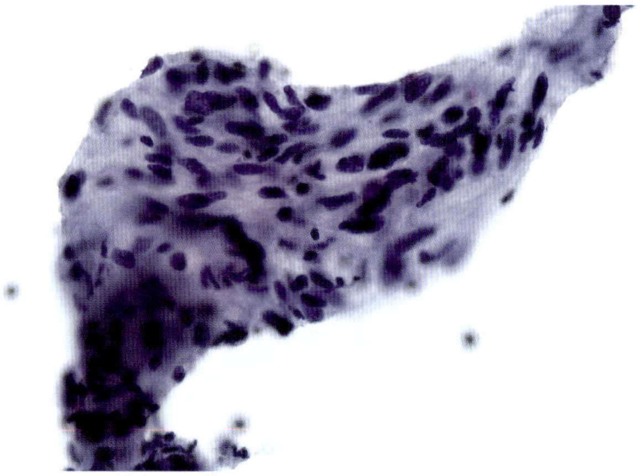

Fig. 7.58 Leiomyosarcoma. Spindle cells in a tissue fragment show a vague fascicular architecture with enlarged, irregular, blunt-ended nuclei (transbronchial FNAB, liquid-based cytopathology, Pap).

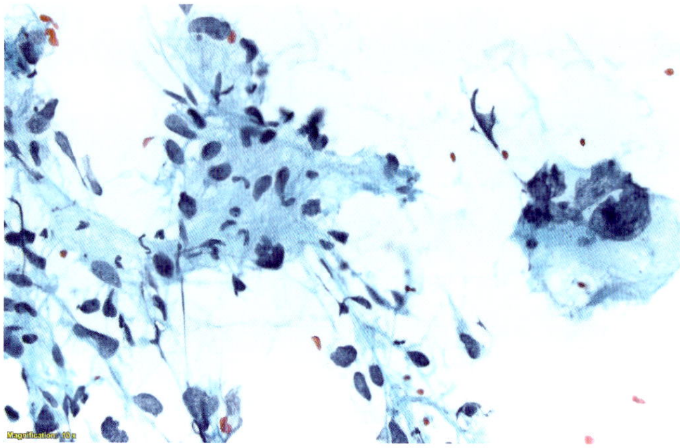

Fig. 7.59 Pulmonary artery intimal sarcoma. Loosely cohesive cells embedded in an extracellular matrix. The cells vary from round to spindle with a variable amount of cytoplasm and poorly defined cell borders. The nuclei are elongated and vary in size, shape, and chromasia. Occasional multinucleated cells with highly atypical nuclei are seen scattered among the spindle cells (Pap).

Monophasic synovial sarcoma consists of monomorphic, delicate, relatively uniform and small spindle cells with a high N:C ratio, sparse cytoplasm, and ovoid hyperchromatic nuclei with inconspicuous nucleoli, arranged in dense cellular sheets or vague fascicles with scant collagen, occasional herringbone architecture, staghorn vascular pattern, and limited myxoid change. Biphasic synovial sarcoma has epithelial and spindle cell components in varying proportions.

Spindle cell melanoma variant is characterized by cells with elongated, narrow, tapering cytoplasmic processes and can have a mix of more typical epithelioid melanoma. Melanin pigment may or may not be present.

Sarcomatoid mesothelioma displays a proliferation of spindle cells arranged in fascicles or in haphazard patterns. The spindle cells are elongated and tapered, with nuclei that range from bland to pleomorphic.

Gastrointestinal stromal tumours consist of spindle cells in sheets or vague storiform arrangements, or epithelioid cells in sclerosing or hypercellular tumours or (on occasion) in mixed tumours. There is usually minimal nuclear pleomorphism, although some cases may show more marked nuclear atypia.

Key diagnostic cytopathological features

In general, the malignant spindle cell tumours produce in FNAB smears greater cell dissociation, cellularity, necrosis, and mitotic activity than benign tumours, which usually show intact tissue fragments with few dispersed cells (see Table 7.06). See also *Spindle cell tumours*, p. 75, in the chapter on the "Benign" diagnostic category.

Discussion and differential diagnosis

The differential diagnosis includes sarcomas of smooth muscle, nerve sheath tumours, myofibroblastic tumours, and other neoplasms of mesenchymal origin, as well as spindle cell carcinoma and spindle cell melanoma. Correlating the patient's history and clinical and imaging features is essential. Metastatic

Table 7.06 Histopathological and cytopathological features and ancillary testing for the differential diagnosis of malignant spindle cell tumours (continued on next page)

Differential diagnosis	Histopathology	Cytopathological features	Immunocytochemistry	Molecular diagnostics
Spindle cell carcinoma	• Consists solely of neoplastic spindle cells • Markedly atypical or deceptively bland {772,980,264}	• Single cells, loose tissue fragments, and poorly formed fascicles • Pleomorphic spindle cells • Necrotic background • Numerous lymphocytes and neutrophils {352,335,147}	Vimentin+, pancytokeratin+/−, TTF1+/−, p40+/− {35}	*MET* exon 14–skipping mutations {906}
Spindle cell neuroendocrine (carcinoid) tumour	• Predominantly or entirely spindle cells • Fairly uniform in length • Organoid pattern or mesenchymal in appearance	• Single cells or loosely cohesive cells, arranged haphazardly • Spindle cells • Cells are curved or form arches • Nuclei predominantly ovoid or spindle • Plexiform vessels (50%) *Typical carcinoid:* • No cytopathological atypia, no necrosis, no mitoses *Atypical carcinoid:* • Mild atypia, focal necrosis or mitosis {564}	Pancytokeratin+/−, CD56+, chromogranin+, synaptophysin+, INSM1+ {734}	Mutations in *MEN1* and in other chromatin-remodelling genes {253}
Pulmonary blastoma	• Primitive mesenchymal cells • Branching glandular structures resembling endometrioid carcinoma • Morule formation	*Mesenchymal component:* • Scattered single cells or cohesive cells • Oval to spindle cells • Uniform nuclei with fine chromatin and indistinct nucleoli *Epithelial component:* • Cohesive tissue fragments • Slightly larger, round to ovoid or columnar cells • Grey-blue or pale cytoplasm {172,519}	*Mesenchymal component:* Vimentin+, SMA+, β-catenin+, pancytokeratin+/−, desmin+/−, S100+/− *Epithelial component:* Pancytokeratin+, CK7+, EMA+, TTF1+, β-catenin+ {1009}	*CTNNB1* exon 3 missense mutations {607}
Pulmonary artery intimal sarcoma	• Poorly differentiated mesenchymal tumours • Fibroblastic and myofibroblastic differentiation • Occasionally leiomyosarcomatous, rhabdomyosarcomatous, or angiosarcomatous differentiation {896,355}	• Loosely cohesive tissue fragments • Spindle cells and epithelioid cells • Varying amount of cytoplasm, poorly defined cell borders • Nuclei of variable size, irregular nuclear membrane • Coarse chromatin, prominent nucleoli {320,111,553,678}	Vimentin+, myogenin+/−, desmin+/−, S100+/−, ERG+/−, CD31+/−, SMA+/− {131,896,355}	*MDM2* amplification, *PDGFRA* amplification {73,211}
Leiomyosarcoma	• Intersecting fascicles of spindle cells • Moderate to abundant eosinophilic cytoplasm • Elongated, blunt-ended (cigar-shaped) nuclei • Cytopathologically high-grade	• Cohesive fascicles and dispersed cells • Different cell types: spindle cells, rounded/polygonal cells, pleomorphic tumour cells • Elongated, blunt-ended (cigar-shaped) nuclei • Enlarged irregular nuclei • Multinucleated tumour cells {218}	Vimentin+, desmin+, SMA+, CD34−, pancytokeratin−, S100−, DOG1− {616}	
Synovial sarcoma	*Monophasic synovial sarcoma:* • Dense fascicles of monomorphic spindle cells • High N:C ratio *Biphasic synovial sarcoma:* • Epithelial and spindle cell components in varying proportions	• High cellularity and uniformity of cells • Cell tissue fragments with irregular borders and dispersed cells • Pericapillary arrangement • Mixture of round, oval, and spindle cells • Mitoses are numerous or occasional {859,1022,872}	BCL2+, pancytokeratin+, EMA+, CD99+, S100+/−, CD34−, SS18::SSX fusion-specific antibody+ {668,41}	t(X;18)(p11.2;q11.2) {668}
Spindle cell melanoma	• Elongated, narrow, tapering cytoplasmic processes	• Cohesive fascicles or whorls intermingled with scattered epithelioid tumour cells • Short or slender cells • Mild or moderate nuclear pleomorphism • Some cells extremely bland and uniform • Melanin pigment intracellular and extracellular {695,957}	S100+, SOX10+, HMB45+/−, melan-A+/−, MART1+ {695,572}	*BRAF* p.V600E {417}

TTF1, thyroid transcription factor 1.

Table 7.06 Histopathological and cytopathological features and ancillary testing for the differential diagnosis of malignant spindle cell tumours (continued)

Differential diagnosis	Histopathology	Cytopathological features	Immunocytochemistry	Molecular diagnostics
Sarcomatoid mesothelioma	• Arranged in fascicles or in haphazard patterns • Elongated and tapered spindle cells • Nuclei that range from bland to pleomorphic	• Hypocellular smears • Few cohesive tissue fragments • Atypical spindle cells • Collagenous stroma +/− • Primarily pleural-based {159}	Pancytokeratin+, calretinin+/−, D2-40+, WT1+/−, vimentin+ {913,890}	Homozygous del(9p21) {158}
Gastrointestinal stromal tumour (GIST)	• Arranged in fascicles or in a nested growth pattern • Hypocellular to densely cellular • Spindle and/or epithelioid cells • Eosinophilic and fibrillary cytoplasm • Elongated nuclei with fine chromatin	• Cohesive tissue fragments • Spindle or epithelioid cells • Moderate amount of cytoplasm • Elongated, blunt-ended nuclei • Minimal nuclear atypia or pleomorphism • Mitoses and necrosis in malignant GIST {237,472}	KIT (CD117)+, DOG1+, SMA+/−, CD34+/− {506}	*KIT* mutations, *PDGFRA* mutation, SDH alteration, *BRAF* p.V600E mutations {985}
Inflammatory myofibroblastic tumour	• Arranged in fascicles • Plump and spindle cells with indistinct cell borders • Chronic inflammatory infiltrate	• Scantly cellular to hypercellular bland, fibroblast-like cells to spindle to epithelioid cells • Prominent atypia and prominent nucleoli • Rich in plasma cells and lymphocytes {287,829,872,78}	SMA+, ALK+ {169}	*ALK* rearrangement {89,24}
Solitary fibrous tumour	• Patternless architecture • Staghorn vessels • Varying cellularity • Uniform fibroblastic spindle cells	• Cellular tissue fragments with irregular fascicles with pink collagenous stroma • Low to moderate cellularity • Bland spindle cells with a fusiform nucleus • Finely dispersed chromatin and inconspicuous nucleolus {893,68}	CD34+, STAT6+ {145,756}	*NAB2::STAT6* gene fusions
Lymphangio-leiomyomatosis	• Variably sized cysts • Spindle cells with fine chromatin, small nucleoli, and granular eosinophilic cytoplasm	• Loosely cohesive tissue fragments consisting of spindle cells with dispersed single spindle cells • Oval nuclei {529}	SMA+, HMB45+, melan-A (MART1)+, ER+, PR+, S100− {77,255}	
Malignant peripheral nerve sheath tumour	• Arranged in fascicles • Alternating cellularity • Densely cellular monomorphic spindle cells	• Moderate to high cellularity • Elongated, slender, or wavy nuclei • Marked nuclear pleomorphism • Less commonly, a delicate, fibrillary, metachromatic stroma {383}	S100+/−, SOX10+/−	
Type A thymoma	• Spindle and/or oval nuclei • Finely dispersed chromatin • Inconspicuous nucleoli	• High cellularity • Elongated or elliptical nuclei in epithelial cells • Relative lack of lymphocytes {954}	Pancytokeratin+, p63+, p40+ {220}	

TTF1, thyroid transcription factor 1.

soft tissue tumours are more common in the lung than primary spindle cell tumours, apart from spindle cell mesothelioma.

Spindle cell carcinoma cannot be diagnosed on the basis of cytopathology specimens, but if poorly differentiated spindle cells showing varying degrees of nuclei atypia are present, it enters the differential diagnosis. However, if cytopathology shows non-small cell carcinoma with a spindle cell carcinoma component, a comment should be made that its presence raises the possibility of a spindle cell carcinoma.

Spindle NETs are usually located peripherally, with bland, elongated nuclei and long, whip-like cytoplasm {677}.

So-called benign metastasizing leiomyoma should be considered if there are multiple lung nodules in women with a previous hysterectomy, and it is otherwise difficult to distinguish from primary low-grade leiomyosarcomas, which have cohesive tissue fragments of cells often arranged in a parallel pattern with oval, blunt-ended to spindle nuclei and spindle cytoplasm. High-grade leiomyosarcoma may have similar more-cellular tissue fragments with more plentiful dispersed single intact cells and may show bland to hyperchromatic pleomorphic nuclei, prominent nucleoli, mitoses, and necrosis. There are epithelioid subtypes.

Metastatic melanoma can enter the differential diagnosis of a spindle cell tumour in a thoracic FNAB. Tumour cells may be misdiagnosed as reactive fibroblasts if they are bland, or as centrocytes of lymph nodes if they are rounded and highly dispersed. If the cells are pleomorphic, the differential diagnosis includes sarcoma, and the presence of pigment in tumour cells (which can be confirmed in cell block material by melanin bleach stains and negative Perls iron stain) and rounded, often pleomorphic nuclei with macronucleoli and nuclear pseudoinclusions may be clues to the diagnosis {957}.

The differential diagnosis of sarcomatoid mesothelioma is primarily with soft tissue sarcomas and spindle cell carcinoma, and requires ICC {533}.

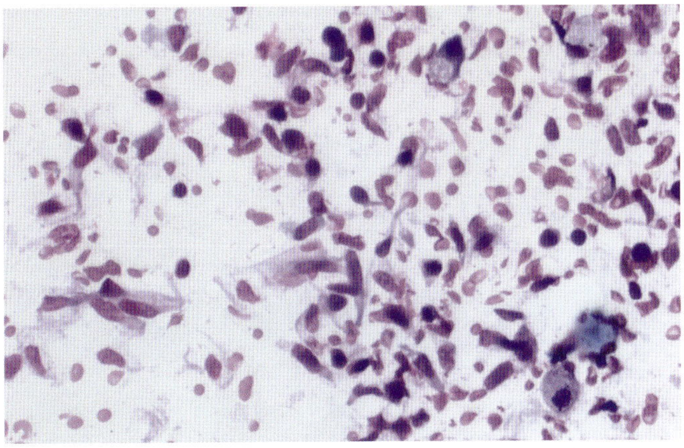

Fig. 7.60 Sarcomatoid mesothelioma. Spindle and occasional polygonal cells are haphazardly dispersed. The nuclei are elongated, vary in size, and exhibit mild pleomorphism and atypia (Giemsa).

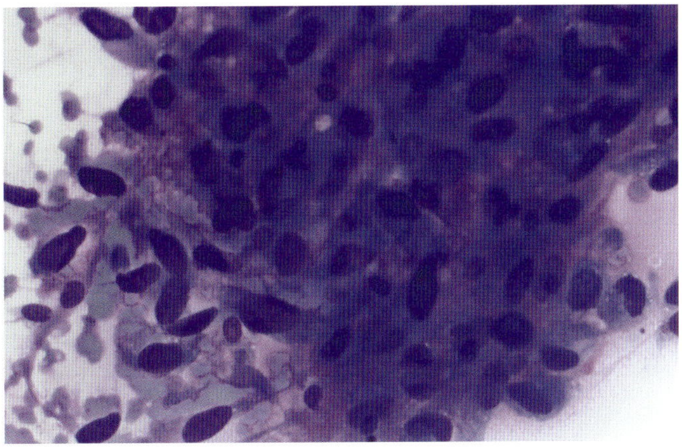

Fig. 7.61 Leiomyosarcoma. Mildly crowded tissue fragment showing spindle cells with elongated and (in many cells) blunt-ended nuclei with variable nuclear pleomorphism embedded in a collagenous matrix (Giemsa).

Gastrointestinal stromal tumour is the most common mesenchymal tumour in the gastrointestinal tract and most often metastasizes to the liver and peritoneum; it rarely metastasizes to lung {660,992}.

Inflammatory myofibroblastic tumour and solitary fibrous tumour may recur or (rarely) metastasize and can be seen in FNAB of the thorax and in the differential diagnosis of low-grade sarcomas. The cytopathology of these tumours is relatively bland, and their diagnosis often relies on the cell block. Inflammatory myofibroblastic tumour exhibits nonspecific features and can be hypocellular to hypercellular with bland, fibroblast-like cells varying to spindle to epithelioid cells with prominent atypia and prominent nucleoli admixed with inflammatory cells {287,829,872,78}. Solitary fibrous tumour shows low to moderate cellularity of mixed oval, elongated, round, and stellate cells with pink (Pap) collagenous stroma and hypercellular tissue fragments with minimal atypia {893,68}. Benign and malignant solitary fibrous tumours have common cytopathological features, and the ability to distinguish between them is limited.

Lymphangioleiomyomatosis, malignant peripheral nerve sheath tumours, and type A thymoma all occur in the thoracic cavity and have been rarely reported in FNAB material. FNAB of lymphangioleiomyomatosis reveals relatively large, monomorphic spindle cells with a moderate N:C ratio both in tissue fragments and as dissociated single cells, with oval nuclei with evenly distributed chromatin {58,529}. Because the cytopathology of malignant peripheral nerve sheath tumour overlaps with that of other sarcomas, the FNAB diagnosis of peripheral nerve sheath tumours is difficult {955}. However, elongated, slender, often wavy nuclei and (less commonly) a delicate, fibrillary, metachromatic stroma are observed in some cases {383}. FNAB of type A thymoma yields highly cellular smears with epithelial cells in tissue fragments and as single cells demonstrating elongated or elliptical cell nuclei with minimal irregularity and bland chromatin, as well as a relative lack of lymphocytes {954}.

Ancillary testing

An initial ICC panel for spindle cell tumours is recommended to include pancytokeratin, vimentin, and at least one marker each for NET, mesothelioma, and melanoma, such as synaptophysin, calretinin, and melan-A (MART1), respectively (see Table 7.06) {856}. For further analysis, the panel might be expanded, especially if there is any history of a previous soft tissue tumour at another site. In spindle cell tumours, specific genetic changes may occur, and appropriate use of sequencing techniques and FISH may make a definite diagnosis possible in these cases (see Table 7.06).

Pulmonary arterial intimal sarcoma should be differentiated from other spindle cell sarcomas and tumours that express MDM2 amplification (e.g. liposarcoma).

SS18::SSX fusion testing is recommended when ICC of cell block material is inconclusive in synovial sarcomas.

Cytoplasmic immunoreactivity for ALK is detectable in 50–60% of cases of inflammatory myofibroblastic tumour and correlates well with the presence of *ALK* gene rearrangement {291,169,89,24}.

Nuclear STAT6 immunoreactivity is a valuable marker for solitary fibrous tumours.

The spindle cells of lymphangioleiomyomatosis are consistently positive for SMA and HMB45; ER, PR, and melan-A (MART1) are also often positive, whereas S100 is negative.

Paragaglioma

Kholova I

Definition

Paraganglioma is a rare neuroendocrine neoplasm arising from the pluripotent neural crest–derived chromaffin cells occurring in extra-adrenal sites.

Clinical features and imaging

Pulmonary paraganglioma is extremely rare. It usually forms a solitary pulmonary mass found close to blood vessels and nerves, and it is often located near the branching pulmonary artery. Paragangliomas are non-functioning or may produce catecholamines {904}.

Histopathology

Paraganglioma is a well-circumscribed, solid tumour with nests or anastomosing trabeculae of tumour cells surrounded by an arching thin fibrovascular network, producing an organoid architecture (Zellballen). The tumour cells are variably sized and shaped: round, polyhedral, or spindle, with moderate to abundant granular, eosinophilic, and pale cytoplasm, and with indistinct borders. The nuclei are round to ovoid with finely granular chromatin, common nuclear pseudoinclusions, and occasional hyperchromasia and binucleation {837,202}.

Key diagnostic cytopathological features

- Cellularity ranges from scant to hypercellular
- Loosely cohesive and often syncytial tissue fragments are 3D with follicular, acinar, and nested architecture and intervening thin fibrovascular strands; papillary-like structures are rare
- Variable single cell dissociation and stripped nuclei are seen
- Often bloody background due to hypervascularity
- Medium-sized epithelioid and/or spindle cells vary in size with poorly defined cell margins when in the tissue fragments, whereas single cells show abundant granular, pale-grey (Pap) cytoplasm with magenta (Giemsa) cytoplasmic granules
- Round to oval nuclei show evenly dispersed chromatin, micronucleoli, and occasional anisonucleosis, with scattered

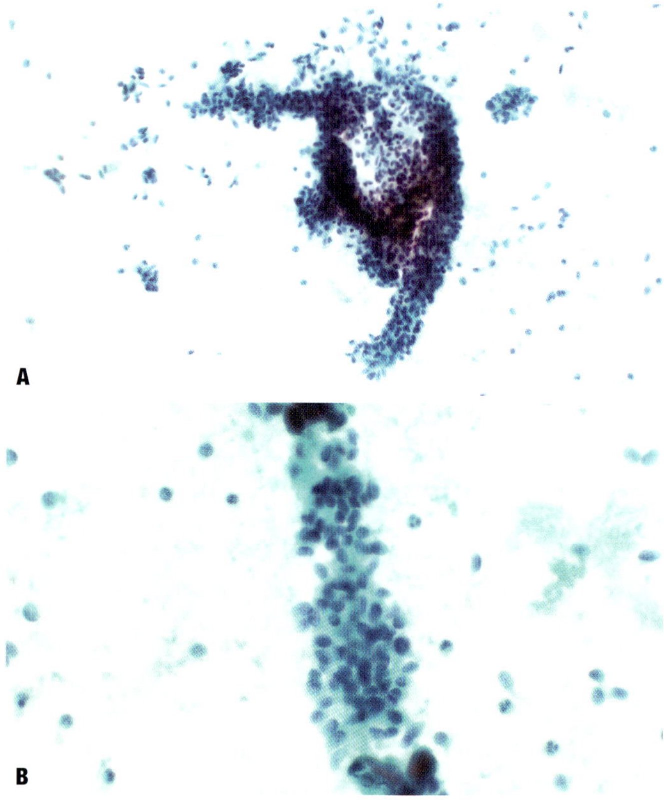

Fig. 7.63 Paraganglioma. **A,B** Cohesive tissue fragment of mildly crowded cells with round to oval, mildly pleomorphic nuclei and poorly delineated cytoplasm. Occasional nuclei are larger and more pleomorphic. Stripped nuclei are in the background (Pap).

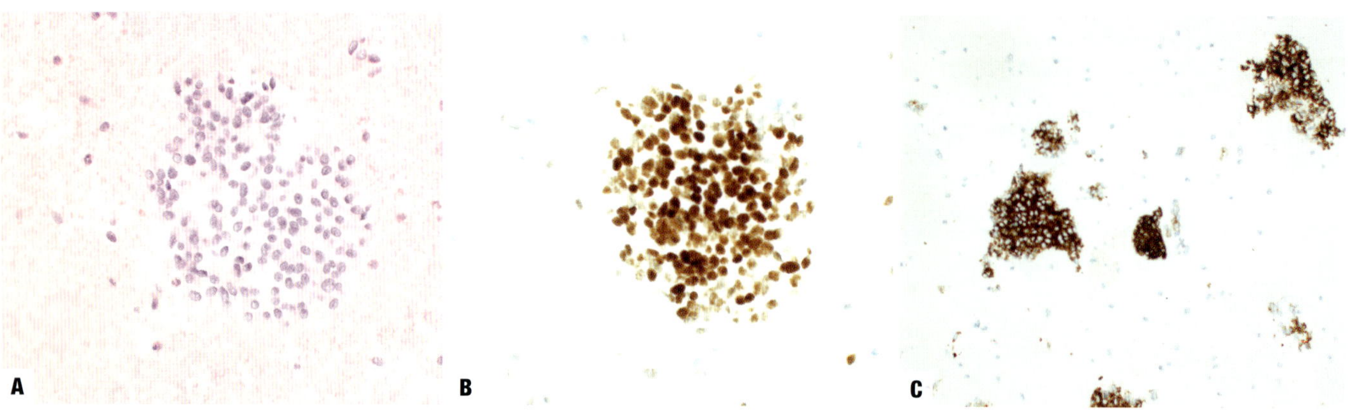

Fig. 7.62 Paraganglioma. **A** Cell block showing cells with ovoid regular nuclei and poorly defined margins (H&E). **B** Cell block showing a tissue fragment with nuclear positivity for INSM1 (ICC). **C** Cell block showing tissue fragments with strong diffuse cytoplasmic positivity for synaptophysin (ICC).

larger cells showing marked pleomorphism, nuclear grooves, intranuclear pseudoinclusions, binucleation, and multinucleation

Reference(s): {418,640,265,385}

Discussion and differential diagnosis

Paraganglioma shows nuclear features reminiscent of an endocrine neoplasm {418,640,265,160}. The differential diagnosis includes cases of primary or metastatic neuroendocrine neoplasms, including neuroendocrine tumours (NETs, or carcinoids), metastatic adrenal cortical carcinomas, melanomas, metastatic renal cell carcinomas, and solid pseudopapillary carcinoma {640,160}. In rare paragangliomas with papillary-like features, sclerosing haemangioma and adenocarcinoma with lepidic pattern are in the differential diagnosis {418}.

Ancillary testing

Paragangliomas in all locations including the lungs are positive in ICC for neuroendocrine markers such as synaptophysin, chromogranin, INSM1, NSE, and CD56, and negative for cytokeratins and thyroid transcription factor 1 (TTF1) {418,837, 764,440}. In ICC, NETs (carcinoids) and other neuroendocrine carcinomas are positive for cytokeratin and TTF1 {228}, in contrast to paraganglioma.

Diffuse pleural mesothelioma

Michael CW
Davidson B
Engels M
Hiroshima K
Önal BÜ
Sauter JL
Welker L

Definition

Diffuse pleural mesothelioma is a tumour of malignant mesothelial cells showing diffuse involvement of the pleura.

Clinical features and imaging

Pleural mesothelioma is a disease primarily caused by asbestos and/or erionite fibre exposure, with male predominance, a median age of 65–69 years, and a latency period of > 30 years between fibre exposure and disease presentation {561,227, 625,1001}. Mesothelioma has a slight predominance in the right pleura and less commonly involves the peritoneum and (rarely) the pericardium {697,227}. Patients present initially with the insidious onset of unilateral recurrent pleural effusions and persistent, slowly increasing non-pleuritic pain, followed by dyspnoea and cough (see Table 7.07). However, a small proportion of patients present with an acute onset of severe pain and dyspnoea, usually secondary to either haemothorax or spontaneous pneumothorax {261}. A definitive diagnosis is usually established 2 months to > 6 months after the onset of symptoms {22}. Assuming a high performance status, < 30% of patients are treated surgically {573}. Tumour seeding may occur in sites of previous invasive procedures {461,560,88}. The 6-month, 1-year, and 5-year overall survival rates are 55%, 33%, and 5%, respectively {573}.

Initial CXR demonstrates a large unilateral pleural effusion, which may obscure the pleural thickening. CT with contrast is more sensitive and often shows the pleural effusion and pleural thickening (which tends to form a rind that encases the lung and often extends into the fissures and along the mediastinal pleura and diaphragm), as well as the size of the lymph nodes. MRI with contrast is more sensitive in identifying invasion of the chest wall and diaphragm. PET is more reliable in detecting contralateral chest involvement and extrathoracic spread, thus facilitating staging, especially for patients who are considered for potential curative surgery {369}.

Table 7.07 Clinical signs found on initial examination of cases, by site of primary tumour (frequency and percentage) {227}

Clinical sign	Site of primary tumour			
	Pleura[a] (*N* = 278)		Peritoneum (*N* = 15)	
	n	%	*n*	%
Pleural effusion	231	83	1	7
Crepitations	77	28	3	20
Hepatomegaly	56	20	2	13
Chest wall tenderness	16	6	0	0
Ascites	3	1	11	73
Lymphadenopathy	11	4	3	20
Pleural rub	12	4	0	0
Abdominal mass	5	2	4	27
Clubbing	5	2	1	7[a]

[a]Includes 2 cases with a pericardial primary tumour.

Histopathology

Diffuse pleural mesotheliomas are divided into epithelioid, biphasic, and sarcomatoid subtypes. Epithelioid mesothelioma is mainly composed of polygonal, rounded cells that infiltrate the pleura most frequently in a tubulopapillary pattern; however a broad range of architectural patterns, including trabecular, solid, micropapillary, and (rarely) adenomatoid and microcystic, may be observed. Cells range from the classic bland cuboidal to deciduoid, rhabdoid, signet ring, small cell, and pleomorphic. Some architectural patterns and cellular features in epithelioid pleural mesothelioma have been shown to have prognostic significance; for example, micropapillary and solid architecture and pleomorphic and rhabdoid cytopathological features

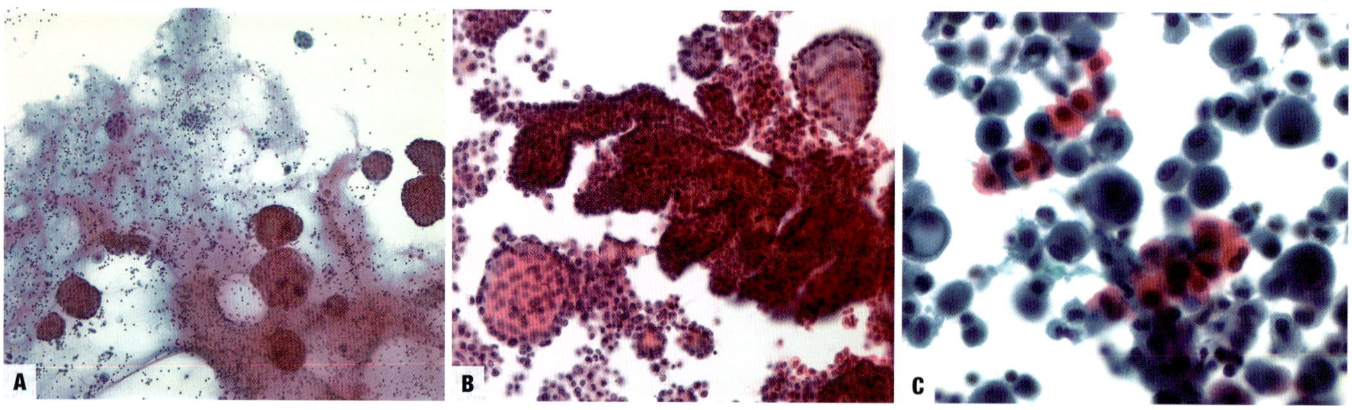

Fig. 7.64 Pleural mesothelioma. **A** Rounded, densely cellular, spherical tissue fragments floating in a mucin-like material representing the high background hyaluronan secreted by the malignant mesothelial cells (Pap). **B** Direct smear showing a complex papillary tissue fragment and other spherical papillae with epithelium surrounding a pink matrix (Pap). **C** Malignant mesothelial cells showing variable size and including pseudokeratotic cells with pyknotic nuclei and orangeophilic cytoplasm (liquid-based cytopathology, Pap).

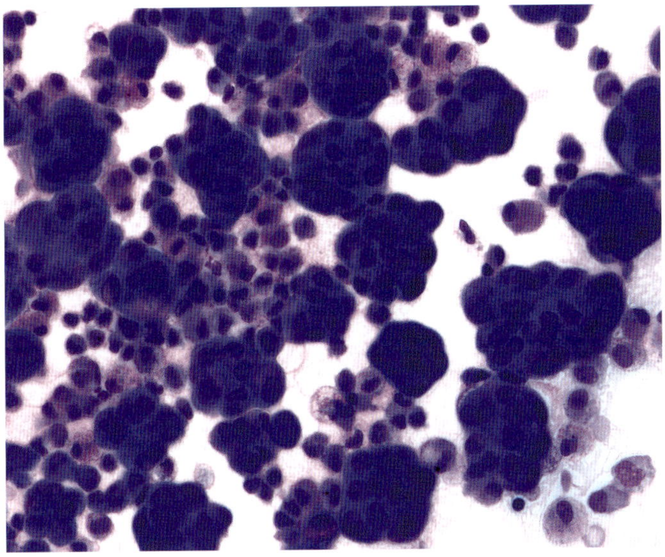

Fig. 7.65 Pleural mesothelioma. Highly cellular direct smear showing plentiful variably sized, berry-like, 3D tissue fragments with scalloped borders (Giemsa).

in epithelioid pleural mesothelioma are associated with an adverse prognosis {394,651,767,649,630}. A nuclear grading system that merges nuclear atypia with mitotic count has been developed for epithelioid mesothelioma and has prognostic significance. Subsequently, a two-tiered grading system incorporating low and high grades and utilizing nuclear grade and the presence of necrosis has been suggested on the basis of data from current multi-institutional studies {393,767,630,1023}.

Key diagnostic cytopathological features

- Often extremely highly cellular FNAB smears with innumerable, often large tissue fragments and or single cells
- Numerous morular (berry-like), papillary, or tubular tissue fragments showing a wide variation in size; papillary fragments may have green (Pap) or magenta (Giemsa) collagen cores
- Enlarged pleomorphic cells with wide variation in size, varying from that of benign mesothelial cells to gigantic cells the size of small morular tissue fragments, and numerous multinucleated cells with more than three nuclei and abundant cytoplasm
- Dense cytoplasm, which can be concentric or eccentric, is green with an outer pale region with intercellular windows (Pap) or shows an inner lighter and outer blue staining (Giemsa); hyaluronan may appear as magenta material in the cytoplasm (Giemsa)
- Enlarged nuclei (although atypia may be subtle) and prominent nucleoli of varying shape and size, including macronucleoli
- Atypical mitoses
- Pseudokeratotic cells with pyknotic nuclei and eosinophilic (Pap) cytoplasm
- Numerous perinuclear lipid vacuoles detected on Giemsa staining and confirmed by Oil Red O staining on a fresh smear
- Abundant hyaluronan is seen as a pink or red granular background (Giemsa) in cytospin preparations, and as mucin-like extracellular matrix in cell blocks and direct smears (H&E, Pap, and Giemsa)

Discussion and differential diagnosis

This section discusses diffuse pleural mesothelioma, and not localized pleural mesothelioma, well-differentiated papillary mesothelial tumour of the pleura, adenomatoid tumour, or mesothelioma in situ, where FNAB cannot make a definitive diagnosis at present. Given that as many as 90% of patients with diffuse pleural mesothelioma present with a pleural effusion, the fluid is usually the first sample acquired in the diagnostic workup. Mesothelioma may also be diagnosed by FNAB of pleural-based masses or metastatic sites. Rare examples have been reported in bronchial samples and sputum samples. For sputum samples, the largest published series contained 5 cases where papillary tissue fragments of malignant cells were seen. In 2 of these patients, infiltration of the mucosa of large bronchi by mesothelioma was found at autopsy {975}. Only rare, mainly single case reports of bronchial washing, bronchoalveolar lavage (BAL), or bronchial brushing have described diffuse pleural mesothelioma seen as single atypical cells and small tissue fragments from pulmonary invasion by mesothelioma {206,516,12}.

Two studies from the 1980s reported 58 cases diagnosed by transthoracic FNAB {894,866}, and a more recent study reported the diagnosis of 4 pleural mesotheliomas by endobronchial ultrasound–directed FNAB {286}. FNAB shows a spectrum of features including cohesive papillary tissue fragments, plentiful

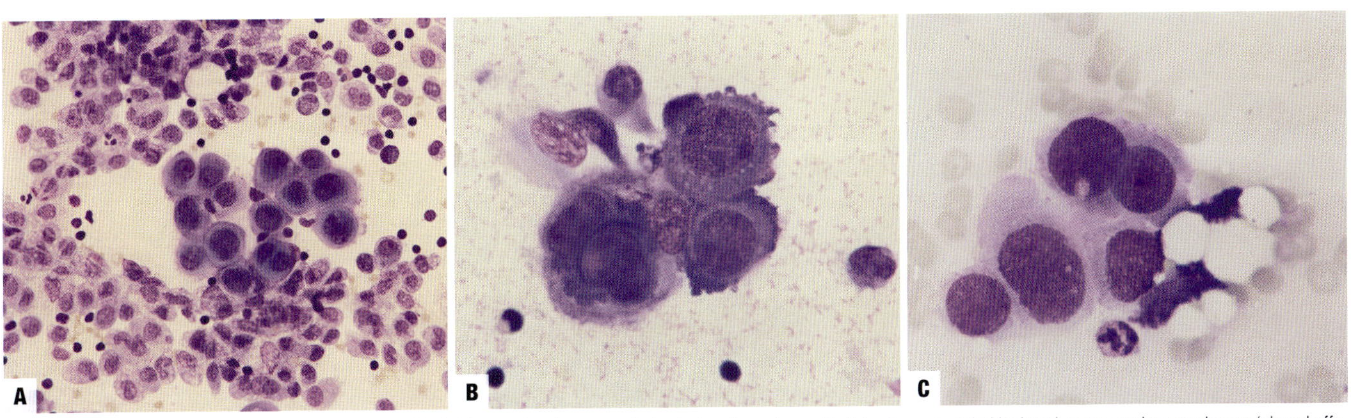

Fig. 7.66 Pleural mesothelioma. **A** Mesothelioma of epithelioid type, showing a small sheet of malignant mesothelial cells surrounded by lymphocytes and macrophages (pleural effusion, Giemsa). **B** Mesothelioma of epithelioid subtype. Minute tissue fragment of malignant mesothelial cells, with pink granular material in the background, suggestive of hyaluronan. Note the cytoplasmic blebs (pleural effusion, Giemsa). **C** Same patient as in Panel B, 2 years later. Metastasis in the thoracic wall in a scar after thoracotomy (transbronchial FNAB, Giemsa).

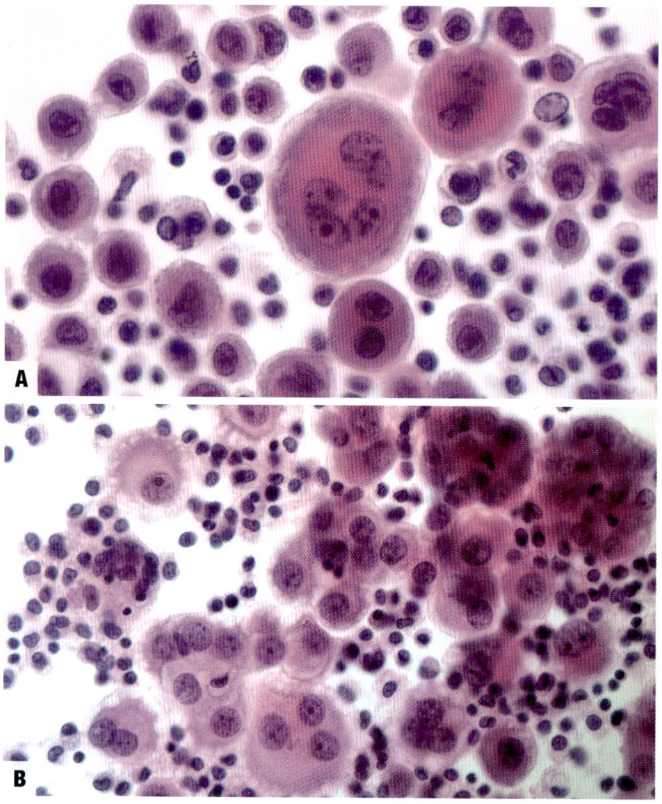

Fig. 7.67 Pleural mesothelioma. **A** Direct smear showing malignant mesothelial cells that vary in size from mildly enlarged to gigantic multinucleated cells, with dense squamoid cytoplasm with a frilly pale margin and marked nuclear pleomorphism (Pap). **B** Variably sized mesothelial cells, seen in small tissue fragments and as single cells, some gigantic in size and multinucleated (Pap).

dispersed single cells, and biphasic or mesenchymal features {866}. In any given case of pleural mesothelioma, the cytomorphology in effusion and that in FNAB usually show some resemblance.

In effusions, only the epithelioid type or epithelioid component of a biphasic type may exfoliate adequate cells for diagnosis {341}. Sarcomatoid mesotheliomas usually present as a bloody effusion but rarely exfoliate any tumour cells. The reported sensitivity ranges from 30% to 75%, with a specificity approaching 99–100% {325,821}. Both the lack of exfoliation in some cases and the subtle cytopathological presentation contribute to the low sensitivity. Grossly, these fluids are very thick in consistency (tar-like), secondary to the hyaluronan secreted by the cells, and they are frequently serosanguineous or bloody. The diagnosis is based on the recognition of the malignant nature of the cytopathology, and this can be supported by molecular surrogate markers {341,340,29}.

Mesothelioma usually presents with marked cellularity that far exceeds any reactive effusion; however, not all cases exfoliate with high cellularity and may overlap with that of reactive processes. Although atypia may be subtle in mesothelioma and significant in reactive lesions, the presence of variably sized and complex tissue fragments and often markedly enlarged mesothelial cells should always raise a concern for mesothelioma. On the other hand, the presence of significant cellular pleomorphism is a feature that favours carcinoma over mesothelioma.

The differential diagnosis of diffuse pleural mesothelioma, whether in effusions or FNAB, includes reactive mesothelial proliferations and metastatic carcinomas (see Table 7.08, p. 160). Carcinomas can show diffuse pleural or pseudomesotheliomatous spread and mimic mesothelioma clinically and on imaging. In rare cases, mesothelioma can present as a predominantly discohesive single cell population, for which melanoma and high-grade lymphoma should also be considered in the differential diagnosis. Metastatic carcinomas often will show a distinct population of malignant cells, usually in tissue fragments in a background of distinctly different mesothelial cells and chronic inflammatory cells.

The differential diagnosis of reactive mesothelial proliferations and mesothelioma can be challenging because reactive mesothelial proliferations can demonstrate striking cytopathological atypia and it is not possible to confirm the presence of invasion in cytopathology. Ancillary testing becomes essential. The Oil Red O stain on fresh fluids highlights the perinuclear fat droplets, which are present in abundance in mesothelioma but of which only few, if any, are seen in reactive mesothelial cells or rare carcinomas.

Mesothelioma in situ (MIS) is an extremely rare entity. It is considered a precursor of pleural mesothelioma, with a published median time to progression of 60 months, occurring in

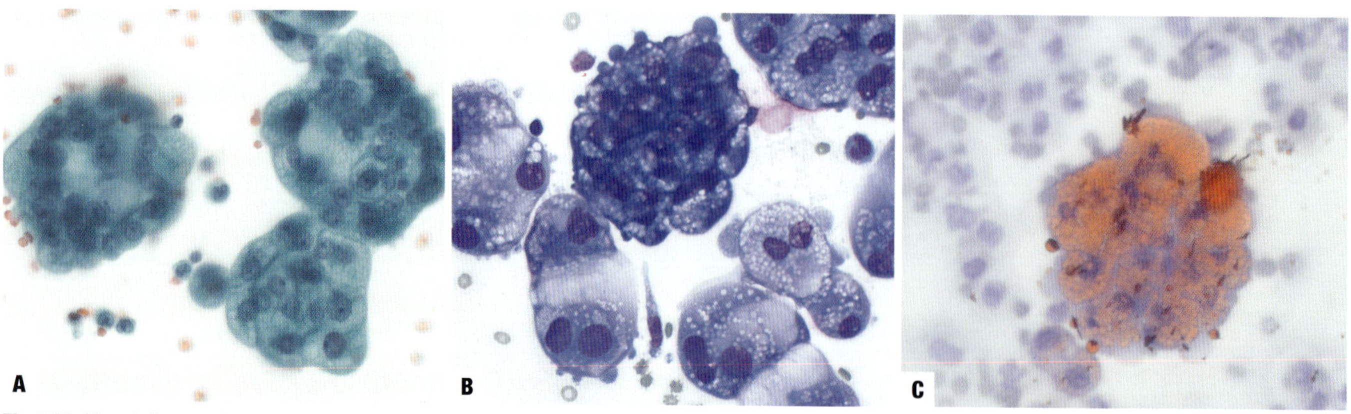

Fig. 7.68 Mesothelioma. **A** Tissue fragments of malignant mesothelial cells with intracytoplasmic lipid vacuoles (lipid-rich mesothelioma) (pleural effusion, Pap). **B** Tissue fragments of mesothelioma with intracytoplasmic lipid vacuoles in the abundant cytoplasm (pleural effusion, Giemsa). **C** Tissue fragment of mesothelioma with intracytoplasmic lipid vacuoles in the abundant cytoplasm (pleural effusion, Oil Red O).

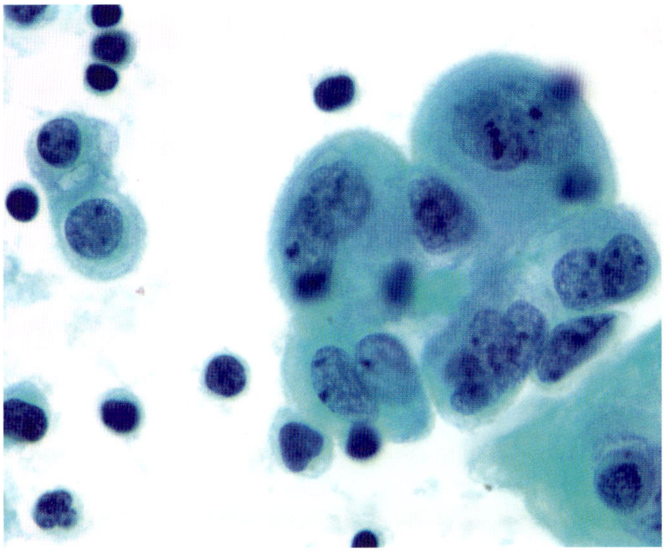

Fig. 7.69 Pleural mesothelioma. Direct smear showing several large multinucleated mesothelioma cells with relatively dense cytoplasm and marked nuclear enlargement and pleomorphism (Pap).

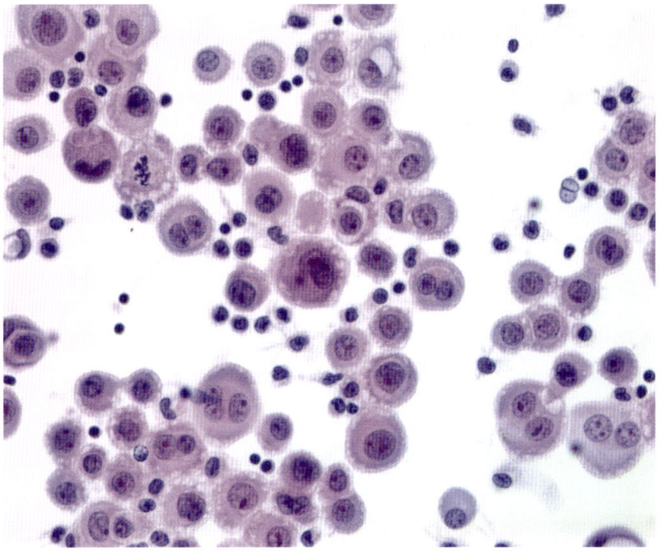

Fig. 7.71 Pleural mesothelioma. The malignant cells are primarily seen as a discohesive population of loosely attached or single cells, many of which have a frilly margin to the denser, more central cytoplasm (Pap).

patients with known asbestos exposure who develop unresolved pleural effusions, yet no mass lesions are seen either by imaging studies or by thoracoscopy {156}. Instead, normal, smooth pleural thickening or tiny nodules may be seen. Histologically, MIS shows a layer of flat or cuboidal cells with or without cytopathological atypia and/or small papillary projections, or small nodules that may show moderate to severe atypia and demonstrate loss of BAP1 and/or MTAP and/or show *CDKN2A* homozygous deletion {155,157}. The role of cytopathology in diagnosing MIS is controversial. Pleural effusion specimens that are cytopathologically concerning for mesothelial malignancy would raise the possibility of MIS, but it is not possible to exclude MIS from early stages of invasive diffuse mesothelioma on cytopathology even with imaging correlation {430}. Although the diagnosis of MIS is not currently recommended

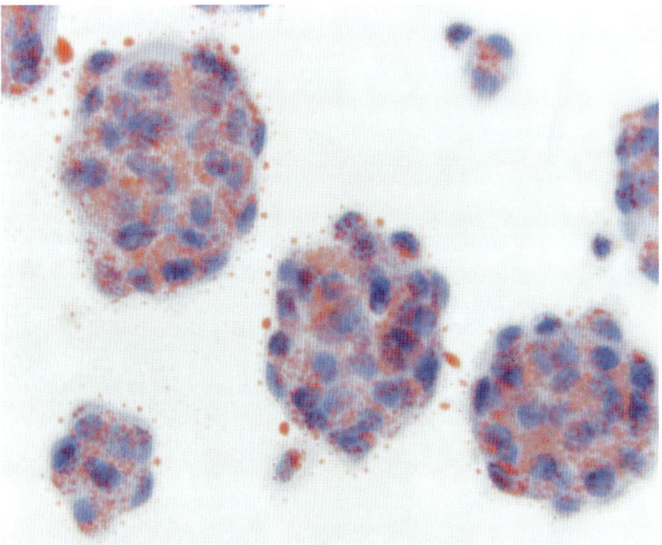

Fig. 7.70 Pleural mesothelioma. Tissue fragments of mesothelioma showing the Oil Red O stain highlighting numerous perinuclear fat droplets in fresh smears.

on cytopathology, a cytopathology specimen may represent the first clue towards the histopathological diagnosis of MIS. The current literature is scarce regarding the cytopathological features of MIS, with only rare cases reported as retrospectively demonstrating loss of BAP1 on pleural fluids originally diagnosed as reactive, but cytopathology will play a role in this diagnosis in the future as more cases of this extremely rare entity are recognized and reported {715,312}.

Ancillary testing

Mesothelioma can show malignant nuclear features and be categorized as "Malignant", but ICC is usually needed to establish a mesothelial origin. However, if the atypia is subtle, or if the cellularity is not striking or only some of the supportive features are noted, ancillary testing is required to establish both the "Malignant" categorization and precise diagnosis. In rare cases where the cytopathology is either diagnostic or very suspicious for pleural mesothelioma with confirmatory surrogate findings (e.g. loss of BAP1 and/or MTAP expression) but the imaging presentation of a typical diffuse pleural mesothelioma is absent, the possibility of early stage mesothelioma should be considered, and rarely, the possibility of a diagnosis of MIS could be raised {312}.

The main roles of ancillary testing are to confirm the mesothelial origin, distinguish epithelioid pleural mesothelioma from adenocarcinoma, and (when relevant) confirm malignancy of a mesothelial proliferation. It is recommended that at least two epithelial and two mesothelial ICC markers should be used {341,192}.

The ability of ICC to distinguish mesotheliomas from carcinomas depends substantially on the origin of the carcinoma, and the differential diagnosis from serous carcinoma of female genital or peritoneal origin is the most challenging. The most robust mesothelial marker is calretinin, but it is not specific and can be expressed (with various percentages) in some carcinomas, such as squamous cell carcinoma and adenocarcinoma of the lung, serous carcinoma of the ovary, and renal cell carcinoma

Table 7.08 Differential diagnosis of mesothelioma

Feature	Mesothelioma	Reactive mesothelium	Carcinoma
Gross examination of pleural fluid:			
Consistency	Thick, tar-like	Thin	Generally thin
Appearance	Serosanguineous or bloody	Serosanguineous	Serosanguineous or bloody
Background:			
Clear	Some cases	Most cases	Some cases
Bloody	Frequently	Rare cases[a]	Most cases
Obscuring matrix	Frequent (hyaluronan)	Absent	In cases with mucin
Inflammation	May be present	Frequent	May be present
Low magnification:			
Cellularity	Strikingly high[b]	Moderate to high	Usually high
Tissue fragments	Plentiful, vary in size	Few, small	May be numerous, little variation in size
Single cells	Alone or combined with tissue fragments	Most cases	Alone or combined with tissue fragments
Populations	Monotonous population of mesothelial cells with wide variation in size	Monotonous population of mesothelial cells with minimal variation in size	Alien population in background of mesothelial cells
Tissue fragments:			
Shape	Predominantly 3D, berry-like morules with scalloped borders or spheres	Predominantly 2D tissue fragments with scalloped borders	3D tissue fragments with common cell borders
Architecture	Variable size and complexity, sometimes very complex branching papillae	Mostly simple and small	Variable complexity depending on primary
Collagenous core	Occasionally present and may be conspicuous	Rare	Uncommon, fibrovascular cores in papillary tumours
Hollow tissue fragments	May be present	Absent	Not characteristic
Cellular features:			
Shape and size	Round, significantly enlarged	Slightly enlarged	Vary by cell origin
Size variation	Varies from benign to gigantic	Minimal variation	Minimal variation
Atypia	Mild to severe	Mild to moderate	Moderate to severe
Nuclei	Markedly enlarged	Slightly enlarged	Markedly enlarged
N:C ratio	Low	Minimally increased	High
Nucleoli	Macronucleoli in many cases	May be prominent	Prominent
Multinucleation	Common	Occasional	Not common
Number of cells	Numerous	Few	
Number of nucleoli	2 to many	2–3	
Cytoplasm	Abundant	Moderate	Scant to moderate

[a]Bloody benign effusion may occur, depending on etiology (e.g. lung infarction). [b]Strikingly high cellularity is a feature of malignancy but may not always be present.

{193,359,648,653,654,652}. WT1 is another sensitive mesothelial marker, with high specificity in some differentials (e.g. against lung adenocarcinoma {714}), but it cannot be used for differentiating mesothelioma from serous carcinoma of female genital origin, which is also positive for WT1. Similarly, D2-40 is a robust mesothelial marker, but it is expressed in the majority of serous carcinomas {45}. CK5/6 is expressed in the majority of mesotheliomas, although it is also present in some carcinomas {714,195,20}. Tenascin X is another marker whose expression has been reported to be specific for mesothelioma {1012}. HEG1 has been recently reported as a highly sensitive marker for mesothelial cells and was only expressed in about 30% of ovarian serous carcinomas {337}.

BerEP4 and MOC31, targeting the surface molecule EpCAM, are among the most widely used carcinoma markers. However, they stain, at least focally, a significant number of mesotheliomas {714}. Claudin-4, CEA, and B72.3 are more specific in this differential diagnosis, with claudin-4 being more sensitive {679,388,642}. Less commonly used markers include CD15 (LeuM1) and BG8. Other potential candidate carcinoma markers that have been reported to be absent in mesothelioma include claudin-1 and claudin-3 {432}, CD24 {191}, and MMP7 {194}.

A summary of selected site-specific markers used to establish a primary origin of malignancy and markers that may be coexpressed with mesothelioma is presented in Table 7.09.

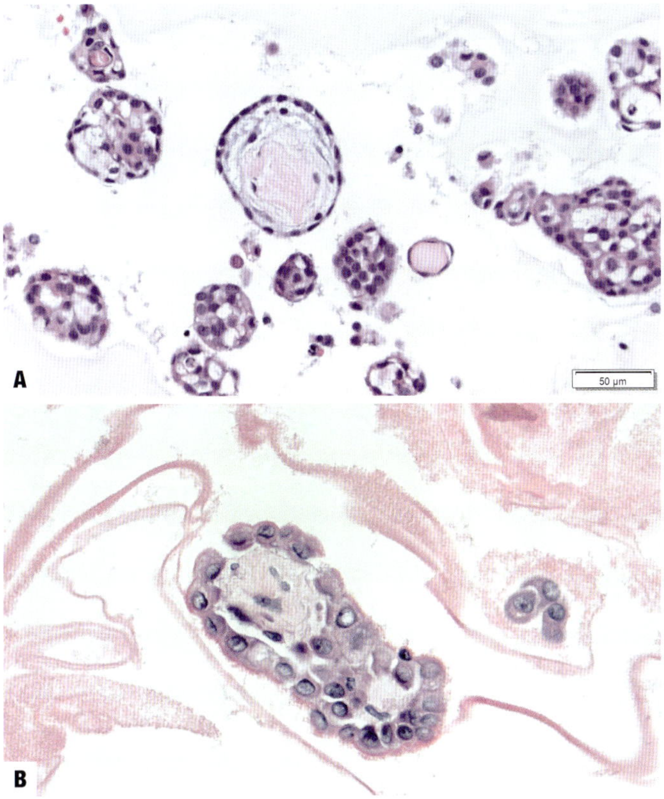

Fig. 7.72 Pleural mesothelioma. **A** Variably sized tissue fragments and spherical papillae with collagenous cores. Some of the spheres are hollow, surrounding a loose pink matrix, or show vacuolization of the cells (cell block, H&E). **B** Papillary tissue fragment with a collagen core and covered in an atypical mesothelial cell layer. Hyaluronan is present, appearing as granular ropy material in the background (cell block, H&E).

Table 7.09 Site-specific markers useful in establishing primary origin of malignancy

Origin of metastasis	Useful markers	Coexpression of markers
Lung	TTF1, napsin A	
Gastrointestinal tract	CDX2, CK20, SATB2	
Ovary	PAX8, ER, WT1	> 90% of mesotheliomas express WT1 Some mesotheliomas express PAX8, especially in the peritoneum and in women {122,525,990} Calretinin is expressed in as many as 30% of serous carcinomas of the ovary {652}
Breast	ER, PR, GATA3, SOX10, GCDFP-15, mammaglobin	> 50% of mesotheliomas express GATA3 {571} 38% of triple-negative breast carcinomas express calretinin {476,566}
Kidney	PAX8, RCCm	
Urothelium	GATA3, p63	> 50% of mesotheliomas express GATA3 {571}
Liver	HepPar1, GPC3, ARG1	
Prostate	PSA, NKX3-1	
Thyroid	TTF1, PAX8	
Squamous cell carcinoma	p40, p63, CK5/6	As many as 40% of squamous carcinomas of the lung focally express calretinin {653}
Melanoma	Melan-A, SOX10, S100, MART1	
Haematopoietic process	CD20, CD45, CD3	

ARG1, arginase-1; GPC3, glypican-3; TTF1, thyroid transcription factor 1.

Loss of nuclear expression of BAP1 by ICC is 55–60% sensitive in distinguishing mesothelioma from benign proliferations {18,195,20,57,333,427,426}. Both MTAP and BAP1 ICC are 100% specific for mesothelioma in the differential diagnosis of benign mesothelial proliferations, but they must only be interpreted in the presence of adequate positive internal controls {57,427,425,426}. Combinations or panels of p16 FISH, merlin (NF2) FISH, BAP1 ICC, and MTAP ICC have been reported to yield a greater sensitivity of 84–98%, which is greater than that of any individual assay {57,333,427,425,426}.

The soluble markers in effusions that have been reported to be the most useful in supporting the diagnosis of mesothelioma compared with metastatic carcinomas and benign effusions are mesothelin and hyaluronan, both overexpressed in mesothelioma {177,597,108,69}, whereas galectin-1 and galectin-3 are overexpressed in lung adenocarcinoma {596,69}.

Homozygous deletion of *CDKN2A* (9p21; encoding p16) detected by p16 FISH distinguishes mesothelioma from benign mesothelial proliferations with a high specificity of 100% and sensitivity of 60–78% {808,333,427,425,426,1006}. But p16 FISH is less sensitive for epithelioid mesothelioma than for biphasic and sarcomatoid types, which are very rare in effusion specimens but may be encountered in FNAB. It is important to emphasize that ICC for p16 is not an acceptable alternative to FISH {154}. Recently, hemizygous *NF2* loss (chromosome 22 monosomy or hemizygous deletion) by FISH has been reported to demonstrate 52–53% sensitivity and 100% specificity in differentiating mesothelioma from reactive mesothelial proliferations {425,426}.

However, FISH can be technically difficult and truncation artefact can be an issue when detecting deletions, and FISH is not widely available worldwide. Cytoplasmic loss of MTAP expression by ICC can serve as a surrogate marker for *CDKN2A* deletions. Because of the proximity of *MTAP* and *CDKN2A* genes on chromosome 9, *MTAP* is codeleted in approximately 90% of tumours with homozygous *CDKN2A* deletion {364}. Cytoplasmic loss of MTAP expression by ICC has been reported to be 42–70% sensitive in distinguishing mesothelioma from benign mesothelial proliferations {57,333,427,425,426}. Rare cases showed a loss of MTAP expression by ICC but no *CDKN2A* deletion by FISH {57}.

Additionally, detection of any of the molecular alterations commonly seen in mesothelioma, including *BAP1*, *CDKN2A*, *NF2*, and *SETD2* by next-generation sequencing can confirm a diagnosis of mesothelioma because these alterations are seen only in malignant processes.

For quality assurance, it is essential that proper validation studies of these methods, particularly in cytopathology

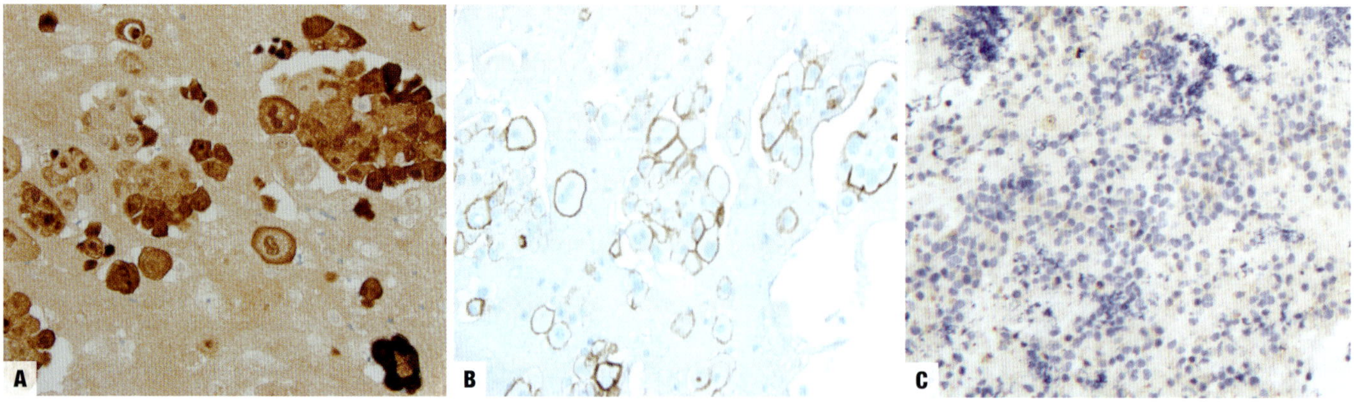

Fig. 7.73 Pleural mesothelioma. **A** Strong nuclear and cytoplasmic positivity for calretinin (cell block, ICC). **B** Pleural mesothelioma showing cytoplasmic marginal D2-40 positivity (cell block, ICC). **C** Pleural mesothelioma cells show loss of MTAP cytoplasmic expression (cell block, ICC).

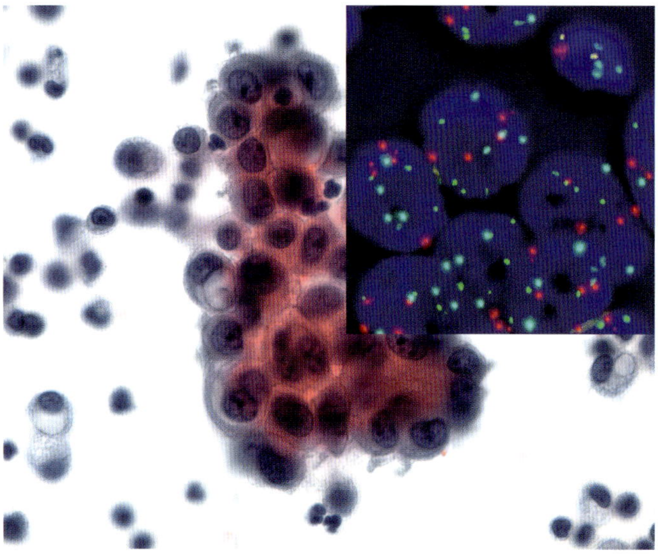

Fig. 7.74 Pleural mesothelioma. Cohesive tissue fragment of mildly crowded malignant mesothelial cells with considerable cytoplasm (Pap). **Inset:** FISH of Pap-stained smear showing homozygous 9p21 deletion: increased copy numbers of chromosomes 3 (red), 7 (green), and 17 (blue), and complete loss of 9p21 (gold); benign reference cell with two intact 9p21 signals in the upper-right corner.

specimens, are performed in laboratories providing these tests. Use of cell block material can be helpful for ICC but it should be noted that fixation differences may cause differences in results and, in particular, issues with false negative staining {95,804}. Cytopathology specimens, including FNAB smears, are well suited for molecular methods {8,779,741A, 347,778}. Formalin fixation is recommended for ICC with BAP1 and MTAP because they are sensitive to fixatives and may be leached with alcohol {154}.

It is important to note that any of these ancillary tests can be used to distinguish mesothelioma from benign mesothelial proliferations but none of them are appropriate for distinguishing mesothelioma from other malignant tumours and should only be used to support a diagnosis of mesothelioma once mesothelial lineage has been established through other ancillary tests.

Primary germ cell tumours of the mediastinum

Engels M
Hiroshima K
Monaco SE

Definition

Primary germ cell tumours of the mediastinum include seminoma and non-seminomatous carcinomas, including yolk sac tumour, choriocarcinoma and mixed germ cell tumour, and have the same morphology and ICC as primary gonadal germ cell tumours.

Seminoma is a malignant neoplasm composed of cells resembling primordial germ cells.

Embryonal carcinoma is a malignant neoplasm composed of large primitive cells of epithelial appearance, resembling cells of the embryonic germ disc.

Yolk sac tumours can occur in extragonadal sites, such as the mediastinum, as a primary or metastatic tumour.

Choriocarcinoma is a highly malignant trophoblastic neoplasm composed of cytotrophoblast, syncytiotrophoblast, and variably intermediate trophoblast.

Teratoma is a germ cell tumour composed of somatic tissues derived from two or three of the germ layers; it may be mature and composed exclusively of mature, adult-type tissues, or immature, containing immature embryonic or fetal tissues either exclusively or in addition to mature tissues.

Mixed germ cell tumours are neoplasms composed of two or more types of germ cell tumours.

Clinical features and imaging

See Table 7.10 (p. 164).

Histopathology

Each of the germ cell tumours can occur in a pure form or in mixed germ cell tumours.

Seminoma is composed of round to polygonal tumour cells with oval, central, non-overlapping nuclei with one or more large central nucleoli, frequently with a lymphoid infiltrate and a granulomatous reaction.

Embryonal carcinoma is composed of solid sheets or tubules or papillae, consisting of large, pleomorphic tumour cells with pleomorphic nuclei and prominent nucleoli, often in a background of haemorrhage and necrosis.

Yolk sac tumours have a variety of morphological growth patterns, most commonly reticular but also including microcystic, macrocystic, solid, glandular/alveolar, endodermal sinus with characteristic Schiller–Duval bodies, papillary, myxomatous, polyvesicular vitelline, hepatoid, and enteric.

Choriocarcinoma consists of cytotrophoblasts and syncytiotrophoblasts typically intermingled in a bilaminar plexiform pattern or in disordered sheets.

Mature teratoma consists of two or three of the mature germ layers throughout the tumour in a haphazard distribution, most commonly skin and cutaneous appendages lining cysts, and also bronchial mucosa, gastrointestinal mucosa, brain tissue, smooth muscle, and adipose tissue. Granulomatous inflammation may be found in association with ruptured cysts.

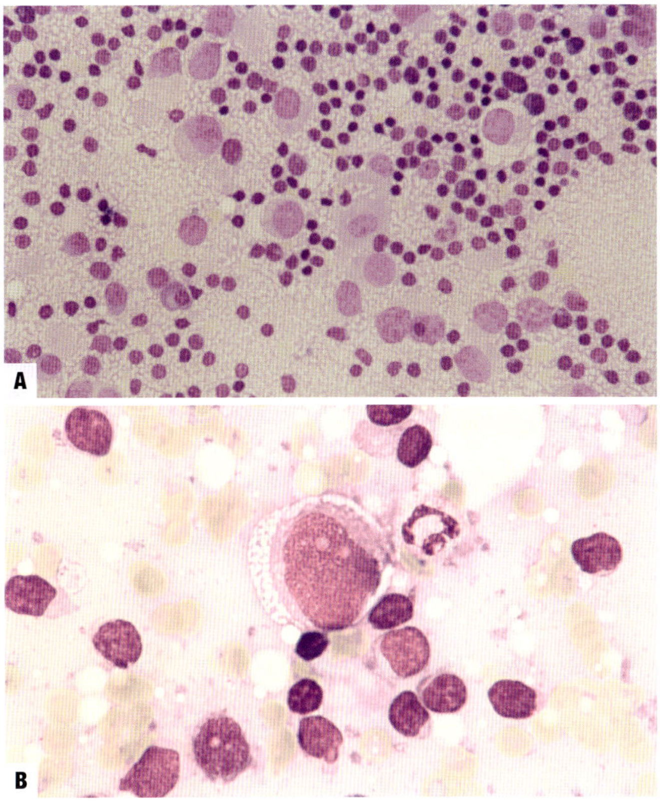

Fig. 7.75 Seminoma. **A** Seminoma as dispersed single cells in a tigroid background with lymphocytes (imprint of a lymph node, Giemsa). **B** Single large cell with a high N:C ratio and an irregular nucleus with two nucleoli, in a background of lymphocytes (imprint of a lymph node, Giemsa).

Immature teratomas contain embryonic tissues derived from the various germ layers such as immature glands, fetal lung, primitive cartilage, rhabdomyoblasts and blastema-like stromal cells, and (most commonly) neuroectodermal tissue.

A germ cell tumour can be accompanied by a non–germ cell or somatic-type malignant component of sarcoma or carcinoma. Somatic-type solid carcinomas and sarcomas occur more commonly in association with mature teratomas and less commonly with immature teratomas, choriocarcinomas, yolk sac tumours, and embryonal carcinomas, but not with seminomas. Rhabdomyosarcoma is the most frequent sarcoma, and carcinomas include adenocarcinoma, adenosquamous carcinoma, and squamous cell carcinoma. A germ cell tumour can be accompanied by haematological malignancies that are clonally related to the underlying germ cell tumours, although these have not been reported in the cytopathology literature.

Key diagnostic cytopathological features

Seminoma

- Moderate to high cellularity with a homogeneous cell population
- Predominantly dispersed malignant cells, some flat sheets

Table 7.10 Clinical and imaging findings and ancillary testing for germ cell tumours

Diagnosis	Clinical findings	Imaging features	Ancillary testing: immunocytochemistry (ICC)
Seminoma	Men in their third or fourth decade of life Most patients symptomatic on presentation Symptoms correlate with tumour size Metastasis in 20–40%, predominantly in cervical lymph nodes Serum AFP and β-hCG normal in pure seminoma, AFP could be elevated with liver metastasis {590,230,889,765,814}	Mass in the anterior mediastinum Homogeneous mass without calcification, indistinguishable from malignant lymphoma {873,765}	Positive for OCT3/4, SALL4, and KIT (CD117) Focal positivity for CAM5.2 keratin in a dot-like pattern Negative for SOX2, AFP, GPC3, CD30, and β-hCG {498,882,370,971}
Embryonal carcinoma	Young male patients Most patients symptomatic on presentation Metastasis in 50%, predominantly pulmonary Elevated serum AFP in all patients Elevated β-hCG in some patients {589,765,814}	Mass in the anterior mediastinum Locally invasive heterogeneous mass {873,765}	Positive for CAM5.2 keratin, OCT3/4, SALL4, SOX2, and CD30 Negative for KIT (CD117) {498,795,763,589}
Yolk sac tumour	Rare in its pure form More commonly occurs as a component of mixed germ cell tumour Metastatic yolk sac tumour found at presentation in 10–20% of children with testicular germ cell tumour, typically with haematogenous spread to the lung Aggressive course Disease monitoring with serum AFP levels Specific chemotherapy treatment regimens {1008,844,44}	Cystic or centrally necrotic mass in the anterior mediastinum Metastatic foci in the thorax Recommended: scrotal or pelvic ultrasound to exclude a primary gonadal tumour {497}	Diffuse strong staining for pancytokeratin, SALL4, and GPC3 Many cases positive for AFP, but AFP is negative in 38% of yolk sac tumours ZBTB16 and HNF1β: sensitive markers for yolk sac tumour Positive for TTF1 and CDX2 in some cases Negative for OCT3/4 {400,970,989,774,844,661}
Choriocarcinoma	Lung: common site for metastases of gestational choriocarcinoma Primary pulmonary choriocarcinoma in male patients is extremely rare Rapid growth of tumour Highly elevated serum β-hCG level {230,847,107,889,407,282,234,1031}	Mass in the anterior and posterior mediastinum {588,1024}	CK7 and β-hCG positive in both tumour subpopulations Cytotrophoblasts: positive for GATA3, SALL4, and p63, and negative for α-inhibin Syncytiotrophoblasts: negative for SALL4 and p63 and positive for α-inhibin, variable staining for GATA3 {759,40,968,841,869,556}
Teratoma	All age groups, predominantly the third and fourth decades of life *Mature teratoma {587,889,763}:* Equal sex distribution Causes minor or no symptoms in many patients Often an incidental finding Benign course in most patients after curative resection, regardless of patient age *Immature teratoma {230,763}:* Benign course in infants and children Aggressive course in adults	Anterior mediastinum *Mature teratoma {765}:* Rounded mass with sharp margination from the lung Calcifications in 20–40% *Immature teratoma {873}:* Solid mass	Useful for characterizing immature components of a teratoma S100 and synaptophysin positive in immature neural components Desmin and myogenin positive in muscle components S100 and GFAP positive in cartilaginous and neurogenic components {763}
Mixed germ cell tumour	Young male patients Most patients symptomatic at presentation Elevated serum tumour markers in 90% {589,765,415,889}	Mass in the anterior mediastinum Locally invasive heterogeneous mass {873,765}	Each single component shows ICC identical to that of the pure form
Germ cell tumour with somatic-type solid malignancy	Young male patients Metastatic at the time of diagnosis Elevated serum tumour markers {295,28,435,810,311}	Mass in the anterior mediastinum	ICC of the corresponding germ cell tumour ICC of the corresponding sarcoma or carcinoma

GPC3, glypican-3; TTF1, thyroid transcription factor 1.

- Large cells with fragile cytoplasm and plentiful stripped large nuclei with prominent nucleoli
- Typical tigroid background consisting of crushed cytoplasm full of glycogen (Giemsa)
- Numerous small mature lymphocytes and small epithelioid histiocytes in a granulomatous background

Reference(s): {143,110,763,370,11}

Embryonal carcinoma

- Often highly cellular smears
- Malignant cells arranged in flat sheets or 3D tissue fragments or papillary or acinar tissue fragments
- Large pleomorphic nuclei with coarse chromatin and prominent nucleoli
- Numerous mitotic figures, may be atypical
- Necrosis and haemorrhage in the background

Reference(s): {763,765,11}

Yolk sac tumour

- Loosely cohesive tissue fragments with occasional alveolar-type spaces, glands or microcysts, and stripped nuclei
- Cytoplasm shows microvacuolization and is fragile
- Round to irregular nuclei, less uniform than seminomas (except for the hepatoid variant), with plentiful stripped nuclei
- Cells lining the spaces tend to have more compressed nuclei or endometrioid features
- Background shows string-like metachromatic material, hyaline globules, and basophilic proteinaceous fluid (Giemsa)
- Syncytiotrophoblast, granulomas, and prominent lymphocytes have only rarely been described

Reference(s): {995,874,186,116}

Choriocarcinoma

- Background of abundant necrosis and inflammatory cells including neutrophils and lymphocytes
- Cytotrophoblast and/or intermediate trophoblast is seen as tissue fragments or isolated medium-sized, mononucleated cells with indistinct cell borders, vesicular (Pap) nuclei showing perinucleolar clearing, prominent nucleoli, and moderate pale cytoplasm
- Syncytiotrophoblast consists of large giant cells with bizarre shapes, hyperchromatic pleomorphic mononucleated or multinucleated nuclei, irregular nuclear membranes, indistinct cell borders, and abundant cytoplasm

Reference(s): {543,270,135}

Mature teratoma

- Usually low cellularity

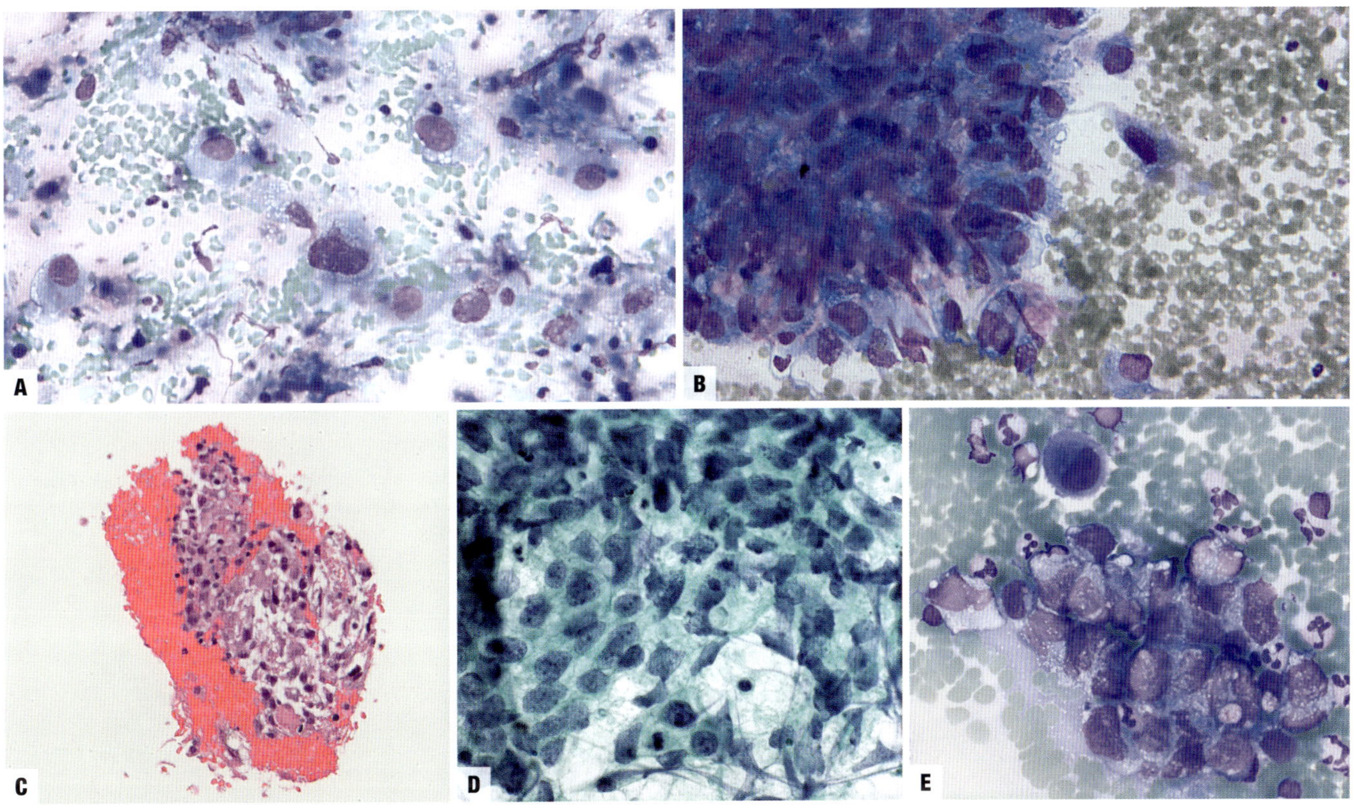

Fig. 7.76 Yolk sac tumour. **A** Metastasis to the lung showing dispersed single cells with marked nuclear pleomorphism, prominent macronucleoli, and moderate cytoplasm containing small, discrete cytoplasmic vacuoles, in a background of metachromatic material and blood (Giemsa). **B** Metastasis to the lung showing a tissue fragment demonstrating crowding, and cells with finely foamy to granular cytoplasm and prominent nuclear pleomorphism in a bloody background (Giemsa). **C** Metastasis to the lung showing a tissue fragment of tumour cells with cytoplasmic clearing, prominent sieve-like spaces, and rare hyaline globules (cell block, H&E). **D** Crowded tissue fragment consisting of tumour cells with enlarged pleomorphic nuclei and pale, glassy cytoplasm with variably defined cell borders. Mitoses are present. Final diagnosis on excision was mixed germ cell tumour with yolk sac tumour and mature teratoma (Pap). **E** Same patient as in Panel D. A crowded tissue fragment of tumour cells with pleomorphic nuclei and a variable amount of finely vacuolated cytoplasm (Giemsa).

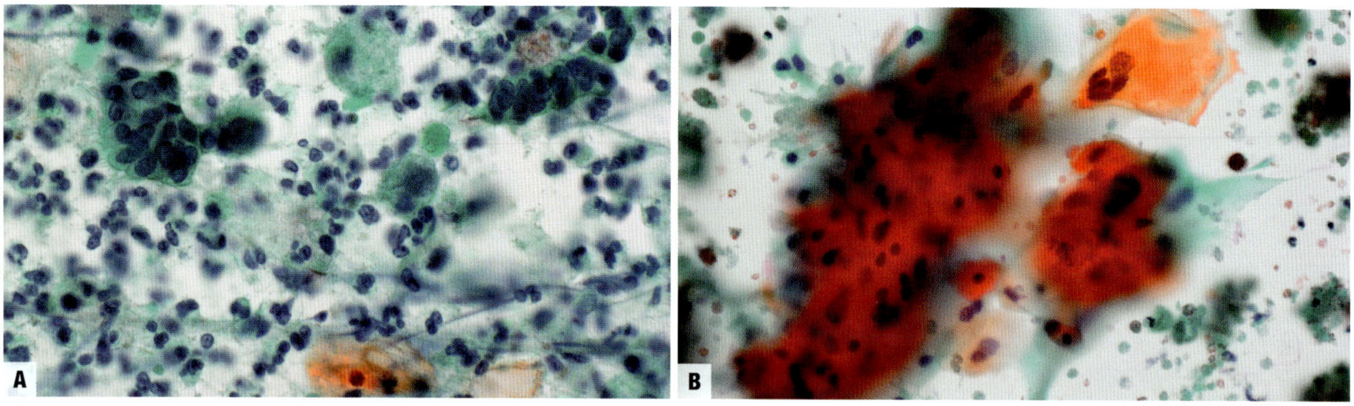

Fig. 7.77 **A** Mature teratoma. Tissue fragments of ciliated columnar bronchial epithelium associated with many inflammatory cells, histiocytes, and occasional keratinized squamous epithelial cells (Pap). **B** Teratoma with somatic-type malignancy. Squamous cell carcinoma present in a teratoma. Tissue fragments and single cells are keratinized, with variably sized hyperchromatic or pyknotic nuclei in a background of cellular debris (Pap).

- Mature squamous epithelium, mature columnar epithelium, cells of choroid and glial tissue, stromal fragments, and adipose tissue
- Background may be mucoid owing to mature mucin-producing glands, or thick and proteinaceous with keratinous debris

Reference(s): {307,763,11}

Immature teratoma

- High cellularity, small blue cell tumour
- Tissue fragments and rosettes
- Small, round to oval tumour cells
- Bland nuclei and high N:C ratio
- Focal neuropil matrix

Reference(s): {724,824,11,121}

Mixed germ cell tumours

- Various types of germ cell tumours in any combination
- Cytomorphology of each single component is identical to that of the pure form

Discussion and differential diagnosis

Seminoma is the second most common mediastinal germ cell tumour, and a pure seminoma has an excellent prognosis. In FNAB, sampling error may pose a problem as other components of a mixed germ cell tumour may be missed. Elevated levels of serum AFP or β-hCG suggest a diagnosis of mixed germ cell tumour. In hypocellular smears the typical tigroid background can be difficult to identify. The differential diagnosis includes melanoma, poorly differentiated large cell carcinoma, and malignant lymphoma. Metastasis of a testicular primary should always be considered {765,590}.

The differential diagnosis of embryonal carcinoma includes poorly differentiated adenocarcinoma, thymic carcinoma, and other malignant germ cell tumours. Distinction from metastatic carcinomas requires clinical, imaging, and serological

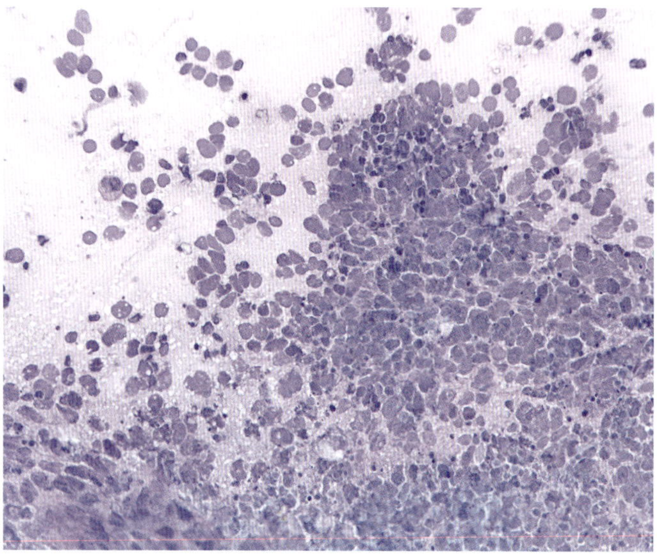

Fig. 7.78 Immature teratoma. Intraoperative touch preparation from metastasis to the pleural cavity and mediastinum, showing sheets of crowded undifferentiated cells with a high N:C ratio and irregular nuclei with granular chromatin, and some apoptosis (touch preparation, Giemsa).

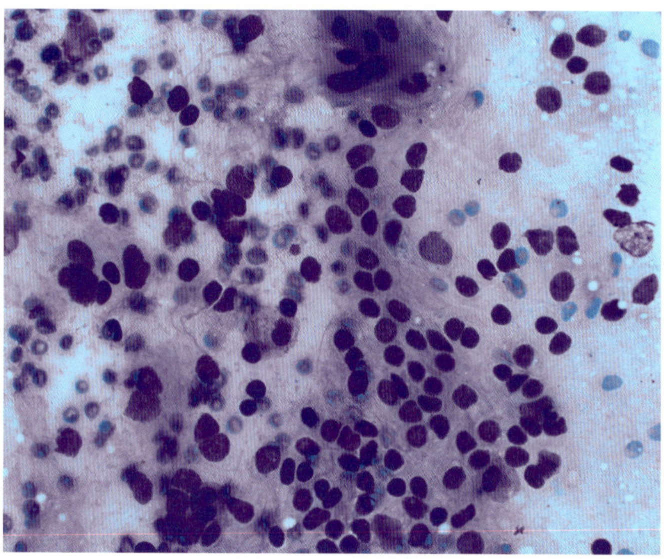

Fig. 7.79 Mixed germ cell tumour. Small blue round cells suspended in a chondromyxoid and fibrillary background, corresponding to the immature teratoma in small biopsy fragments within the cell block. Other areas showed basaloid cells and crush artefact corresponding to the embryonal carcinoma (touch preparation, Giemsa).

correlation. Elevated levels of AFP and β-hCG suggest an embryonal carcinoma {11,589}.

The differential diagnosis of yolk sac tumours includes other subtypes of germ cell tumours, such as yolk sac tumours with a hepatoid pattern or a lymphoid background mimicking seminomas {929,928,116,400}. The hyaline globules and ICC help to identify yolk sac tumours {929}. Rare forms of yolk sac tumours with a sarcomatoid pattern can occur after prior treatment {928}. A glandular pattern in yolk sac tumours can closely resemble the endometrioid, intestinal/enteric, or alveolar morphology seen in other tumours, but adenocarcinomas tend to be more mucinous {518}. The ropy metachromatic (Giemsa) material in yolk sac tumours mimics that seen in mesenchymal tumours, renal cell carcinomas, and salivary gland–type tumours {581}.

Choriocarcinoma can mimic sarcomatoid carcinomas with giant cell features, but giant cell carcinomas show a continuum between smaller or medium-sized tumour cells and the larger giant cells rather than the dual presence of cytotrophoblast and syncytiotrophoblast.

Teratoma is the most common mediastinal germ cell tumour. Mature teratomas are easily diagnosed in cases with squamous cells, columnar cells, stromal fragments, and adipose tissue. If a cystic component of a mature teratoma is sampled, the cyst fluid may be hypocellular and the diagnosis may be missed. A ruptured cyst in a mature teratoma containing squamous epithelium may lead to a granulomatous reaction. Important differential diagnoses are other cystic lesions of the mediastinum. If the diagnosis of a mature teratoma is considered, the slides should be searched carefully for any immature component. The cytopathological findings should be correlated with clinical, imaging, and serological findings. Immature teratoma has a differential diagnosis of a small blue cell tumour, and in the paediatric age group, neuroblastoma, embryonal rhabdomyosarcoma, Wilms tumour, Ewing sarcoma, and malignant lymphoma have to be excluded {307,824}.

Mixed germ cell tumours may be missed in cytopathology if only one of the components is sampled, and thorough sampling of different areas of the tumour, if possible, is required. If two or more subtypes of germ cell tumour are found in FNAB or there are elevated serum markers that are discordant from the cytomorphological findings, a mixed germ cell tumour should be strongly considered. For example, elevated serum AFP in a patient with a diagnosis of seminoma should lead to a review of all slides and correlation to clinical and imaging findings {121,862,11}.

Somatic-type solid malignancies found combined with germ cell tumours may not be distinguishable in FNAB cytopathology from metastatic carcinoma or sarcoma from a different primary site {334}.

Ancillary testing

See Table 7.10 (p. 164).

With limited material, a panel including pancytokeratin, OCT3/4, glypican-3 (GPC3), and AFP is recommended. A seminomatous component is positive for OCT3/4 and negative for AFP and GPC3, whereas a yolk sac tumour component is positive for AFP and GPC3 and negative for OCT3/4. KIT (CD117) can stain yolk sac tumours and is not a reliable marker to distinguish yolk sac tumours from seminoma.

Primary angiosarcoma of the lung

Geisinger KR
Monaco SE

Definition

Primary angiosarcoma of the lung is a very rare high-grade malignant soft tissue tumour with vasoformative features or endothelial differentiation.

Clinical features and imaging

Almost all primary and metastatic angiosarcomas occur in adults. Manifestations include haemoptysis, cough, shortness of breath, and chest pain. In the thorax, angiosarcomas may occur in association with chronic lymphoedema or after radiation exposure, particularly in the setting of prior breast carcinoma {433}. Rare cases of angiosarcoma involving the pleura or pericardium have been described {86,727}. Most angiosarcomas in the lung represent metastases from previously diagnosed tumours.

The most common imaging finding is that of multiple nodules, often bilateral, which may include calcifications or cavitation. Less often, a solitary nodule or mass is identified. In either case, extension to the pleura is common. Very infrequently, a dominant pattern of air space infiltration is recognized. On MRI, these tumours may appear bright on T1- and T2-weighted images, depending on the amount of haemorrhage.

Histopathology

Angiosarcomas are high-grade neoplasms that need to be distinguished from lower-grade epithelioid haemangioendothelioma. At low magnification, a spectrum of vasoformative features is usually present, from obvious small-calibre vessels to slit-like spaces to large blood-containing spaces, and papillary and micropapillary growth may also be present. But in some instances, a solid architecture is present. The cells may be predominantly epithelioid or spindle or an admixture of the two, and cytoplasmic lumina are characteristic. Nuclei tend to be elongated and show marked hyperchromasia and pleomorphism.

Key diagnostic cytopathological features

- Variable cellularity; may be low if blood lakes or necrotic foci are sampled
- Single cells, loosely cohesive tissue fragments with irregular outlines, and tissue fragments with irregular vascular spaces
- Spindle, elongated tumour cells with oval nuclei and indistinct borders can be seen arranged in very poorly formed fascicles in solid areas
- Epithelioid polygonal tumour cells with moderate to plentiful cytoplasm and more distinct borders; may appear plasmacytoid and have cytoplasmic lumina
- Nuclei are round, elongated to pleomorphic, with coarse chromatin
- Characteristically, irregular nucleoli are oval or bar-shaped and possess delicate chromatin extensions connecting

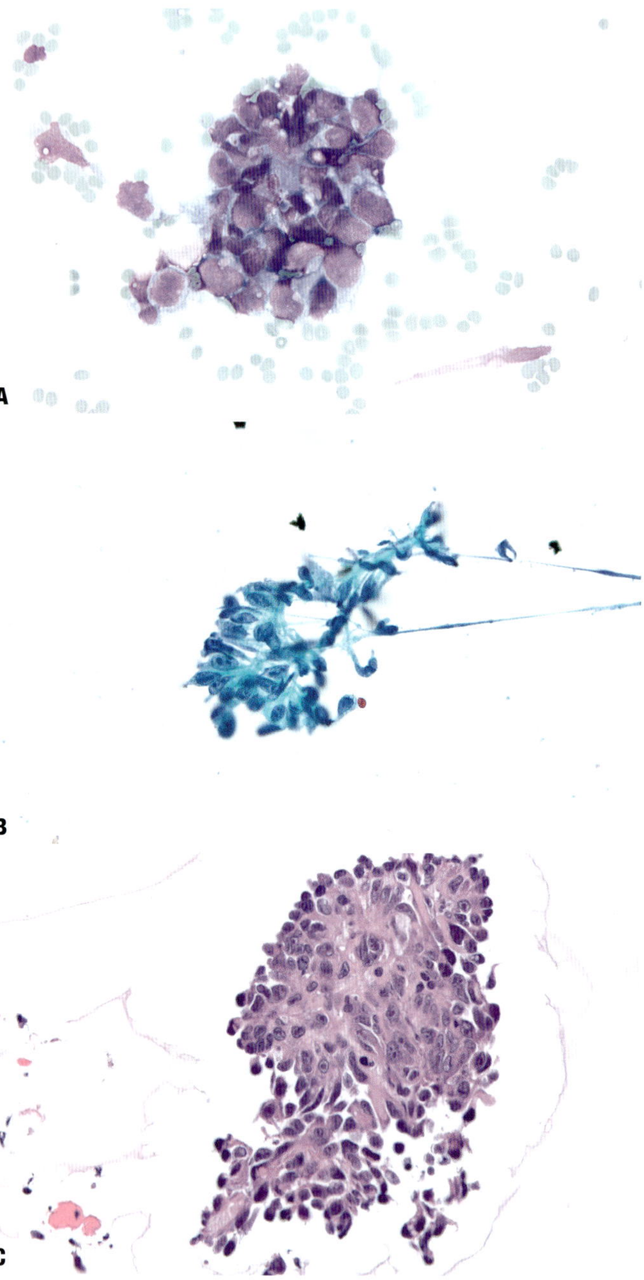

A B C

Fig. 7.80 Angiosarcoma. **A** Small crowded tissue fragment of cells that are relatively uniform in size, with a high N:C ratio and single, highly pleomorphic nuclei with fine chromatin, variably prominent nucleoli, and a suggestion of nuclear pseudoinclusions in some nuclei. The pale blue eccentric cytoplasm in some cells is vacuolated (Giemsa). **B** Tissue fragment consisting of cells that range from polygonal to spindle, with large ovoid to elongated, highly pleomorphic nuclei with finely granular chromatin and often prominent and large nucleoli (Pap). **C** Tissue fragment shows crowded, often epithelioid cells with relatively dense cytoplasm that in some cells contains vacuoles or rudimentary lumina. The nuclei are large and highly pleomorphic, with large nucleoli (cell block, H&E).

to the nuclear membrane, imparting a spider-like nuclear appearance
- Cytoplasmic vacuoles may contain erythrocytes or segmented leukocytes
- Haemosiderophages

Reference(s): {86,939,283}

Discussion and differential diagnosis

The differential diagnosis includes both carcinomas and other sarcomas, especially those with a spindle cell component. The epithelioid forms need to be distinguished from non-small cell carcinomas, especially those with slit-like luminal spaces seen in tissue fragments. Epithelioid haemangioendothelioma has lower-grade nuclei and lacks large irregular nucleoli, whereas abnormal mitotic figures favour angiosarcoma. Melanoma and plasmablastic lymphomas enter the differential diagnosis especially with angiosarcomas that show prominent discohesion and single cells, although these entities show prominent nucleoli that tend to be round and centrally placed.

Ancillary testing

Angiosarcoma expresses endothelial markers, including CD31, CD34, ERG, and FLI1, but may be positive for pankeratin, which is a potential pitfall in the differential diagnosis from carcinoma. Angiosarcoma is negative for CAMTA1, which is typically positive in epithelioid haemangioendothelioma, due to the *CAMTA1::WWTR1* translocation.

Pulmonary and thoracic metastases

Baloch ZW
Geisinger KR

Definition

Pulmonary and thoracic metastases represent spread to the lungs and thorax of malignancies that arise in other sites.

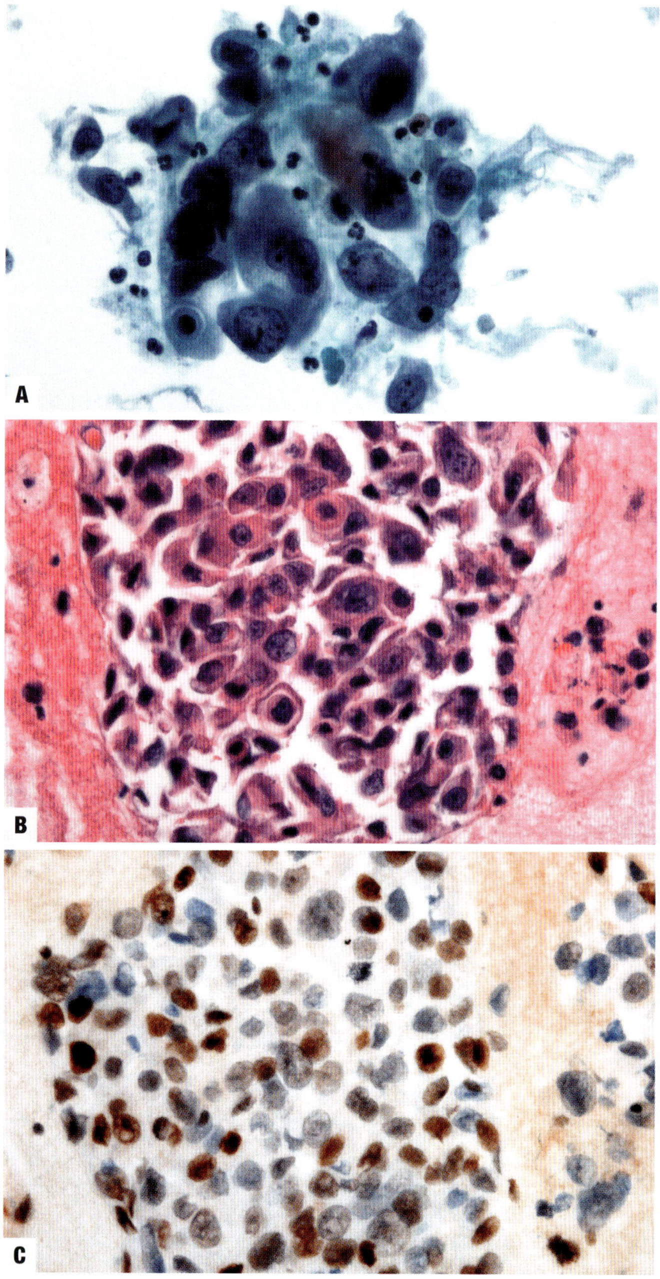

Fig. 7.81 Metastatic breast carcinoma. **A** Discohesive tissue fragment of pleomorphic tumour cells (Pap). **B** Tissue fragment of tumour cells with marked nuclear pleomorphism and no glandular architecture (cell block, H&E). **C** Tissue fragment showing positive nuclear immunostain for GATA3, confirming the diagnosis of metastatic breast carcinoma to lung (cell block).

Clinical features and imaging

Although primary pulmonary carcinomas are common lethal neoplasms, metastases to the lungs are much more frequent occurrences and are associated with very high mortality rates. When assessing any carcinoma of the lung, the cytomorphology and ICC findings should always be correlated assiduously with the clinical history of any previous carcinoma or other malignancy, as well as with the imaging. Adenocarcinomas are the most common histopathological type of metastasis to the lung, including breast, colorectal, and renal cell, and along with head and neck carcinomas are the most frequent sites of origin to produce metastatic deposits, but essentially any type of cancer may spread to involve lungs in all age groups. Many patients with pulmonary metastases are asymptomatic and the lung lesions are initially detected via staging or surveillance imaging. However, in other patients the presenting symptoms most commonly include cough, chest pain, and shortness of breath, and less commonly include haemoptysis and pneumothorax, thus mirroring the manifestations of primary tumours. Most metastases evolve through haematogenous spread in variably sized veins of the caval system, but less often lymphatic vessels or arteries are the routes.

The classic and most common imaging findings are peripherally located multiple, bilateral nodules of variable size with rather smooth, rounded contours. However, it must be remembered that primary carcinomas may spread, producing multiple masses, and patients may, rarely, have two synchronously developed lung primaries {254,540,404,899}. The lower lung fields are preferentially involved. Imaging may show a solitary mass, which may appear solid with or without foci of necrosis {272}, and metastases (most often from a squamous cell carcinomas primary in the head and neck) may appear cavitated {299}. The metastatic nodules can be associated with a prominent feeding vessel {272}. Typically, metastatic nodules are smaller than a primary mass but grow more rapidly than non-small cell carcinomas. When tumour spread occurs largely or exclusively in small blood vessels or lymphatics, imaging identifies linear densities rather than a mass. In contrast to primary tumours, which classically manifest a spiculated imaging, metastases have smooth contours. Metastases are usually not associated with hilar adenopathy. For some patients, pleural effusions are the dominant imaging feature.

Histopathology

The morphology of pulmonary metastases generally mirrors that of the primary neoplasm.

Key diagnostic cytopathological features

- Breast carcinomas commonly present as poorly differentiated adenocarcinomas, with minute tissue fragments arranged in single file or in small nests, and (frequently) single cell dispersal; the cells often have a high N:C ratio and eccentric cytoplasm, with some showing vacuoles

- Gastric adenocarcinomas tend to be moderately to poorly differentiated with less well formed glands, and more diffuse types may show signet-ring cells with large single vacuoles in the eccentric cytoplasm impinging on the nucleus
- Colorectal carcinoma is typically moderately differentiated, with distinct glandular structures consisting of oriented columnar cells with elongated pleomorphic nuclei in a background of necrosis and mucin
- Pancreatic adenocarcinomas tend to be poorly differentiated, with poorly formed glands and high-grade pleomorphic nuclei, vacuoles, necrosis, and mucin
- Renal cell carcinoma is most commonly of the clear cell type, with large cells that have abundant eosinophilic or variably vacuolated cytoplasm and large, often central, round to pleomorphic nuclei with prominent single nucleoli
- Prostate adenocarcinoma usually shows an acinar pattern, with cuboidal cells and peripherally sited, round to mildly pleomorphic nuclei, but nuclear grade can be high with prominent single nucleoli
- Urothelial carcinoma is usually poorly differentiated, with cells showing prominent eosinophilic cytoplasm that can resemble squamous cells with large pleomorphic nuclei
- Papillary thyroid carcinoma can display a spectrum of cytopathological features often encountered in well-differentiated pulmonary adenocarcinoma; the cells from both can show round to oval nuclei, powdery chromatin, small and eccentrically placed nucleoli, and intranuclear grooves and pseudoinclusions; in addition, psammoma bodies can be seen in both papillary thyroid carcinoma and well-differentiated pulmonary adenocarcinoma; thyroid transcription factor 1 (TTF1) will be expressed in both tumours, but PAX8 and thyroglobulin are positive in the thyroid metastasis
- Melanoma metastases usually show high cellularity with single dispersed cells that typically are plasmacytoid, with large nuclei that vary from round to highly pleomorphic with plentiful binucleation, parachromatin clearing, and intranuclear cytoplasmic pseudoinclusions; melanin pigment in tumour cells is variably present and must be distinguished from haemosiderin pigment in macrophages; rare cases of metastatic melanoma, especially amelanotic types, can demonstrate a rich capillary framework and papillary formations leading to an expanded differential including primary and metastatic neoplasms of lung with papillary growth architecture

Reference(s): {153,742,465,800,360}

Discussion and differential diagnosis

Metastatic adenocarcinomas to the lung originating from various extrapulmonary sites are known to mimic primary lung adenocarcinomas. Metastatic adenocarcinoma from the breast, prostate, gastrointestinal tract, colorectum, and kidney can be easily mistaken for primary lung adenocarcinoma, but there are some cytopathological clues that suggest particular adenocarcinomas.

It is virtually impossible to distinguish between primary and metastatic squamous cell carcinoma of the lung by cytomorphology and ICC. This requires a thorough clinical and imaging correlation.

Adenoid cystic carcinoma, with its classic features of basaloid cells arranged in a cribriform growth pattern with globules of basement membrane–like material, can be easily recognized as a metastatic tumour in a patient with a known history. However, the high-grade forms of this tumour may be challenging to differentiate from primary adenocarcinomas of lung and from the very rare primary adenoid cystic carcinoma of lung.

Primary pulmonary lymphoid neoplasms are rare and account for < 1% of all lung tumours. Lung involvement by lymphomas from the haematopoietic system are far more common and spread via haematogenous dissemination from other sites or through direct invasion from involved hilar or mediastinal lymph nodes. When a lymphoproliferative disorder is suspected, an aliquot of the specimen should be submitted for flow cytometry and FISH {794,702}.

In the paediatric population, > 95% of all malignant pulmonary tumours represent metastases from non-pulmonary tumours. The list includes adrenocortical carcinoma, thyroid carcinoma, germ cell tumours, neuroblastoma, nephroblastoma, and osteosarcoma. Some of these tumours display small blue cell morphology and can mimic primary neuroendocrine tumours (NETs) of the lung {973}.

Some primary tumours may manifest a histopathological spectrum of differentiation, with only a certain clonal fraction

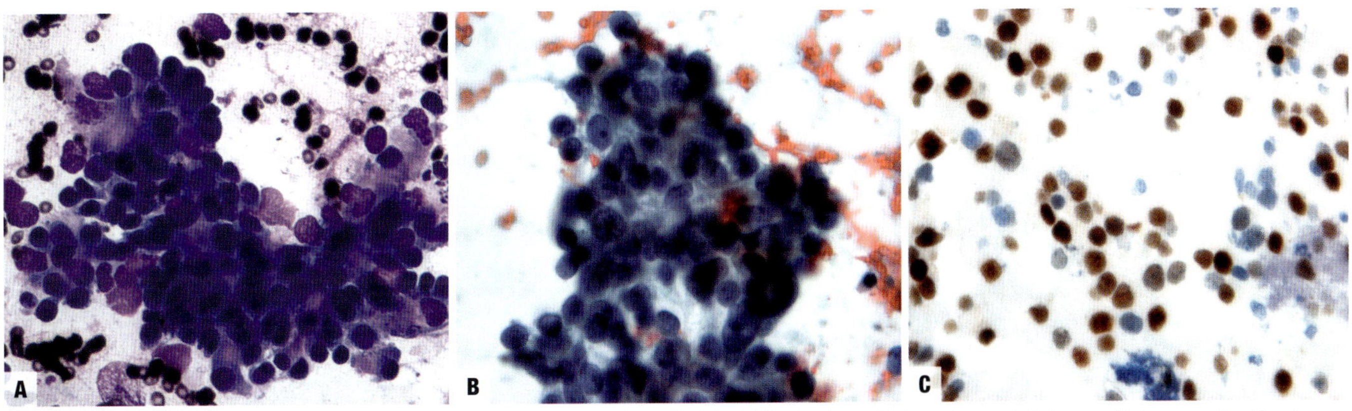

Fig. 7.82 Metastatic prostate adenocarcinoma. **A** FNAB of lung nodule in a patient with rising PSA, showing a 3D tissue fragment of pleomorphic tumour cells with acinar architecture (Giemsa). **B** Tumour fragment showing round, moderately pleomorphic tumour cells with prominent nucleoli and an acinar architecture (Pap). **C** Cell block preparation showing nuclear expression of NKX3-1, confirming prostate origin.

Table 7.11 Immunocytopathology of pulmonary metastases {825,490,399,945,865,168}

Site of origin	Immunocytochemistry profile[a]
Gastrointestinal tract	
Oesophagus (adenocarcinoma)	CK7+, CK20−, TTF1−, CDX2+/−, CEA+, EMA (MUC1)−/+, MUC5AC−/+, SATB2−
Stomach	CK7+, CK20+, TTF1−, CEA+, CDX2−/+, EMA (MUC1)−/+, MUC5AC−/+
Colon and rectum	CK7−, CK20+, CDX2+, SATB2+, MOC31+
Breast	CK7+, CK20−, GATA3+, mammaglobin+/−, GCDFP-15−/+, ER+, PR+, TTF1
Melanoma	SOX10+, melan-A+, MART1+, S100+, HMB45+, CK7−, CK20−
Pancreas (adenocarcinoma)	CK7+, CK20+, SMAD4 (DPC4)−/+, CK17+/−, VHL protein−, maspin+, S100+, MOC31+, MUC5AC+
Liver (hepatocellular)	CK7−, CK20−, HepPar1+, AFP+, GPC3+, ARG1+, CD10+, polyclonal CEA+, monoclonal CEA−
Genitourinary tract	
Urinary bladder (urothelial)	CK7+, CK20+/−, GATA3+, p63+, p40+, CK5/6+, S100+, 34βE12 (CK903)+, uroplakin+, thrombomodulin+
Prostate (adenocarcinoma)	CK7−, CK20−, PSA+, NKX3-1+, PAP+, AMACR (P504S)+
Ovary (serous)	CK7+, CK20−, PAX8+, ER+, WT1+, TTF1−, TFF3−, GATA3−
Ovary (clear cell)	CK7+, CK20−, VHL protein+, napsin A+, WT1−, ER−, AFP−
Ovary (mucinous)	CK7+, CK20−, SMAD4 (DPC4)+, CA125+, CDX2+/−
Endometrium	CK7+, CK20−, ER+, PR+, PAX8+, CEA+ (foci of squamous metaplasia)
Uterine cervix (adenocarcinoma)	CK7+, CK20−, p16+, CEA+, PR−, PAX8+/−
Kidney	
Clear cell	CK7−, PAX8+, PAX2+, CAIX+, CD10+, RCCm+, AE1/AE3+, CAM5.2+, EMA+, AMACR+/−, GATA3−, TTF1−
Clear cell papillary	CK7+, PAX8+, CAIX+, CD10−, RCCm+/−, AMACR−, GATA3−/+ (rare cases)
Papillary renal cell	CK7+, PAX8+, CAIX+/−, CD10+, RCCm+, AMACR+, GATA3−
Thyroid	
Papillary or follicular	CK7+, CK20−, TTF1+, PAX8+, thyroglobulin+
Medullary	CK7+, TTF1+, PAX8−, calcitonin+, CEA+, synaptophysin+, chromogranin+, thyroglobulin−
Germ cell tumours	KIT (CD117)+, OCT4+, CD30+, GPC3+, PLAP+, SALL4+

ARG1, arginase-1; GPC3, glypican-3; TTF1, thyroid transcription factor 1.
[a]It is preferable that all immunostains be validated on cytopathology preparations.

spreading and developing metastases. Thus, whenever prior histopathological, cytopathological, or ICC slides exist, it is prudent to review the preceding slides or digital images when evaluating a new lung lesion, and always to closely check the patient's history for previous malignancies.

Although rare, some primary tumours are known to frequently metastasize to lungs, including choriocarcinoma, uterine leiomyosarcoma, Ewing sarcoma, osteosarcoma, and germ cell tumours.

Ancillary testing

In the majority of cases, the cytomorphological findings and ICC utilizing cell block material will elucidate the type and origin of tumour in the lung {471} (see Table 7.11).

Gastrointestinal adenocarcinoma producing copious amounts of mucin and containing mucinous cells can be impossible to differentiate from mucinous well-differentiated adenocarcinoma of lung. In some cases the ICC may be of little value, because TTF1 can be negative in a subset of mucinous adenocarcinomas of lung, which, however, are usually positive for napsin A. Both tumours will show positive CK20, CDX2, and MOC31 ICC.

Metastatic melanoma can be confirmed by positive S100, HMB45, melan-A (MART1), and SOX10.

There may be a role for p16 in distinguishing HPV-related head and neck squamous cell carcinomas from lung primaries, which are negative.

A panel of TTF1, CK7, KIT (CD117), and napsin A often proves helpful in arriving at a definite diagnosis to separate metastatic adenoid cystic carcinoma from a primary lung adenocarcinoma, which will be positive for TTF1 and napsin A and negative for KIT (CD117) and myoepithelial markers such as p63.

Sample reports: Malignant

Field AS
Bubendorf L

The sample reports provided here are based on the standardized cytopathology report in the *Diagnostic categories and report structure* (p. 8) section of the first chapter. See that section for a discussion on the structure and components.

These are sample reports that include the components required in one possible format; the final report format will depend on local practice and local laboratory information system requirements. For brevity, demographics and information on the macroscopic features and rapid onsite evaluation (ROSE) are not presented here.

Each institution should select a term for the main heading of the diagnostic summary, such as "Diagnostic summary" (as used in the examples below), "Diagnosis", or "Final diagnosis", and use it consistently.

Sample report 1

Type of specimen:
Sputum sample.

Clinical and imaging information:
30 mm mass in left upper lobe. No definite hilar lymphadenopathy. Smoker.

Diagnostic summary:
Category: Malignant
Diagnosis: Adenocarcinoma

Microscopic description:
Occasional crowded tissue fragments of large cells with large, highly pleomorphic nuclei and prominent single nucleoli, and with eccentric, pale, occasionally vacuolated cytoplasm, are present. Small bronchial sheets, siderophages, histiocytes, neutrophils, and squamous cells are also present. There is no mucin in the background.
Comment: Poorly differentiated adenocarcinoma is present. Correlation with imaging and clinical history is required. Further workup with FNAB is recommended to enable classification of the carcinoma.

Sample report 2

Type of specimen:
Bronchial brush.

Clinical and imaging information:
Smoker. Poorly defined mass in right middle lobe on routine CXR with hilar lymphadenopathy. Bronchial brush right middle lobe bronchus.

Diagnostic summary:
Bronchial brush right middle lobe bronchus
Category: Malignant
Diagnosis: Non-small cell carcinoma NOS

Microscopic description:
These highly cellular smears show occasional tissue fragments of intermediate-sized to large cells with variable (often high) N:C ratios, large pleomorphic nuclei, prominent nucleoli, and pale cytoplasm, with no definite squamous or glandular differentiation. Plentiful bronchial epithelial tissue fragments, neutrophils, and histiocytes, with some carbon-laden macrophages, are also present.
Comment: A poorly differentiated carcinoma is present, suggesting a non-small cell carcinoma of lung of uncertain type. There is no cell block available for ICC. FNAB is recommended to provide material for typing, staging, and ancillary tests.

Editorial note:
The diagnostic summary includes the specific information regarding the site of the lesion from the request form and specimen container of any needle-rinsing material.

Sample report 3

Type of specimen:
Endobronchial ultrasound–guided FNAB right upper lobe and subcarinal lymph node.

Clinical and imaging information:
Right upper lobe 30 mm mass FNAB. Lesion seen on CXR. Hilar lymphadenopathy. History of colonic cancer.

Diagnostic summary:

Specimen 1:
Subcarinal lymph node FNAB
Category: Malignant
Diagnosis: Metastatic small cell carcinoma

Specimen 2:
Right upper lobe 30 mm mass FNAB
Category: Malignant
Diagnosis: Small cell carcinoma of the lung

Microscopic description:

Specimen 1: These moderately cellular smears show metastatic small cell carcinoma in a lymphoid background.

Specimen 2: These moderately cellular smears show small cell carcinoma with tissue fragments of intermediate-sized cells with a high N:C ratio, pleomorphic nuclei showing finely dispersed chromatin and occasional small nucleoli, and poorly defined cytoplasm. There is chromatinic smearing and apoptosis is prominent. Occasional mitoses are seen.
Comment: Features are those of small cell carcinoma of lung.

Supplementary report 1:
Specimen 2: ICC on the cell block shows the carcinoma to be positive for thyroid transcription factor 1 (TTF1), chromogranin, and synaptophysin, and negative for p40, confirming small cell carcinoma of lung.

Editorial note:
The diagnostic summary includes the specific information regarding the site of the lesion from the request form and specimen container of any needle-rinsing material.
There has been a supplementary report on the ICC for this case performed subsequently on a cell block, and this is included in the single integrated report.

Sample report 4

Type of specimen:
Transthoracic FNAB left upper lobe of lung.

Clinical and imaging information:
Left upper lobe 30 mm solid mass transthoracic FNAB. Presented with haemoptysis. Prior history of colorectal carcinoma. ? metastasis.

Diagnostic summary:
Left upper lobe 30 mm solid mass transthoracic FNAB
Category: Malignant
Diagnosis: Adenocarcinoma of the lung

Microscopic description:
These highly cellular smears show moderately differentiated adenocarcinoma consisting of crowded sheets of large cells with a moderate N:C ratio and occasional vacuoles in the eccentric cytoplasm. There is no prominent necrosis or mucin.
Comment: Adenocarcinoma is present. ICC is underway on the cell block.

Supplementary report 1:
The adenocarcinoma in the cell block is positive for thyroid transcription factor 1 (TTF1), negative for p40, and negative for CDX2. Predictive biomarker analysis including PDL1 ICC and next-generation sequencing is underway.
Supplementary report 2:
The adenocarcinoma is negative for EGFR. PDL1 to follow.

Editorial note:
The diagnostic summary includes the specific information regarding the site of the lesion from the request form and specimen container of any needle-rinsing material.
There has been a supplementary report on the ICC for this case performed subsequently on a cell block, and a further supplementary report on the next-generation sequencing, and these are included in the single integrated report (for brevity, the full next-generation sequencing report has not been included here). If a further study such as a PDL1 is underway, this is noted in this report to alert the clinical team that a further report will be issued as an integrated report.

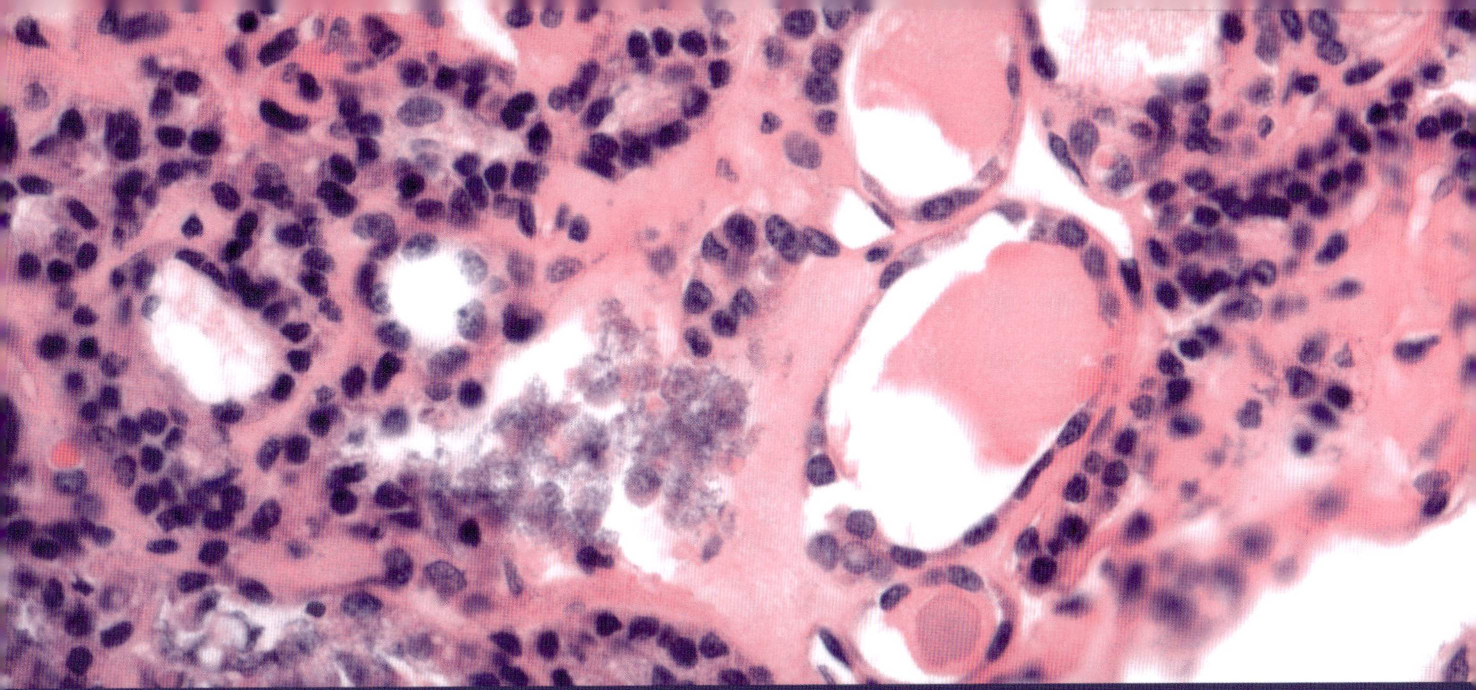

8

Management recommendations for each diagnostic category

Edited by: Chandra A, Field AS, Layfield LJ, Pitman MB, Satoh Y

Introduction

Bubendorf L
Engels M

Cytopathology plays a crucial role in the management of patients with symptomatology or imaging findings that suggest lung infection or carcinoma, particularly because lung infections do not require surgery and most patients with lung cancer present with advanced disease where surgical management is not appropriate {849}. Cytopathological samples and, where necessary, core needle biopsies or forceps biopsies are often the only material available for diagnosis, ICC, and predictive marker molecular studies. Cytopathology offers a variety of complementary sampling techniques that are often used in combination for the evaluation of patients with lung symptomatology and lesions seen on imaging {736,850}. In addition, cytopathological evaluation of intrathoracic lymph nodes utilizing endobronchial ultrasound guidance during bronchoscopy at the same time as FNAB of the mass lesion in the lung is an efficient and safe method for the staging of lung carcinoma, which in turn determines clinical management and prognosis. Evaluation of pleural effusion is also used for determining stage IV in lung cancer.

Appropriate management of cell material, methods, and procedures in patients who are suspected on clinical or imaging findings to have lung cancer is an important task for cytotechnologists and cytopathologists. The aims are the precise cytopathology and ICC diagnosis and accurate assessment of predictive biomarkers, to be achieved in the least invasive and most cost-effective manner, usually in a situation of a limited amount of material {93,778,940}. Notably, lung cytopathology does not only aim to diagnose or exclude lung cancer but can also serve as an important method for the rapid and inexpensive diagnosis of infectious diseases in all countries, especially in countries with low levels of medical infrastructure {257}. Recently published guidelines on the collection and handling of thoracic small biopsy and cytopathology specimens serve as a useful resource for the management of cytopathological specimens {778}.

Effective management of the patient depends not only on categorizing the findings and providing a precise cytopathological diagnosis, but also on the material type, the cellularity of individual specimens, and clinical factors such as general health status and correlation with imaging or microbiological findings {940}. The ability of the cytopathologist to communicate with clinicians and proceduralists in the real-time setting of rapid onsite evaluation (ROSE), or by phone or at the multidisciplinary conference, is the key to optimizing management. The multidisciplinary team meeting to discuss the clinical, imaging, and cytopathological findings (including ICC and next-generation sequencing results) of individual patients is a crucial requirement in the best-practice management of patients with lung tumours. Direct access to the clinical and imaging database can also greatly facilitate interpretation and deciding on the next diagnostic steps.

It is important to realize that in many instances, cytopathology, core needle biopsy, or forceps biopsy specimens are sampled during the same procedure, and this requires systematic correlation between these sample types. This necessitates a tight collaboration between cytopathologists and histopathologists. Ideally, one single team of (cyto-)pathologists oversees all respiratory specimens from the same patient. Uncertainty in a cytopathology specimen can often be resolved by clear findings in a concurrent small biopsy, or vice versa.

Once there is an established categorization of "Malignant", further management aims at ensuring the selection and reporting of the appropriate predictive biomarkers, which will depend on the histopathological lung cancer subtype and tumour stage. In the other categories, the risk of malignancy is the key determinant for defining the further diagnostic strategy and the diagnostic workup for each individual patient.

The WHO Reporting System for Lung Cytopathology includes recommendations for the diagnostic workup of patients with particular categories of cytopathology reports and specific diagnoses. It is recognized that the availability of local expertise and laboratories, as well as radiological and other imaging modalities, will be major determinants in the actual diagnostic workup of individual patients. Local circumstances and resources may well modify these recommendations, and this is most obviously the case in low- and middle-income countries. Therefore, it is not intended that these recommendations are mandatory in any way. It is clear that local practice and cytopathologists may be challenged by the recommendations, and it is expected that this reporting system will generate considerable debate and further research which will improve the overall management of lung disease.

The intention of this chapter is to bring all the recommendations for diagnostic management of each category into one place, so as to assist clinicians and their use of the WHO Reporting System.

Category: Insufficient/Inadequate/Non-diagnostic

Canberk S
Bongiovanni M
Raymond WA

The causes of insufficient/inadequate/non-diagnostic cytopathology specimens include a paucity of cellular material; extensive necrosis; poor preparation, fixation, or staining; and obscuring of potentially diagnostic material by blood, inflammatory cells, mucus, or other material. The reasons for an inadequate specimen should be documented in the report. If there is any atypical material, however scant, in a cytopathology specimen – even if the slides are otherwise insufficient – the case is immediately categorized as "Atypical" rather than "Insufficient".

Integration into a multidisciplinary evaluation of clinical, imaging, and cytopathological features plays a crucial role in assessing sample adequacy {675,465}. It is recognized that in some low- and middle-income country settings there may not be any imaging available with which to correlate the cytological sample.

Any specimen can be regarded as adequate if the material demonstrates a pathological process consistent with the clinical and imaging findings and can be appropriately categorized as "Benign", "Atypical", "Suspicious for malignancy", or "Malignant". However, if nonspecific benign cytopathological material is present on the slides and does not correlate with the suspicious lesion seen on imaging, a malignant process cannot be excluded and the implication is that further biopsy or repeat sampling of the lesion or other investigation will be required. Cytopathologists can decide to report these cases as "Benign", with a clear description of the material found on the cytopathological preparations, and add a caveat statement in the report conclusion that "the material may not represent the target lesion on imaging and further biopsy is recommended", or they can report the material as "Non-diagnostic". Each cytopathologist and institution will determine how they report these cases, depending on local historical usage, the availability of imaging to allow for correlation, and billing concerns related to the terms "Insufficient" and "Inadequate", and they should be consistent and clearly communicate with their clinicians.

The term "Non-diagnostic" is not recommended to be used for cases where there is good benign cytopathological material that does not correlate with a pulmonary nodule or other suspicious imaging, and at the same time, "Insufficient" or "Inadequate" is used to categorize cases where there is a lack of cellular material, poor smearing, poor fixation with artefact and

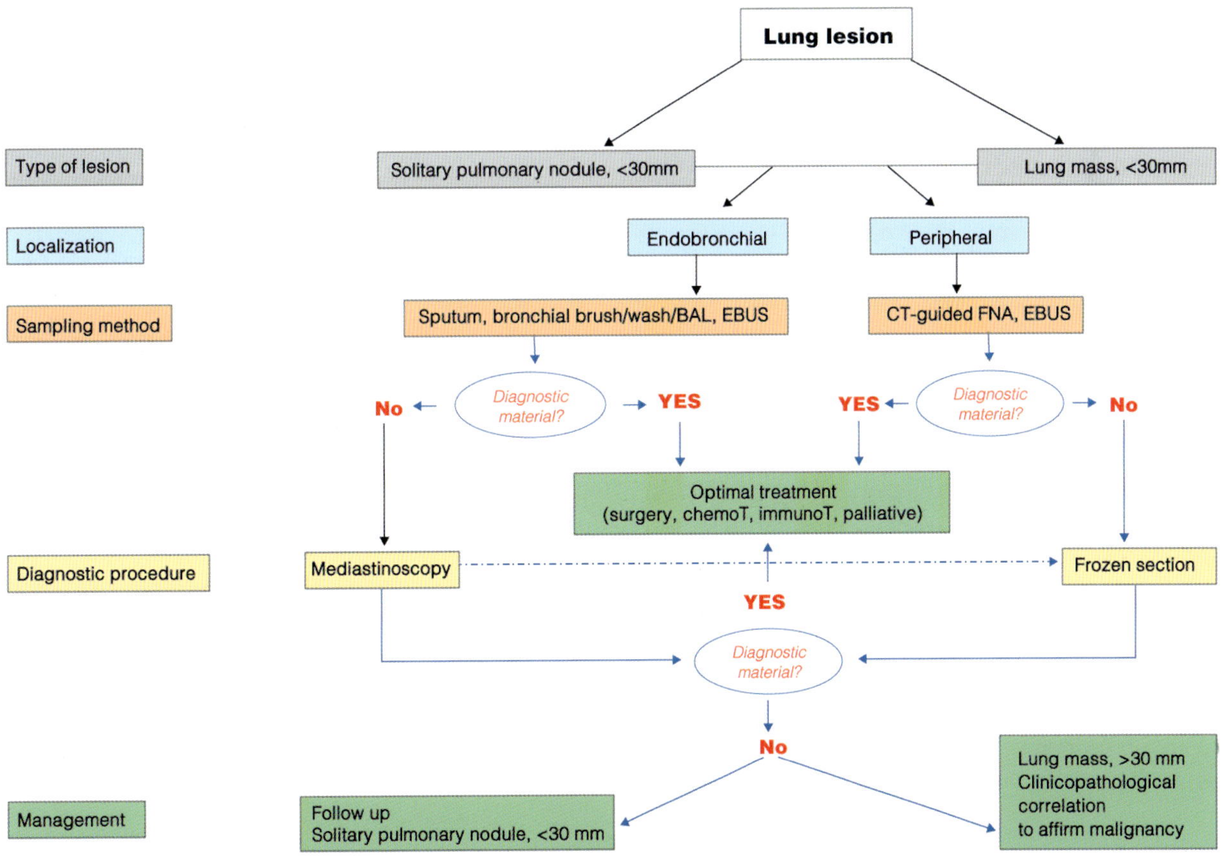

Fig. 8.01 The "Insufficient/Inadequate/Non-diagnostic" category. Management algorithm. Diagnostic management recommendations in "Insufficient/Inadequate/Non-diagnostic" cytopathological specimens. chemoT, chemotherapy; EBUS, endobronchial ultrasound; immunoT, immunotherapy.

poor staining, or inflammation or other material obscuring the cytopathological material.

Reporting the reasons for inadequacy in a specimen can contribute to improving the diagnostic yield of a repeat examination; for example, to perform an adequate deep cough to produce a sputum sample after a previous "Insufficient" report due to a predominantly buccal sampling, or to control or cease anticoagulant therapy in the case of a pure bloody specimen {338}. In the case of an endobronchial brush or FNAB of an endobronchial mass that yields only normal bronchial cells, which is most likely due to a submucosal location or a fibrotic tumour, the proceduralist can change the approach and perform an FNAB under ultrasound assistance or add a core needle biopsy.

After unsuccessful non-invasive or minimally invasive procedures such as sputum sampling or bronchial washing (BW) and bronchial brushing (BB), FNAB can be used under EUS direction, known as endobronchial ultrasound–guided transbronchial FNAB (EBUS-TBFNAB), or using CT guidance and a transthoracic approach or an exploratory mediastinoscopy may be appropriate.

In principle, a lung mass on imaging that is > 30 mm in diameter is considered malignant {318,515}. If an "Insufficient" result is obtained after several attempts to get a cytopathological and core needle biopsy diagnosis, then a final clinical and imaging correlation is required, and the management decision must be based on other diagnostic modalities, such as open surgical biopsy where intraoperative frozen sectioning can guide the extent of surgery.

It is recommended that cytopathology services regularly audit their "Insufficient" rates to highlight problems with the procurement of the specimens and the reporting of these cases. The risk of malignancy varies with the mode of cytopathological sampling and the imaging characteristics of the lung lesion; it is reported as 40% for EBUS-TBFNAB, as high as 60% for transthoracic FNAB, and > 60% for exfoliative samples {465,318, 515,466,117,105} (see Table 1.04, p. 11, and Table 1.05, p. 12, in Chapter 1: *Introduction to the WHO Reporting System for Lung Cytopathology*).

If a sputum sample is "Insufficient", the clinical and imaging findings can be reviewed and the sputum sample repeated. This applies both in low- and middle-income countries and in better-resourced countries. If the imaging is suspicious and further biopsy is required, BW/BB, EBUS-TBFNAB, or transthoracic FNAB or mediastinoscopy can be used to obtain material, depending on the site of the lesion (see Table 1.05, p. 12, in Chapter 1: *Introduction to the WHO Reporting System for Lung Cytopathology*). If these procedures are not available in a low- or middle-income country, then there may be a need to proceed to biopsy of another site, such as a left supraclavicular lymph node if enlarged, or an open wedge surgical biopsy.

If a BW/BB is "Insufficient", correlation with clinical and imaging findings is recommended, but in almost all cases, repeat BW/BB or EBUS-TBFNAB or transthoracic FNAB with or without a core needle biopsy will be required (see Table 1.05, p. 12, in Chapter 1: *Introduction to the WHO Reporting System for Lung Cytopathology*). Some clinical teams will have mediastinoscopy available.

If an EBUS-TBFNAB or transthoracic FNAB is "Insufficient" at rapid onsite evaluation (ROSE), as many as four or five repeat passes are recommended {647}. If the specimen is still "Insufficient", or if the diagnosis of inadequacy is reported without ROSE at a later date, repeat FNAB with or without core needle biopsy is recommended and again correlation with the imaging findings is required. Mediastinoscopy may be available. Ancillary testing on the cell block may provide diagnostic material, which can allow the initial cytopathology report to be changed to a "Benign", "Atypical", "Suspicious for malignancy", or "Malignant" category. The multidisciplinary clinical team may decide to progress to lung wedge biopsy and/or lobectomy, with frozen section providing information to determine the extent of surgery (see Table 1.04, p. 11, in Chapter 1: *Introduction to the WHO Reporting System for Lung Cytopathology*).

Category: Benign

Engels M
Navani N

The published risk of malignancy for pulmonary cytopathology cases categorized as "Benign" is highly variable and differs somewhat between the different types of cytopathology specimens: 0–42% for sputum, 32–42% for bronchial washing (BW) and bronchial brushing (BB), and 19–64% for FNAB specimens {574,465,65,105,467,338}.

The "Benign" cytopathology report should always be correlated with the clinical and imaging features. The aim of the cytopathology study is to exclude malignancy and diagnose infections, various inflammatory processes, and benign neoplasms. If the cytopathology report correlates with the clinical and imaging findings, and confirms an inflammatory process or a benign neoplasm, then recommended routine follow-up may be to review the patient in 3–6 months after treatment of any infection, or to get an immediate surgical assessment if the patient has symptoms related to the neoplasm, such as respiratory obstruction (see Table 1.04, p. 11, and Table 1.05, p. 12, in Chapter 1: *Introduction to the WHO Reporting System for Lung Cytopathology*).

If a sputum sample "Benign" report does not correlate with the clinical and/or imaging findings, then BW, BB, and FNAB should be considered to further define the lesion, depending on the site of the lesion and the status of the patient (see Table 1.04, p. 11, in Chapter 1: *Introduction to the WHO Reporting System for Lung Cytopathology*). These techniques have a combined sensitivity of 88% {569,858}.

Infectious or granulomatous entities require the cytopathologist or cytotechnologist at rapid onsite evaluation (ROSE) or in the laboratory to triage the sample for further workup, including cultures, drug sensitivities, and PCR molecular testing, and to possibly recommend serological analysis {290}. BW and BB have a low diagnostic yield for detecting granulomatous disease; however, BW when combined with sputum sampling has a sensitivity of 88% for detecting acid-fast bacilli. Postbronchoscopy sputum samples can also be collected, with a sensitivity of 35%. Unless the samples are transferred immediately, they should be kept at −4°C.

Bronchoalveolar lavage (BAL) is the method of choice for the diagnosis of a wide range of interstitial lung disease, with a sensitivity of 85% alone and 94% when combined with biopsy {162,569}. If a BW, BB, or BAL "Benign" report does not correlate with the clinical and/or imaging findings, then endobronchial ultrasound–guided transbronchial FNAB or transthoracic FNAB should be considered (see Table 1.04, p. 11, in Chapter 1: *Introduction to the WHO Reporting System for Lung Cytopathology*).

In general, endobronchial ultrasound–guided FNAB is best for central submucosal lesions, and transthoracic FNAB is best for peripheral lesions {569,568}. CT-directed sampling can be performed for well-defined nodules or non-infectious tumour-like lesions. Benign lesions account for 30% of transthoracic FNAB specimens {465}. If an FNAB does not correlate with the clinical and/or imaging findings, transbronchial core needle biopsy should be considered immediately if ROSE has been performed, or at a later procedure (see Table 1.05, p. 12, in Chapter 1: *Introduction to the WHO Reporting System for Lung Cytopathology*). If transbronchial core needle biopsy is not available, open surgical biopsy should be considered. ROSE plays a pivotal role in the workup of both infectious and neoplastic lesions. It allows efficient and cost-effective triage of the sample and has been demonstrated to reduce the need for subsequent procedures {568,778,290}.

Category: Atypical

Raymond WA

The risk of malignancy of the "Atypical" category in the literature is highly variable, ranging from 62% to 100% for exfoliative specimens and from 46% to 55% for FNAB {105,338,467}, and not all studies distinguish between the categories of "Atypical" and "Suspicious for malignancy" (see Table 1.04, p. 11, and Table 1.05, p. 12, in Chapter 1: *Introduction to the WHO Reporting System for Lung Cytopathology*). The value of an "Atypical" category in a hierarchical system is to maintain a high negative predictive value of a "Benign" categorization and a high positive predictive value of a "Malignant" categorization. A lesion categorized as "Atypical" is more likely than not to be benign, whereas one categorized as "Suspicious for malignancy" is more likely than not to be malignant, and the risk of malignancy increases in a stepwise fashion from "Benign" through "Atypical" to "Suspicious for malignancy" and "Malignant". The use of the "Atypical" category should be kept to a minimum, and the features of the atypical material should always be stated in the report.

The cytopathologist's approach to atypical cytopathology is often a two-step process: the first step being the identification of the atypical cells and the second an attempt to resolve the diagnosis by repeating the sample or preparing a cell block and performing appropriate ancillary tests. However, performing ancillary tests on FNAB cases with scant atypical cells is not recommended {185,372,347}.

If additional laboratory studies resolve the dilemma, the "Atypical" case may be downgraded to "Benign" or upgraded to "Suspicious for malignancy" or "Malignant". If the additional workup is inconclusive because of a paucity of available material, inherent ambiguous cytopathological features, or equivocal ancillary test results, the case remains categorized as "Atypical". Adequately cellular specimens consisting of atypical lymphoid cells should be submitted for flow cytometric analysis to further characterize the lymphoid population. The availability of such ancillary tests in low- and middle-income countries will impact this process.

The initial management of cases categorized as "Atypical" is similar for all respiratory cytopathology samples: correlation with the clinical and imaging findings. If the clinical and imaging features are atypical or suspicious for malignancy, further investigation by the same or a different cytopathological modality, with core needle biopsy as required, is recommended. However, if the imaging and clinical features are consistent with or explain the atypia, either a repeat sample may be obtained or the patient may be clinically observed for a period of time. An "Atypical" sputum sample can be repeated or bronchial brushing/washing or FNAB can be performed, depending on the lesion's nature and site. If a bronchial brushing/washing sample is "Atypical", then it could be repeated or FNAB performed (see Table 1.04, p. 11, in Chapter 1: *Introduction to the WHO Reporting System for Lung Cytopathology*). An "Atypical" FNAB after correlation with imaging could be repeated, or the patient could be monitored (see Table 1.05, p. 12, in Chapter 1: *Introduction to the WHO Reporting System for Lung Cytopathology*).

Category: Suspicious for malignancy

Moreira AL
Field AS

The category "Suspicious for malignancy" is used in respiratory cytopathology for cases with adequate material, which the cytopathologist assesses as most likely malignant but where there is a degree of uncertainty as to a definitive diagnosis of malignancy {465,338,463}. The majority of cases categorized as "Suspicious for malignancy" will have core needle biopsy or surgical excision follow-up showing malignant lesions; the risk of malignancy of the "Suspicious for malignancy" category is 75–100% for exfoliative specimens and 75–88% for FNAB {465,105,338,467}.

This category is used when there is insufficient quality or quantity of cellular material in an adequate smear for a definite diagnosis of malignancy, and it has a high rate of interobserver variability; therefore, consultation with more experienced cytopathologists is recommended when assessing cases with a limited cellularity, obscuring or technical problems, or with cytopathological features that may be shared by inflammatory reactive epithelium and carcinoma {468}. It is mandatory to review the clinical presentation and any imaging that is available, ideally in a multidisciplinary setting, before proceeding to further diagnostic steps or definitive management.

The high rate of interobserver disagreement varies because the threshold for the diagnosis of malignancy depends on the cytopathologist's experience, the type of cytopathological preparation, and the degree of cellular atypia. The category is used particularly to avoid a false positive diagnosis of malignancy (which may lead to unnecessary intervention) and so maintain the high positive predictive value of a "Malignant" categorization. Rapid onsite evaluation (ROSE) has been shown to reduce the rate of "Suspicious for malignancy" {306,372,568}, but limiting factors related to the intrinsic cytopathological characteristics of the tumour and technical problems remain. Necrosis, obscuring inflammatory changes, fibrosis, tumour cytopathology that may overlap with benign reactive processes, and prior radiation and/or chemotherapy (particularly for lung carcinomas) may all contribute to a "Suspicious for malignancy" categorization. Tumour size < 20 mm, the location of the targeted nodule, and the experience of the interventionalist procuring the biopsy may result in low cellularity and an inability to give an unequivocal diagnosis of malignancy {656,815,1021,753}.

The categorization of a case as "Suspicious for malignancy" should not be used as the sole basis for therapy and is not equivalent to a final diagnosis of malignancy {463,591,338}. It is imperative to have good communication with the members of the clinical team (with review of all relevant clinical and imaging information) for the determination of a management plan, in order to avoid unnecessary additional risks and costs.

The "Suspicious for malignancy" category can be applied to any malignant tumour type, including non-small cell carcinoma, neuroendocrine (carcinoid) tumours, small cell carcinoma, large cell neuroendocrine carcinoma (LCNEC), lymphoma, sarcoma, and metastatic carcinomas, and the type of tumour or a differential diagnosis of the suspected tumour types should always be stated in the cytopathology report. The category is equally applicable to any cytopathological study, including sputum sampling, bronchial washing, bronchial brushing, CT-guided transthoracic FNAB, and endobronchial ultrasound–guided transbronchial FNAB.

If a sputum sample is "Suspicious for malignancy", it can be repeated or the patient can proceed to bronchoscopy with bronchial washing and bronchial brushing or endobronchial ultrasound–guided transbronchial FNAB with or without core needle biopsy (see Table 1.04, p. 11, and Table 1.05, p. 12, in Chapter 1: *Introduction to the WHO Reporting System for Lung Cytopathology*). Transthoracic FNAB for peripheral lesions or where bronchoscopy is not available in low- and middle-income countries is an option. If the bronchial washing/brushing and/or FNAB are benign and correlate with benign clinical and imaging findings, routine follow-up with imaging at 3–6 months can be recommended.

If the cytopathology remains "Suspicious for malignancy" and the clinical and imaging findings are suspicious, repeat FNAB (preferably with ROSE) is recommended and core needle biopsy can be added, although proceeding to surgical biopsy (with or without frozen sectioning) should be considered on the basis of the overall findings (see Table 1.04, p. 11, and Table 1.05, p. 12, in Chapter 1: *Introduction to the WHO Reporting System for Lung Cytopathology*).

Ancillary techniques, particularly ICC, may make a specific malignant diagnosis possible, but in many cases the quality and quantity of the suspicious cells may prevent further definition of the diagnosis. Thyroid transcription factor 1 (TTF1) as a marker of lung adenocarcinoma and p40 as a marker of squamous differentiation are often used for further classification of non-small cell carcinomas, but these markers are also expressed in reactive cells and do not separate benign from malignant.

Category: Malignant

Bubendorf L
Navani N

The management of all specimens in the "Malignant" category depends on correlation with the clinical and imaging findings and on the specific type of malignant tumour. In patients for whom potential surgical intervention is possible, staging of mediastinal lymph nodes by endobronchial ultrasound–guided transbronchial FNAB may be required, and distant metastases should be confirmed or excluded by FNAB and, where necessary, core needle biopsies in patients with suspicious imaging findings. After a diagnosis of advanced, inoperable non-small cell lung carcinoma, priority should be given to securing sufficient tumour for molecular biomarker testing {778}. When there is insufficient tumour material after review of all available specimens including cytopathology and biopsies, rebiopsy may be required, preferably targeting the easiest accessible tumour lesion. In rare situations, where rebiopsy is impossible owing to the high risk of complications or poor health status of the patient, serological liquid biopsies for the detection of predictive DNA alterations are an option {4}. Direct access to the electronic medical record may facilitate interpretation and decisions on the next diagnostic steps. In patients with a high suspicion of metastatic disease, or if the diagnostic material proves an advanced stage of primary carcinoma such as in the case of a malignant effusion, reflex molecular and biomarker testing can accelerate the process and reduce the time to systemic treatment.

The reported risk of malignancy for a sputum sample categorized as "Malignant" is 100%. The sensitivity of sputum sample cytopathology has been reported to be as low as 5%, particularly for more peripheral lung cancers, and ranges in other reports from 34% to 97%, with an average of 66% {292, 599} (see Table 1.04, p. 11, in Chapter 1: *Introduction to the WHO Reporting System for Lung Cytopathology*). If a sputum sample is "Malignant", the next step should be white-light bronchoscopy to identify central lesions and imaging including CXR and CT for peripheral lesions {791}. Lesions detected can then undergo endobronchial ultrasound–guided transbronchial FNAB or transthoracic FNAB depending on their site and the available biopsy expertise. In addition to white-light bronchoscopy, autofluorescence bronchoscopy has improved the detection of preinvasive and malignant endobronchial lesions, and narrow-band imaging is useful for detecting the microvascular network of bronchial mucosa {362,838}. Close follow-up of initially undetectable cases with repeat sputum sample studies and imaging is required to localize carcinoma in cases with positive sputum sample cytopathology.

A bronchial brushing, bronchial washing, or bronchoalveolar lavage (BAL) is typically performed for the evaluation of peripheral lung lesions, which are usually small in size, solitary, and not visible on bronchoscopy {754}. The reported risk of malignancy for exfoliative cytopathology (bronchial washing/brushing) is 94–100% (see Table 1.04, p. 11, in Chapter 1: *Introduction to the WHO Reporting System for Lung Cytopathology*). For a peripheral non-small cell lung carcinoma without evidence of distant metastasis, further management is dependent on imaging: a small primary tumour (< 30 mm) without evidence of mediastinal lymph node involvement can directly undergo surgical resection if not contraindicated by poor lung function or comorbidities.

The reported risk of malignancy for FNAB specimens categorized as "Malignant" at endobronchial ultrasound is 87–100% {467,105} (see Table 1.05, p. 12, in Chapter 1: *Introduction to the WHO Reporting System for Lung Cytopathology*). The cytopathology specimen frequently provides material for further specific diagnosis by ICC, FISH, and next-generation sequencing performed on cell block and direct smear slide scrapings, and if there is correlation between the clinical, imaging, and cytopathology findings, the decision to proceed to definitive treatment may be made. If there is insufficient material for ancillary testing or if there is no correlation that the lesion is malignant, then repeat FNAB with or without core needle biopsy should be considered. Each case should, as far as possible, be reviewed with full correlation and discussion in a multidisciplinary setting to establish treatment.

Mediastinal staging by endobronchial ultrasound–guided transbronchial FNAB is indicated in cases where there are enlarged mediastinal or hilar lymph nodes measuring > 10 mm in their short axis on CT or there is abnormal uptake on FDG PET, or where the primary tumour is > 30 mm {709}. If the FNAB does not yield a diagnosis, transthoracic FNAB and/or core needle biopsy or surgical resection (depending on site and size of the lesion) are recommended.

Contributors

BALOCH, Zubair Wahid
Hospital of the University of Pennsylvania, Perelman School of Medicine
6 Founders, Rm 6.043, 3400 Spruce St
Philadelphia PA 19104-4283

BELLEVICINE, Claudio
University of Naples Federico II
Via Sergio Pansini, 5
80138 Naples

BONGIOVANNI, Massimo
Synlab Pathology
Rue du Liseron 5
1006 Lausanne

BUBENDORF, Lukas*
Institute of Medical Genetics and Pathology
Schönbeinstrasse 40
4031 Basel

CANBERK, Sule
i3S - Instituto de Investigação e Inovação em Saúde da Universidade do Porto
Rua Alfredo Allen
4200-135 Porto

CHANDRA, Ashish
Guy's and St Thomas' NHS Foundation Trust
Westminster Bridge Rd
London SE1 7EH

CHEN, Longwen
Mayo Clinic Arizona
13400 E Shea Blvd
Scottsdale AZ 85259

CREE, Ian A.
International Agency for Research on Cancer
25 Av. Tony Garnier, CS 90627
69366 Lyon, CEDEX 07

DALURZO, Mercedes Liliana
Hospital Italiano de Buenos Aires
Tte. Gral. Juan Domingo Perón 4190
1181 Buenos Aires

DAVIDSON, Ben
Oslo University Hospital, University of Oslo
Ullernchausseen 70
0310 Oslo

ENGELS, Marianne
Institute of Pathology
University Hospital Cologne
Kerpener Str. 62
50937 Cologne

FIELD, Andrew S.
University of NSW Sydney and
University of Notre Dame Medical Schools
Department of Anatomical Pathology
St Vincent's Hospital Sydney
Victoria St
2010 Darlinghurst NSW

FONSECA, Anil Felix Angelo
Gandhi Medical College/TIMS
Hyderabad, Telangana

GEISINGER, Kim R.*
Joint Pathology Center
606 Stephen Sitter Ave
Silver Spring MD 20910

GOLDMAN-LÉVY, Gabrielle
International Agency for Research on Cancer
25 Av. Tony Garnier, CS 90627
69366 Lyon, CEDEX 07

HABA, Reiji
Kagawa University Hospital
Miki-cho
Kagawa 761-0793

HEINE, Ralf
Krankenhaus St. Elisabeth und St. Barbara
Halle (Saale)
Mauerstraße 5
06110 Halle (Saale)

HIROSHIMA, Kenzo
Chiba University Graduate School of Medicine
1-8-1 Inohana, Chuo-ku
Chiba 260-8670

JAIN, Deepali
All India Institute of Medical Sciences
Ansari Nagar
New Delhi 110029

KAWAHARA, Kunimitsu
Osaka Habikino Medical Center
3-7-1 Habikino
Habikino, Osaka 583-8588

KHOLOVA, Ivana
Tampere University and Fimlab Laboratories
Arvo Ylpön katu
33520 Tampere

LAYFIELD, Lester J.
University of Missouri
1 Hospital Dr
Columbia MO 65212

LIN, Oscar*
Memorial Sloan Kettering Cancer Center
1275 York Ave
New York NY 10065

LLOVERAS, Belen
Hospital del Mar
Pg. Marítim de la Barceloneta, 25-29
08003 Barcelona

LOKUHETTY, Dilani
University of Colombo
25 Kynsey Rd
Colombo 00800

LOZANO, María D.
University of Navarra
Av. de Pío XII, 36
31008 Pamplona

MALEKI, Zahra
Johns Hopkins Hospital
600 N Wolfe St, Pathology 304A
Baltimore MD 21287

McLEAN, Emma
Guy's and St Thomas' NHS Foundation Trust
Westminster Bridge Rd
London SE1 7EH

MEHROTRA, Ravi
Centre for Health Innovation and Policy
361, Sector 15A
Noida 20301

MICHAEL, Claire W.*
University Hospitals Cleveland Medical Center / Case Western Reserve University
11100 Euclid Ave, MSPTH 5077
Cleveland OH 44106

MONACO, Sara E.
Geisinger Medical Center
100 N Academy Ave, MC 19-20
Danville PA 17822

MOREIRA, Andre L.*
New York University Langone Health
560 1st Ave, TH4-15B
New York NY 10016

NAVANI, Neal
University College London
Rayne Institute, 5 University St
London WC1E 6JF

* Indicates disclosure of interests (see p. 187).

ÖNAL, Binnur Ü.
Acıbadem Healthcare Group
Central Pathology Laboratory
Kayışdağı Cd. No:32, Atasehir
34752 Istanbul

OSAMURA, Robert Y.
Nippon Koukan Hospital and
Keio University School of Medicine
1-2-1 Koukan-dori, Kawasaki-ku, Kawasaki-shi
Kanagawa 210-0852

PANTANOWITZ, Liron
University of Michigan
NCRC Building 35, Room 36-1221-35
2800 Plymouth Rd
Ann Arbor MI 48109-2800

PAPOTTI, Mauro*
University of Turin
Via Santena, 7
10126 Turin TO

PIJUAN, Lara
Hospital del Mar
Pg. Marítim de la Barceloneta, 25-29
08003 Barcelona

PITMAN, Martha Bishop
Harvard Medical School,
Massachusetts General Hospital
55 Fruit St
Boston MA 02114

RAYMOND, Wendy A.
Department of Surgical Pathology,
Flinders Medical Centre, Flinders University
of South Australia, and Clinpath Pathology
Flinders Dr, Bedford Park 5042
Adelaide SA

REKHTMAN, Natasha
Memorial Sloan Kettering Cancer Center
1275 York Ave
New York NY 10065

ROY-CHOWDHURI, Sinchita
University of Texas
MD Anderson Cancer Center
1515 Holcombe Blvd, Unit 85
Houston TX 77030

SATOH, Yukitoshi
Kitasato University School of Medicine
1-15-1 Kitasato, Minami-ku
Sagamihara, Kanagawa 252-0374

SAUTER, Jennifer L.
Memorial Sloan Kettering Cancer Center
1275 York Ave
New York NY 10044

SAVIC PRINCE, Spasenija*
University Hospital Basel
Schönbeinstrasse 40
4031 Basel

SCAGLIOTTI, Giorgio V.*
University of Turin
Regione Gonzole, 10
10043 Orbassano TO

SCHMITT, Fernando
CINTESIS@RISE (Health Research Network);
Medical Faculty of the University of Porto;
Molecular Pathology Unit, Ipatimup
Rua Júlio Amaral de Carvalho 45
4200-135 Porto

SHEAFF, Michael T.*
Barts Health NHS Trust
80 Newark St
London E1 2ES

STOLZ, Daiana*
University Hospital Basel
Petersgraben 4
4031 Basel

TRAVIS, William D.
Memorial Sloan Kettering Cancer Center
1275 York Ave
New York NY 10065

TRONCONE, Giancarlo
University of Naples Federico II
Via Sergio Pansini, 5
80128 Naples

VanderLaan, Paul A.
Beth Israel Deaconess Medical Center
330 Brookline Ave
Boston MA 02215

VIGLIAR, Elena
University of Naples Federico II
Via Sergio Pansini, 5
80131 Naples

VIVERO, Marina
Brigham and Women's Hospital
75 Francis St
Boston MA 02145

WELKER, Lutz
UKE Hamburg, Institute of Pathology
Martinistraße 52
20246 Hamburg

ZAKOWSKI, Maureen F.
Mount Sinai Medical Center
1468 Madison Ave
New York NY 10029

* Indicates disclosure of interests (see p. 187).

Declaration of interests

Dr Bubendorf reports that his unit at University Hospital Basel benefited from research funding from Roche and MSD.

Dr Geisinger reports having provided medicolegal expert opinion in relation to lung cancer cases, including defence work in tobacco exposure cases.

Dr Lin reports receiving personal consultancy fees from Hologic and Janssen.

Dr Michael reports providing expert opinion on behalf of several legal firms in relation to litigation for plaintiffs in asbestos exposure cases.

Dr Moreira reports having received personal consultancy fees from Olympus Corporation in his capacity as an advisory board participant.

Dr Papotti reports receiving honoraria from Lilly, Roche, and Pfizer.

Dr Savic Prince reports having received personal consultancy fees from MSD Merck Sharp & Dohme for medical, scientific, and usability-related assistance with an open-source PDL1 online platform, and receiving honoraria from Diaceutics Ireland Limited, MSD, AstraZeneca, Boehringer Ingelheim, Roche, Pfizer, Bristol Myers Squibb, Abbott, and Thermo Fisher Scientific.

Dr Scagliotti reports receiving honoraria from Lilly, Roche, Pfizer, AstraZeneca, Novartis, and MSD.

Dr Sheaff reports providing expert opinion on behalf of plaintiffs in connection with medicolegal reports in relation to asbestos-induced thoracic disease.

Dr Stolz reports receiving personal consultancy fees from Chiesi, Novartis, GSK, AstraZeneca, Vifor, AG Pharma, MSD, and Sanofi, and that her unit at University Hospital Basel benefits from research funding from ResMed, Weinmann, AG Pharma, and AstraZeneca.

Sources

Note: For any figure, table, or box not listed below, the original source is this volume; the suggested source citation is

International Academy of Cytology – International Agency for Research on Cancer – World Health Organization Joint Editorial Board. WHO Reporting System for Lung Cytopathology. Lyon (France): International Agency for Research on Cancer; 2022. (IAC-IARC-WHO cytopathology reporting systems series, 1st ed.; vol. 1). https://publications.iarc.fr/620.

Figures

Figure	Source
2.01A–C	Heine R
2.02	Heine R
2.03A–C	Engels M
2.04A	Jain D
2.04B	Heine R
2.05A,B	Engels M
2.06	Kholova I
2.07	Heine R
2.08A–C	Heine R
2.09A,B	Kholova I
2.10	Pitman MB
2.11	Jain D
2.12A,B	Heine R
2.13A,B	Engels M
2.14	Engels M
2.15	Heine R
2.16	Jain D
2.17	Heine R
2.18A,B	Jain D
2.19	Michael CW
2.20A,B	Michael CW
2.20C	Bubendorf L
2.21A–C	Bubendorf L
2.22A,B	Bubendorf L
2.23A,B	Lozano MD
2.24A,B	Lozano MD
2.25	Bubendorf L
2.26A–D	Lozano MD
2.27A,B	Lozano MD
2.28A,B	Lozano MD
2.29	Lozano MD
3.01	Maleki Z
3.02	Maleki Z
3.03	Raymond WA
4.01	Satoh Y
4.02A–C	Engels M
4.03A–C	Engels M
4.04A–C	Bubendorf L
4.05A,B	Savic Prince S
4.06A,B	Engels M
4.07	Engels M
4.08A	Engels M
4.08B	Engels M; Welker L
4.09A,B	Engels M
4.10A,B	Engels M
4.11A,B	Engels M
4.12A,B	Engels M
4.13A,C,D	Engels M
4.13B	Jain D
4.14A,B	Engels M
4.15A,B	Engels M
4.16A,B	Engels M
4.17A,B	Engels M
4.18	Engels M
4.19A	Pijuan L
4.19B,C	VanderLaan PA
4.20A–C	Engels M
4.21A–D	Engels M
4.22	Engels M
4.23A,B	Chen L
4.23C	Matthew A. Zarka, Department of Pathology, Mayo Clinic, Phoenix AZ
4.23D	Pijuan L
4.24A,B	Zakowski MF
4.25A,B	Zakowski MF
4.25C	Maleki Z
4.26A–D	Zakowski MF
4.27A–C	Zakowski MF
4.28A–C	Baloch ZW
4.29A,B	Baloch ZW
4.30A,B	Momin T. Siddiqui, Department of Pathology and Laboratory Medicine, Cornell Medical School, New York NY
4.31	Momin T. Siddiqui, Department of Pathology and Laboratory Medicine, Cornell Medical School, New York NY
4.32A–C	Hiroshima K
4.33A,B	Pitman MB
4.33C	Satoh Y
4.34	VanderLaan PA
4.35A,B	Pitman MB
4.36	Baloch ZW
4.37	Baloch ZW
5.01	Chandra A
5.02A,B	Raymond WA
5.03	Baloch ZW
5.04A,B	Baloch ZW
5.05A–C	Baloch ZW
5.06	Chandra A
5.07	Baloch ZW
6.01A–C	Raymond WA
6.02A	Moreira AL
6.02B,C	Reiji Haba, Department of Diagnostic Pathology, Kagawa University Hospital, Miki-cho, Kagawa-ken
7.01A–C	Baloch ZW
7.02A–D	Baloch ZW
7.03A–C	Baloch ZW
7.04A–C	Baloch ZW
7.05A,B	Baloch ZW
7.06A,B	Bubendorf L
7.07A,B	Satoh Y
7.08A	Satoh Y
7.08B	Bubendorf L
7.09	Bubendorf L
7.10A–D	Engels M
7.11A,B	Engels M
7.12A,B	Engels M
7.13A,B	Engels M
7.14	Engels M
7.15A–D	Jain D
7.16	Chandra A
7.17A–C	Bubendorf L
7.18A	Bubendorf L
7.18B	Engels M
7.19	Bubendorf L
7.20	Engels M
7.21A	Chandra A
7.21B	Bubendorf L
7.22	Engels M
7.23A–C	Bubendorf L
7.24A–C	Bubendorf L
7.25A,B	Bubendorf L
7.26A–C	Zakowski MF
7.27A,B	Baloch ZW
7.28A–C	Baloch ZW
7.29A,B	Maleki Z
7.30A,B	Engels M
7.31A,B	Engels M
7.32A,B	Engels M

7.33A,B Engels M
7.34A,B Bubendorf L
7.35A,B Bubendorf L
7.36A,B VanderLaan PA
7.37 WHO Classification of Tumours Editorial Board. Thoracic tumours. Lyon (France): International Agency for Research on Cancer; 2021. (WHO classification of tumours series, 5th ed.; vol. 5). https://publications.iarc.fr/595.
7.38A,B Jain D
7.39A,B Jain D
7.40A–C Jain D
7.41A–D Jain D
7.42A,C,E Brie Kezlarian, Department of Pathology and Laboratory Medicine, Memorial Sloan Kettering Cancer Center, New York NY
7.42B,D Jain D
7.43A,B Osamura RY
7.43C,D Michael CW
7.44A,B Michael CW
7.45A,B Michael CW
7.46A–C Engels M
7.47A Engels M
7.47B Osamura RY
7.48A,B Michael CW
7.49A–C Osamura RY
7.50 Michael CW
7.51 Michael CW
7.52A,D Engels M; and 48th Annual Meeting of the German Division of IAP, 24–26 February 2012 in Bonn, Course: Lung cytology, Case 20.2; and 385th Tutorial Lung Cytology, 15 December 2012 in Bonn, Case 20.3; and 52nd Annual Meeting of the German Division of IAP, 4–6 March 2016 in Bonn, Course: Cytological, histological and molecular pathological diagnosis of lung tumors, Case 12.4; and 54th Annual Meeting of the German Division of IAP, 23–25 February 2018 in Bonn, Course: Cytological, histological and molecular pathological diagnosis of lung tumors, Case 12.
7.52B,C Engels M
7.53A,C Engels M; and 48th Annual Meeting of the German Division of IAP, 24–26 February 2012 in Bonn, Course: Lung cytology, Case 20.2; and 385th Tutorial Lung Cytology, 15 December 2012 in Bonn, Case 20.3; and 52nd Annual Meeting of the German Division of IAP, 4–6 March 2016 in Bonn, Course: Cytological, histological and molecular pathological diagnosis of lung tumors, Case 12.4; and 54th Annual Meeting of the German Division of IAP, 23–25 February 2018 in Bonn, Course: Cytological, histological and molecular pathological diagnosis of lung tumors, Case 12.
7.53B Engels M
7.54A,B VanderLaan PA
7.55A,B VanderLaan PA
7.56 Monaco SE
7.57 Monaco SE
7.58 Engels M
7.59 Michael CW
7.60 Michael CW
7.61 Michael CW
7.62A–C Kholova I
7.63A,B Kholova I
7.64A–C Michael CW
7.65 Michael CW
7.66A–C Engels M
7.67A,B Michael CW
7.68A–C Bubendorf L
7.69 Michael CW
7.70 Michael CW
7.71 Michael CW
7.72A Michael CW
7.72B Önal BÜ
7.73A,B Michael CW
7.73C Sauter JL
7.74 Bubendorf L
7.75A,B Engels M
7.76A–C Monaco SE
7.76D,E Masayuki Ota, Department of Diagnostic Pathology, Graduate School of Medicine, Chiba University, Chuo-ku, Chiba City; and Hiroshima K
7.77A,B Masayuki Ota, Department of Diagnostic Pathology, Graduate School of Medicine, Chiba University, Chuo-ku, Chiba City; and Hiroshima K
7.78 Monaco SE
7.79 Monaco SE
7.80A–C Monaco SE
7.81A–C Baloch ZW
7.82A–C Baloch ZW

8.01 Canberk S

Tables

1.01 Adapted, with permission from Elsevier, from: Travis WD, Brambilla E, Noguchi M, et al. International Association for the Study of Lung Cancer/American Thoracic Society/European Respiratory Society international multidisciplinary classification of lung adenocarcinoma. J Thorac Oncol. 2011 Feb;6(2):244–85. PMID:21252716. Copyright 2011; and Travis WD, Brambilla E, Burke AP, et al., editors. WHO classification of tumours of the lung, pleura, thymus and heart. Lyon (France): International Agency for Research on Cancer; 2015. (WHO classification of tumours series, 4th ed.; vol. 7). https://publications.iarc.fr/17; and Adapted, with permission from the American Registry of Pathology, from: Table 1.2-2 of Travis WD, Nicholson AG, Geisinger KR, et al. Tumors of the lower respiratory tract. Washington, DC: American Registry of Pathology; 2019. (AFIP atlas of tumor pathology, series 4; fascicle 29); and WHO Classification of Tumours Editorial Board. Thoracic tumours. Lyon (France): International Agency for Research on Cancer; 2021.

	(WHO classification of tumours series, 5th ed.; vol. 5). https://publications.iarc.fr/595.
1.02	Field AS
1.03	Moreira AL
1.04	Field AS
1.05	Field AS
2.01	Jain D
2.02	Heine R
2.03	Jain D
2.04	Michael CW
2.05	Lozano MD
2.06	Roy-Chowdhuri S
2.07	Lozano MD
4.01	Engels M
4.02	Engels M
4.03	Engels M
7.01	Engels M
7.02	Michael CW
7.03	Michael CW
7.04	Michael CW
7.05	Michael CW
7.06	Engels M; Hiroshima K
7.07	Welker L
7.08	Michael CW
7.09	Michael CW
7.10	Engels M; Hiroshima K; Monaco SE
7.11	Baloch ZW

Boxes

1.01	Adapted, with permission from Elsevier, from: Travis WD, Brambilla E, Noguchi M, et al. International Association for the Study of Lung Cancer/ American Thoracic Society/ European Respiratory Society international multidisciplinary classification of lung adenocarcinoma. J Thorac Oncol. 2011 Feb;6(2):244–85. PMID:21252716. Copyright 2011; and With permission from the Archives of Pathology & Laboratory Medicine: Travis WD, Brambilla E, Noguchi M, et al. Diagnosis of lung cancer in small biopsies and cytology: implications of the 2011 International Association for the Study of Lung Cancer/ American Thoracic Society/ European Respiratory Society classification. Arch Pathol Lab Med. 2013 May;137(5):668–84. PMID:22970842. Copyright 2013 College of American Pathologists; and Travis WD, Brambilla E, Burke AP, et al., editors. WHO classification of tumours of the lung, pleura, thymus and heart. Lyon (France): International Agency for Research on Cancer; 2015. (WHO classification of tumours series, 4th ed.; vol. 7). https://publications.iarc.fr/17; and WHO Classification of Tumours Editorial Board. Thoracic tumours. Lyon (France): International Agency for Research on Cancer; 2021. (WHO classification of tumours series, 5th ed.; vol. 5). https://publications.iarc.fr/595.
2.01	Jain D
2.02	Jain D
2.03	Bubendorf L
2.04	Bubendorf L
3.01	Raymond WA
5.01	Chandra A; VanderLaan PA

Images on the cover

Top left	Fig. 7.10D: Engels M
Bottom left	Fig. 4.23B: Chen L
Top centre	Fig. 7.17B: Bubendorf L
Bottom centre	Fig. 2.26D: Lozano MD
Top right	Fig. 7.46C: Engels M
Bottom right	Fig. 2.21C: Bubendorf L

Images on the chapter title pages

Chapter 1	Fig. 4.05A: Savic Prince S
Chapter 2	Fig. 2.13B: Engels M
Chapter 3	Fig. 3.03: Raymond WA
Chapter 4	Fig. 4.23D: Pijuan L
Chapter 5	Fig. 5.02B: Raymond WA
Chapter 6	Fig. 6.02A: Moreira AL
Chapter 7	Fig. 7.44A: Michael CW
Chapter 8	Fig. 4.37: Baloch ZW

References

1. Abbott GF, Rosado-de-Christenson ML, Franks TJ, et al. From the archives of the AFIP: pulmonary Langerhans cell histiocytosis. Radiographics. 2004 May-Jun;24(3):821–41. PMID:15143231
2. Adachi Y, Kitamura Y, Nakamura H, et al. Benign clear (sugar) cell tumor of the lung with CD1a expression. Pathol Int. 2006 Aug;56(8):453–6. PMID:16872440
3. Agarwal P, Toi PC, Subramaniam H, et al. Prospective comparison of cytological specimen adequacy assessment by different rapid staining techniques for rapid on-site evaluation in fine needle aspiration cytology and their cost-effectiveness. Diagn Cytopathol. 2019 May;47(5):469–74. PMID:30585436
4. Aggarwal C, Rolfo CD, Oxnard GR, et al. Strategies for the successful implementation of plasma-based NSCLC genotyping in clinical practice. Nat Rev Clin Oncol. 2021 Jan;18(1):56–62. PMID:32918064
5. Agustí C, Xaubet A, Montón C, et al. Induced sputum in the diagnosis of peripheral lung cancer not visible endoscopically. Respir Med. 2001 Oct;95(10):822–8. PMID:11601749
6. Ahn D, Lee GJ, Sohn JH, et al. Fine-needle aspiration cytology versus core-needle biopsy for the diagnosis of extracranial head and neck schwannoma. Head Neck. 2018 Dec;40(12):2695–700. PMID:30457183
7. Ahrens P, Noll C, Kitz R, et al. Lipid-laden alveolar macrophages (LLAM): a useful marker of silent aspiration in children. Pediatr Pulmonol. 1999 Aug;28(2):83–8. PMID:10423306
8. Aisner DL, Sams SB. The role of cytology specimens in molecular testing of solid tumors: techniques, limitations, and opportunities. Diagn Cytopathol. 2012 Jun;40(6):511–24. PMID:22619126
9. Akata S, Okada S, Maeda J, et al. Computed tomographic findings of large cell neuroendocrine carcinoma of the lung. Clin Imaging. 2007 Nov-Dec;31(6):379–84. PMID:17996599
10. Akbulut M, Zekioglu O, Kapkac M, et al. Fine needle aspiration cytology of glycogen-rich clear cell carcinoma of the breast: review of 37 cases with histologic correlation. Acta Cytol. 2008 Jan-Feb;52(1):65–71. PMID:18323277
11. Akhtar M, al Dayel F. Is it feasible to diagnose germ-cell tumors by fine-needle aspiration biopsy? Diagn Cytopathol. 1997 Jan;16(1):72–7. PMID:9034742
12. Akinfolarin J, Black A, Al-Abbadi M. Pulmonary mesothelioma in bronchioalveolar lavage: a case report. Diagn Cytopathol. 2008 Mar;36(3):190–2. PMID:18232009
13. Alcala N, Leblay N, Gabriel AAG, et al. Integrative and comparative genomic analyses identify clinically relevant pulmonary carcinoid groups and unveil the supra-carcinoids. Nat Commun. 2019 Aug 20;10(1):3407. PMID:31431620
14. Aldera AP, Schubert PT. Endobronchial masses encountered on fine-needle aspiration biopsy: a focus on unusual entities. Diagn Cytopathol. 2020 Aug;48(8):807–12. PMID:32329967
15. Allison DB, Simner PJ, Ali SZ. Identification of infectious organisms in cytopathology: a review of ancillary diagnostic techniques. Cancer Cytopathol. 2018 Aug;126 Suppl 8:643–53. PMID:30156776
16. Almarzooqi S, Kahwash SB. Detached respiratory cilia: an organism mimicker in BAL specimens. Adv Anat Pathol. 2011 Sep;18(5):414. PMID:21841409
17. Alsharif M, Andrade RS, Groth SS, et al. Endobronchial ultrasound-guided transbronchial fine-needle aspiration: the University of Minnesota experience, with emphasis on usefulness, adequacy assessment, and diagnostic difficulties. Am J Clin Pathol. 2008 Sep;130(3):434–43. PMID:18701418
18. Althakfi W, Gazzo S, Blanchet M, et al. The value of BRCA-1-associated protein 1 expression and cyclin-dependent kinase inhibitor 2A deletion to distinguish peritoneal malignant mesothelioma from peritoneal location of carcinoma in effusion cytology specimens. Cytopathology. 2020 Jan;31(1):5–11. PMID:31713897
19. Anderson C, Ludwig ME, O'Donnell M, et al. Fine needle aspiration cytology of pulmonary carcinoid tumors. Acta Cytol. 1990 Jul-Aug;34(4):505–10. PMID:2375219
20. Andrici J, Sheen A, Sioson L, et al. Loss of expression of BAP1 is a useful adjunct, which strongly supports the diagnosis of mesothelioma in effusion cytology. Mod Pathol. 2015 Oct;28(10):1360–8. PMID:26226841
21. Ang KL, Dhannapuneni VR, Morgan WE, et al. Primary pulmonary pleomorphic adenoma. An immunohistochemical study and review of the literature. Arch Pathol Lab Med. 2003 May;127(5):621–2. PMID:12708911
22. Antman K, Shemin R, Ryan L, et al. Malignant mesothelioma: prognostic variables in a registry of 180 patients, the Dana-Farber Cancer Institute and Brigham and Women's Hospital experience over two decades, 1965-1985. J Clin Oncol. 1988 Jan;6(1):147–53. PMID:3335886
23. Antonescu CR, Owosho AA, Zhang L, et al. Sarcomas with CIC-rearrangements are a distinct pathologic entity with aggressive outcome: a clinicopathologic and molecular study of 115 cases. Am J Surg Pathol. 2017 Jul;41(7):941–9. PMID:28346326
24. Antonescu CR, Suurmeijer AJ, Zhang L, et al. Molecular characterization of inflammatory myofibroblastic tumors with frequent ALK and ROS1 gene fusions and rare novel RET rearrangement. Am J Surg Pathol. 2015 Jul;39(7):957–67. PMID:25723109
25. Araujo RW, Paiva V, Gartner F, et al. Fine needle aspiration as a tool to establish primary human breast cancer cultures in vitro. Acta Cytol. 1999 Nov-Dec;43(6):985–90. PMID:10578968
26. Archie PH, Beasley MB, Ross HJ. Biphasic pulmonary blastoma with germ cell differentiation in a 36-year-old man. J Thorac Oncol. 2008 Oct;3(10):1185–7. PMID:18827617
27. Arora R, Mathur SR, Aron M, et al. Oncocytic carcinoid tumor of the lung: a case report of diagnostic pitfall in filter membrane preparation of bronchial washings. Acta Cytol. 2007 Nov-Dec;51(6):907–10. PMID:18077984
28. Asakura K, Izumi Y, Ikeda T, et al. Mediastinal germ cell tumor with somatic-type malignancy: report of 5 stage I/II cases. Ann Thorac Surg. 2010 Sep;90(3):1014–6. PMID:20732540
29. Ascoli V, Murer B, Nottegar A, et al. What's new in mesothelioma. Pathologica. 2018 Mar;110(1):12–28. PMID:30259910
30. Auger M, Brimo F, Kanber Y, et al. A practical guide for ancillary studies in pulmonary cytologic specimens. Cancer Cytopathol. 2018 Aug;126 Suppl 8:599–614. PMID:30156772
31. Aumann K, Kayser G, Amann D, et al. The format type has impact on the quality of pathology reports of oncological lung resection specimens. Lung Cancer. 2013 Sep;81(3):382–7. PMID:23790451
32. Awasthi A, Malhotra P, Gupta N, et al. Pitfalls in the diagnosis of Wegener's granulomatosis on fine needle aspiration cytology. Cytopathology. 2007 Feb;18(1):8–12. PMID:17250597
33. Bacci E, Cianchetti S, Paggiaro PL, et al. Comparison between hypertonic and isotonic saline-induced sputum in the evaluation of airway inflammation in subjects with moderate asthma. Clin Exp Allergy. 1996 Dec;26(12):1395–400. PMID:9027440
34. Baehner FL, Ng B, Sudilovsky D. Metastatic balloon cell melanoma: a case report. Acta Cytol. 2005 Sep-Oct;49(5):543–8. PMID:16334034
35. Baldovini C, Rossi G, Ciarrocchi A. Approaches to tumor classification in pulmonary sarcomatoid carcinoma. Lung Cancer (Auckl). 2019 Dec 5;10:131–49. PMID:31824199
36. Ball A, Bromley A, Glaze S, et al. A rare case of NUT midline carcinoma. Gynecol Oncol Case Rep. 2012 Oct 8;3:1–3. PMID:24371650
37. Baloch Z, Mete O, Asa SL. Immunohistochemical biomarkers in thyroid pathology. Endocr Pathol. 2018 Jun;29(2):91–112. PMID:29744727
38. Balwan A, Bixby B, Grotepas C, et al. Core needle biopsy with endobronchial ultrasonography: single center experience with 100 cases. J Am Soc Cytopathol. 2020 Jul-Aug;9(4):249–53. PMID:32451285
39. Ban X, Shen X, Hu H, et al. Predictive CT features for the diagnosis of primary pulmonary mucoepidermoid carcinoma: comparison with squamous cell carcinomas and adenocarcinomas. Cancer Imaging. 2021 Jan 6;21(1):2. PMID:33407915
40. Banet N, Gown AM, Shih IeM, et al. GATA-3 expression in trophoblastic tissues: an immunohistochemical study of 445 cases, including diagnostic utility. Am J Surg Pathol. 2015 Jan;39(1):101–8. PMID:25188865
41. Baranov E, McBride MJ, Bellizzi AM, et al. A novel SS18-SSX fusion-specific antibody for the diagnosis of synovial sarcoma. Am J Surg Pathol. 2020 Jul;44(7):922–33. PMID:32141887
42. Barbieri A, Prasad ML, Gilani SM. Thyroid tissue outside the thyroid gland: differential diagnosis and associated diagnostic challenges. Ann Diagn Pathol. 2020 Oct;48:151584. PMID:32871503
43. Barkan GA, Wojcik EM, Pambuccian SE. A tale of atypia: What can we learn from this? Cancer Cytopathol. 2018 Jun;126(6):376–80. PMID:29757490
44. Barman DC, Halder A, Bhattacharya S, et al. Yolk sac tumour of the cryptorchid testis, with an unusual presentation - diagnosed by fine needle aspiration cytology. J Clin Diagn Res. 2013 Jul;7(7):1444–6. PMID:23998088
45. Bassarova AV, Nesland JM, Davidson B. D2-40 is not a specific marker for cells of mesothelial origin in serous effusions. Am J Surg Pathol. 2006 Jul;30(7):878–82. PMID:16819331
46. Basu A, Moreira AL, Simms A, et al. Sarcomatoid carcinoma in cytology: report of a rare entity presenting in pleural and pericardial fluid preparations. Diagn Cytopathol. 2019 Aug;47(8):813–6. PMID:30908904
47. Bauer DE, Mitchell CM, Strait KM, et al. Clinicopathologic features and long-term outcomes of NUT midline carcinoma. Clin Cancer Res. 2012 Oct 15;18(20):5773–9. PMID:22896655
48. Baughman RP. Technical aspects of bronchoalveolar lavage: recommendations for a standard procedure. Semin Respir Crit Care Med. 2007 Oct;28(5):475–85. PMID:17975775
49. Bavikatty NR, Michael CW. Cytologic features of small-cell carcinoma on ThinPrep. Diagn Cytopathol. 2003 Jul;29(1):8–12. PMID:12827707
50. Bayrak BY, Paksoy N, Vural Ç. Diagnostic utility of fine needle aspiration cytology and core biopsy histopathology with or without immunohistochemical staining in the subtyping of the non-small cell lung carcinomas: experience from an academic centre in Turkey. Cytopathology. 2021 May;32(3):331–7. PMID:33145811
51. Bean SM, Baker A, Eloubeidi M, et al. Endoscopic ultrasound-guided fine-needle aspiration of intrathoracic and intra-abdominal spindle cell and mesenchymal lesions. Cancer Cytopathol. 2011 Feb 25;119(1):37–48. PMID:20967877
52. Bechert CJ, Schnadig V, Nawgiri R. The Merkel cell carcinoma challenge: a review from the fine needle aspiration service. Cancer Cytopathol. 2013 Apr;121(4):179–88. PMID:23225406
53. Bedrossian CW, Warren CJ, Ohar J, et al. Amiodarone pulmonary toxicity: cytopathology, ultrastructure, and immunocytochemistry. Ann Diagn Pathol. 1997 Oct;1(1):47–56. PMID:9869825
54. Bellevicine C, Malapelle U, Vigliar E, et al. How to prepare cytological samples for molecular testing. J Clin Pathol. 2017 Oct;70(10):819–26. PMID:28739858
55. Belli C, Penault-Llorca F, Ladanyi M, et al. ESMO recommendations on the standard methods to detect RET fusions and mutations in daily practice and clinical research. Ann Oncol. 2021 Mar;32(3):337–50. PMID:33455880
56. Bellizzi AM, Bruzzi C, French CA, et al. The cytologic features of NUT midline carcinoma. Cancer. 2009 Dec 25;117(6):508–15. PMID:19795508
57. Berg KB, Dacic S, Miller C, et al. Utility of methylthioadenosine phosphorylase compared with BAP1 immunohistochemistry, and CDKN2A and NF2 fluorescence in situ hybridization in separating reactive mesothelial proliferations from epithelioid malignant mesotheliomas. Arch Pathol Lab Med. 2018 Dec;142(12):1549–53. PMID:30059257
58. Berner A, Franzen S, Heilo A. Fine needle aspiration cytology as a diagnostic approach to lymphangioleiomyomatosis. A case report. Acta Cytol. 1997 May-Jun;41(3):877–9. PMID:9167718
59. Bertario L, Russo A, Sala P, et al. Genotype and phenotype factors as determinants of desmoid tumors in patients with familial adenomatous polyposis. Int J Cancer. 2001 Mar 20;95(2):102–7. PMID:11241320
60. Betz BL, Dixon CA, Weigelin HC, et al. The use of stained cytologic direct smears

for ALK gene rearrangement analysis of lung adenocarcinoma. Cancer Cytopathol. 2013 Sep;121(9):489–99. PMID:23536384

61. Bezel P, Tischler V, Robinson C, et al. Diagnostic value of bronchoalveolar lavage for diagnosis of suspected peripheral lung cancer. Clin Lung Cancer. 2016 Sep;17(5):e151–6. PMID:26831835

62. Bhadani PP, Agarwal A, Sah SP, et al. Fine needle aspiration diagnosis of ectopic thyroid with laboratory features of hyperthyroidism. Acta Cytol. 2005 Mar-Apr;49(2):228–30. PMID:15839636

63. Bhalla AS, Goyal A, Guleria R, et al. Chest tuberculosis: radiological review and imaging recommendations. Indian J Radiol Imaging. 2015 Jul-Sep;25(3):213–25. PMID:26288514

64. Bhatti V, Kwatra KS, Puri S, et al. Histopathological spectrum and immunohistochemical profile of lung carcinomas: a 9-year study from a tertiary hospital in north India. Int J Appl Basic Med Res. 2019 Jul-Sep;9(3):169–75. PMID:31392181

65. Binesh F, Pirdehghan A, Mirjalili MR, et al. Comparative assessment of the diagnostic value of transbronchial lung biopsy and bronchoalveolar lavage fluid cytology in lung cancer. Asian Pac J Cancer Prev. 2015;16(1):201–4. PMID:25640352

66. Bishop JA, French CA, Ali SZ. Cytopathologic features of NUT midline carcinoma: a series of 26 specimens from 13 patients. Cancer Cytopathol. 2016 Dec;124(12):901–8. PMID:27400194

67. Bishop JA, Ogawa T, Chang X, et al. HPV analysis in distinguishing second primary tumors from lung metastases in patients with head and neck squamous cell carcinoma. Am J Surg Pathol. 2012 Jan;36(1):142–8. PMID:22173119

68. Bishop JA, Rekhtman N, Chun J, et al. Malignant solitary fibrous tumor: cytopathologic findings and differential diagnosis. Cancer Cytopathol. 2010 Apr 25;118(2):83–9. PMID:20209623

69. Blanquart C, Gueugnon F, Nguyen JM, et al. CCL2, galectin-3, and SMRP combination improves the diagnosis of mesothelioma in pleural effusions. J Thorac Oncol. 2012 May;7(5):883–9. PMID:22729037

70. Boccalatte LA, Higuera F, Gómez NL, et al. Usefulness of 18F-fluorocholine positron emission tomography-computed tomography in locating lesions in hyperparathyroidism: a systematic review. JAMA Otolaryngol Head Neck Surg. 2019 Aug 1;145(8):743–50. PMID:31145436

71. Böcking A, Biesterfeld S, Chatelain R, et al. Diagnosis of bronchial carcinoma on sections of paraffin-embedded sputum. Sensitivity and specificity of an alternative to routine cytology. Acta Cytol. 1992 Jan-Feb;36(1):37–47. PMID:1546511

72. Bocklage TJ, Dail D, Colby TV. Primary lung tumors infiltrated by osteoclast-like giant cells. Ann Diagn Pathol. 1998 Aug;2(4):229–40. PMID:9845743

73. Bode-Lesniewska B, Zhao J, Speel EJ, et al. Gains of 12q13-14 and overexpression of mdm2 are frequent findings in intimal sarcomas of the pulmonary artery. Virchows Arch. 2001 Jan;438(1):57–65. PMID:11213836

74. Boland JM, Colby TV, Folpe AL. Intrathoracic peripheral nerve sheath tumors-a clinicopathological study of 75 cases. Hum Pathol. 2015 Mar;46(3):419–25. PMID:25595633

75. Boland JM, Lee HE, Barr Fritcher EG, et al. Molecular genetic landscape of sclerosing pneumocytomas. Am J Clin Pathol. 2021 Feb 11;155(3):397–404. PMID:33145590

76. Boler AK, Banu N, Bose K, et al. Reproducibility of "the Papanicolaou Society of Cytopathology system for reporting respiratory cytology" - a retrospective analysis of 101 cases of CT-guided FNAC. Diagn Cytopathol. 2020 Aug;48(8):701–5. PMID:32353212

77. Bonetti F, Chiodera PL, Pea M, et al. Transbronchial biopsy in lymphangiomyomatosis of the lung. HMB45 for diagnosis. Am J Surg Pathol. 1993 Nov;17(11):1092–102. PMID:8214254

78. Borak S, Siegal GP, Reddy V, et al. Metastatic inflammatory myofibroblastic tumor identified by EUS-FNA in mediastinal lymph nodes with ancillary FISH studies for ALK rearrangement. Diagn Cytopathol. 2012 Aug;40 Suppl 2:E118–25. PMID:21472870

79. Borczuk AC. Benign tumors and tumorlike conditions of the lung. Arch Pathol Lab Med. 2008 Jul;132(7):1133–48. PMID:18605767

80. Borczuk AC. Neoplastic and nonneoplastic benign mass lesions of the lung. Arch Pathol Lab Med. 2012 Oct;136(10):1227–33. PMID:23020728

81. Borczuk AC. Uncommon types of lung carcinoma with mixed histology: sarcomatoid carcinoma, adenosquamous carcinoma, and mucoepidermoid carcinoma. Arch Pathol Lab Med. 2018 Aug;142(8):914–21. PMID:30040455

82. Borie R, Wislez M, Antoine M, et al. Pulmonary mucosa-associated lymphoid tissue lymphoma revisited. Eur Respir J. 2016 Apr;47(4):1244–60. PMID:26797028

83. Borie R, Wislez M, Thabut G, et al. Clinical characteristics and prognostic factors of pulmonary MALT lymphoma. Eur Respir J. 2009 Dec;34(6):1408–16. PMID:19541720

84. Bosken CH, Myers JL, Greenberger PA, et al. Pathologic features of allergic bronchopulmonary aspergillosis. Am J Surg Pathol. 1988 Mar;12(3):216–22. PMID:3344888

85. Bothamley GH, Ditiu L, Migliori GB, et al. Active case finding of tuberculosis in Europe: a Tuberculosis Network European Trials Group (TBNET) survey. Eur Respir J. 2008 Oct;32(4):1023–30. PMID:18550615

86. Boucher LD, Swanson PE, Stanley MW, et al. Cytology of angiosarcoma. Findings in fourteen fine-needle aspiration biopsy specimens and one pleural fluid specimen. Am J Clin Pathol. 2000 Aug;114(2):210–9. PMID:10941336

87. Boulagnon-Rombi C, Fleury C, Fichel C, et al. Immunohistochemical approach to the differential diagnosis of meningiomas and their mimics. J Neuropathol Exp Neurol. 2017 Apr 1;76(4):289–98. PMID:28340171

88. Boutin C, Rey F, Viallat JR. Prevention of malignant seeding after invasive diagnostic procedures in patients with pleural mesothelioma. A randomized trial of local radiotherapy. Chest. 1995 Sep;108(3):754–8. PMID:7656629

89. Bridge JA, Kanamori M, Ma Z, et al. Fusion of the ALK gene to the clathrin heavy chain gene, CLTC, in inflammatory myofibroblastic tumor. Am J Pathol. 2001 Aug;159(2):411–5. PMID:11485898

90. Brightman I, Morgan JA, von Zwehl D, et al. Cytological appearances of a solitary squamous cell papilloma with associated mucous gland adenoma in the lung. Cytopathology. 1992;3(4):253–7. PMID:1421008

91. Bruno R, Fontanini G. Next generation sequencing for gene fusion analysis in lung cancer: a literature review. Diagnostics (Basel). 2020 Jul 27;10(8):521. PMID:32726941

92. Bryan A, Kurian S, Flowers AB, et al. Intratracheal parathyroid gland: an unexpected diagnosis. BMJ Case Rep. 2021 Feb 12;14(2):e239435. PMID:33579799

93. Bubendorf L, Lantuejoul S, de Langen AJ, et al. Nonsmall cell lung carcinoma: diagnostic difficulties in small biopsies and cytological specimens: Number 2 in the Series "Pathology for the clinician" Edited by Peter Dorfmüller and Alberto Cavazza. Eur Respir Rev. 2017 Jun 28;26(144):170007. PMID:28659503

94. Bulman W, Saqi A, Powell CA. Acquisition and processing of endobronchial ultrasound-guided transbronchial needle aspiration specimens in the era of targeted lung cancer chemotherapy. Am J Respir Crit Care Med. 2012 Mar 15;185(6):606–11. PMID:22071327

95. Buonocore DJ, Konno F, Jungbluth AA, et al. CytoLyt fixation significantly inhibits MIB1 immunoreactivity whereas alternative Ki-67 clone 30-9 is not susceptible to the inhibition: critical diagnostic implications. Cancer Cytopathol. 2019 Oct;127(10):643–9. PMID:31398281

96. Burrah R, Kini U, Correa M, et al. Pulmonary oncocytoma: a rare case. Asian Cardiovasc Thorac Ann. 2006 Dec;14(6):e113–4. PMID:17130314

97. Busmanis I, Harney M, Hellyar A. Nocardiosis diagnosed by lung FNA: a case report. Diagn Cytopathol. 1995 Feb;12(1):56–8. PMID:7789248

98. Butt YM, Smith ML, Tazelaar HD, et al. Pathology of vaping-associated lung injury. N Engl J Med. 2019 Oct 31;381(18):1780–1. PMID:31577870

99. Cai Q, Zhang R, Wu G, et al. Adenoid cystic carcinoma of submandibular salivary gland with late metastases to lung and choroid: a case report and literature review. J Oral Maxillofac Surg. 2014 Sep;72(9):1744–55. PMID:25043143

100. Caliò A, Mengoli MC, Cavazza A, et al. Cathepsin K expression in clear cell "sugar" tumor (PEComa) of the lung. Virchows Arch. 2018 Jul;473(1):55–9. PMID:29516164

101. Cameron SE, Andrade RS, Pambuccian SE. Endobronchial ultrasound-guided transbronchial needle aspiration cytology: a state of the art review. Cytopathology. 2010 Feb;21(1):6–26. PMID:20015257

102. Camidge DR, Doebele RC, Kerr KM. Comparing and contrasting predictive biomarkers for immunotherapy and targeted therapy of NSCLC. Nat Rev Clin Oncol. 2019 Jun;16(6):341–55. PMID:30718843

103. Camidge DR, Otterson GA, Clark JW, et al. Crizotinib in patients with MET-amplified NSCLC. J Thorac Oncol. 2021 Jun;16(6):1017–29. PMID:33676017

104. Canberk S, Engels M. Cytology samples and molecular biomarker testing in lung cancer-advantages and challenges. Virchows Arch. 2021 Jan;478(1):45–57. PMID:33389149

105. Canberk S, Montezuma D, Aydın O, et al. The new guidelines of Papanicolaou Society of Cytopathology for respiratory specimens: assessment of risk of malignancy and diagnostic yield in different cytological modalities. Diagn Cytopathol. 2018 Sep;46(9):725–9. PMID:30051969

106. Canberk S, Tischler V, Engels M. Current topics and practical considerations of cytology practice in lung cancer: reflexions from the lung symposium at the 42nd European Congress of Cytology, Malmö, 2019. Acta Cytol. 2020;64(5):463–70. PMID:32259828

107. Candes FP, Ajinkya MS. Primary mediastinal choriocarcinoma (a case report). J Postgrad Med. 1987 Oct;33(4):219–21. PMID:3449627

108. Canessa PA, Franceschini MC, Ferro P, et al. Evaluation of soluble mesothelin-related peptide as a diagnostic marker of malignant pleural mesothelioma effusions: its contribution to cytology. Cancer Invest. 2013 Jan;31(1):43–50. PMID:23249166

109. Caplin ME, Baudin E, Ferolla P, et al. Pulmonary neuroendocrine (carcinoid) tumors: European Neuroendocrine Tumor Society expert consensus and recommendations for best practice for typical and atypical pulmonary carcinoids. Ann Oncol. 2015 Aug;26(8):1604–20. PMID:25646366

110. Caraway NP, Fanning CV, Amato RJ, et al. Fine-needle aspiration cytology of seminoma: a review of 16 cases. Diagn Cytopathol. 1995 Jun;12(4):327–33. PMID:7544720

111. Caraway NP, Salina D, Deavers MT, et al. Pulmonary artery intimal sarcoma diagnosed using endobronchial ultrasound-guided transbronchial needle aspiration. Cytojournal. 2015 Feb 18;12:3. PMID:25745502

112. Cardoso AV, Neves I, Magalhães A, et al. The value of rapid on-site evaluation during EBUS-TBNA. Rev Port Pneumol (2006). 2015 Sep-Oct;21(5):253–8. PMID:25926258

113. Carlson JW, Fletcher CD. Immunohistochemistry for beta-catenin in the differential diagnosis of spindle cell lesions: analysis of a series and review of the literature. Histopathology. 2007 Oct;51(4):509–14. PMID:17711447

114. Carral F, Jiménez AI, Tomé M, et al. Safety and diagnostic performance of parathyroid hormone assay in fine-needle aspirate in suspicious parathyroid adenomas. Endocrinol Diabetes Nutr (Engl Ed). 2021 Aug-Sep;68(7):481–8. PMID:34863413

115. Celik B, Bulut T, Khoor A. Subtyping of non-small cell lung cancer by cytology specimens: a proposal for resource-poor hospitals. Cytojournal. 2019 Apr 22;16:8. PMID:31080486

116. Ceyhan K, Utkan G, Dincol D, et al. Fine needle aspiration biopsy features with histologic correlation in mediastinal hepatoid yolk sac tumor presenting with sternum metastasis: a case report. Acta Cytol. 2007 Jul-Aug;51(4):610–5. PMID:17718136

117. Chae KJ, Hong H, Yoon SH, et al. Non-diagnostic results of percutaneous transthoracic needle biopsy: a meta-analysis. Sci Rep. 2019 Aug 27;9(1):12428. PMID:31455841

118. Chamberlain BK, McClain CM, Gonzalez RS, et al. Alveolar soft part sarcoma and granular cell tumor: an immunohistochemical comparison study. Hum Pathol. 2014 May;45(5):1039–44. PMID:24746209

119. Chamberlain DW, Braude AC, Rebuck AS. A critical evaluation of bronchoalveolar lavage. Criteria for identifying unsatisfactory specimens. Acta Cytol. 1987 Sep-Oct;31(5):599–605. PMID:3673466

120. Chang M, Lim D, Genovesi M. Clear cell "sugar" tumor of the lung: a case report and review of the literature. AME Case Rep. 2018 Aug 24;2:40. PMID:30363768

121. Chao TY, Nieh S, Huang SH, et al. Cytology of fine needle aspirates of primary extragonadal germ cell tumors. Acta Cytol. 1997 Mar-Apr;41(2):497–503. PMID:9100787

122. Chapel DB, Husain AN, Krausz T, et al. PAX8 expression in a subset of malignant peritoneal mesotheliomas and benign mesothelium has diagnostic implications in the differential diagnosis of ovarian serous carcinoma. Am J Surg Pathol. 2017 Dec;41(12):1675–82. PMID:28877056

123. Chatterjee D, Dey P. Tuberculosis revisited: cytological perspective. Diagn Cytopathol. 2014 Nov;42(11):993–1001. PMID:24975566

124. Chatzopoulos K, Boland JM. Update on genetically defined lung neoplasms: NUT carcinoma and thoracic SMARCA4-deficient undifferentiated tumors. Virchows Arch. 2021 Jan;478(1):21–30. PMID:33409598

125. Chatzopoulos K, Fritchie KJ, Aubry MC, et al. Loss of succinate dehydrogenase B immunohistochemical expression distinguishes pulmonary chondromas from hamartomas. Histopathology. 2019 Dec;75(6):825–32. PMID:31236950

126. Chau NG, Ma C, Danga K, et al. An anatomical site and genetic-based prognostic model for patients with nuclear protein in testis (NUT) midline carcinoma: analysis of 124 patients. JNCI Cancer Spectr. 2019 Nov 6;4(2):pkz094. PMID:32328562

127. Chaudhry AP, Jacobs MS, SunderRaj M, et al. A clinico-pathologic study of 50 adult oral granular cell tumors. J Oral Med. 1984 Apr-Jun;39(2):97–103, 118. PMID:6330328
128. Chebib I, Hornicek FJ, Nielsen GP, et al. Cytomorphologic features that distinguish schwannoma from other low-grade spindle cell lesions. Cancer Cytopathol. 2015 Mar;123(3):171–9. PMID:25641870
129. Chen AC, Pastis NJ Jr, Mahajan AK, et al. Robotic bronchoscopy for peripheral pulmonary lesions: a multicenter pilot and feasibility study (BENEFIT). Chest. 2021 Feb;159(2):845–52. PMID:32822675
130. Chen CC, Chi CY. Biosafety in the preparation and processing of cytology specimens with potential coronavirus (COVID-19) infection: perspectives from Taiwan. Cancer Cytopathol. 2020 May;128(5):309–16. PMID:32259402
131. Chen D, Zhu G, Wang D, et al. Clinicopathological and immunohistochemical features of pulmonary artery sarcoma: a report of three cases and review of the literature. Oncol Lett. 2016 Apr;11(4):2820–6. PMID:27073558
132. Chen KT. Cytodiagnostic pitfalls in pulmonary coccidioidomycosis. Diagn Cytopathol. 1995 Mar;12(2):177–80. PMID:7774502
133. Chen KT. Cytology of bronchial benign granular-cell tumor. Acta Cytol. 1991 Jul-Aug;35(4):381–4. PMID:1927170
134. Chen L, Jing H, Gong Y, et al. Diagnostic efficacy and molecular testing by combined fine-needle aspiration and core needle biopsy in patients with a lung nodule. Cancer Cytopathol. 2020 Mar;128(3):201–6. PMID:31913583
135. Chen X, Wright JD, Abellar RG, et al. Cytological features of choricarcinoma in a Pap smear: a case report and literature review. Diagn Cytopathol. 2016 Apr;44(4):324–8. PMID:26712464
136. Chen YH, Gong Y. Cytopathology in the diagnosis of lymphoma. Cancer Treat Res. 2014;160:211–40. PMID:24092372
137. Cheng AP, Dong MJ, Fu LP, et al. A rare case of pulmonary malignant granular cell tumor detected with 18F-FDG PET/CT imaging. Clin Nucl Med. 2014 Sep;39(9):816–8. PMID:24300348
138. Cheng H, Yang L, Xiong J, et al. Multiple thyroid nodules in the lung: metastasis or ectopia? Diagn Pathol. 2015 Jun 6;10:61. PMID:26047938
139. Cheng L, Jiang X, Jiang Y. Ectopic thyroid as multiple nodules in bilateral lung lobes: a case report. Gland Surg. 2020 Jun;9(3):806–11. PMID:32775272
140. Cheng Y, Zhang Y, Yuan Y, et al. The comprehensive analyses of genomic variations and assessment of TMB and PD-L1 expression in Chinese lung adenosquamous carcinoma. Front Genet. 2021 Feb 17;11:609405. PMID:33679868
141. Cheuk W, Kwan MY, Suster S, et al. Immunostaining for thyroid transcription factor 1 and cytokeratin 20 aids the distinction of small cell carcinoma from Merkel cell carcinoma, but not pulmonary from extrapulmonary small cell carcinomas. Arch Pathol Lab Med. 2001 Feb;125(2):228–31. PMID:11175640
142. Chhieng DC. Cytology of bronchial associated lymphoid tissue lymphoma. Diagn Cytopathol. 2008 Oct;36(10):723–8. PMID:18773446
143. Chhieng DC, Lin O, Moran CA, et al. Fine-needle aspiration biopsy of nonteratomatous germ cell tumors of the mediastinum. Am J Clin Pathol. 2002 Sep;118(3):418–24. PMID:12219784
144. Chiosea SI, Miller M, Seethala RR. HRAS mutations in epithelial-myoepithelial carcinoma. Head Neck Pathol. 2014 Jun;8(2):146–50. PMID:24277618
145. Chmielecki J, Crago AM, Rosenberg M, et al. Whole-exome sequencing identifies a recurrent NAB2-STAT6 fusion in solitary fibrous tumors. Nat Genet. 2013 Feb;45(2):131–2. PMID:23313954
146. Cho YA, Choi YL, Hwang I, et al. Clinicopathological characteristics of primary lung nuclear protein in testis carcinoma: a single-institute experience of 10 cases. Thorac Cancer. 2020 Nov;11(11):3205–12. PMID:33009876
147. Choi HS, Seol H, Heo IY, et al. Fine-needle aspiration cytology of pleomorphic carcinomas of the lung. Korean J Pathol. 2012 Dec;46(6):576–82. PMID:23323109
148. Choi SM, Lee AR, Choe JY, et al. Adequacy criteria of rapid on-site evaluation for endobronchial ultrasound-guided transbronchial needle aspiration: a simple algorithm to assess the adequacy of ROSE. Ann Thorac Surg. 2016 Feb;101(2):444–50. PMID:26431922
149. Choi YD, Han CW, Kim JH, et al. Effectiveness of sputum cytology using ThinPrep method for evaluation of lung cancer. Diagn Cytopathol. 2008 Mar;36(3):167–71. PMID:18232006
150. Chong CR, Wirth LJ, Nishino M, et al. Chemotherapy for locally advanced and metastatic pulmonary carcinoid tumors. Lung Cancer. 2014 Nov;86(2):241–6. PMID:25218177
151. Chopra A, Nautiyal A, Kalkanis A, et al. Drug-induced sarcoidosis-like reactions. Chest. 2018 Sep;154(3):664–77. PMID:29698718
152. Choudhury M, Singh S, Agarwal S. Efficacy of bronchial brush cytology and bronchial washings in diagnosis of non neoplastic and neoplastic bronchopulmonary lesions. Turk Patoloji Derg. 2012;28(2):142–6. PMID:22627632
153. Chrabańska M, Środa M, Kiczmer P, et al. Lung cancer cytology: Can any of the cytological methods replace histopathology? J Cytol. 2020 Jul-Sep;37(3):117–21. PMID:33088028
154. Churg A, Colby TV, Cagle P, et al. The separation of benign and malignant mesothelial proliferations. Am J Surg Pathol. 2000 Sep;24(9):1183–200. PMID:10976692
155. Churg A, Dacic S, Galateau-Salle F, et al. Malignant mesothelioma in situ: clinical and pathologic implications. J Thorac Oncol. 2020 Jun;15(6):899–901. PMID:32307274
156. Churg A, Galateau-Salle F, Roden AC, et al. Malignant mesothelioma in situ: morphologic features and clinical outcome. Mod Pathol. 2020 Feb;33(2):297–302. PMID:31375770
157. Churg A, Hwang H, Tan L, et al. Malignant mesothelioma in situ. Histopathology. 2018 May;72(6):1033–8. PMID:29350783
158. Churg A, Sheffield BS, Galateau-Salle F. New markers for separating benign from malignant mesothelial proliferations: Are we there yet? Arch Pathol Lab Med. 2016 Apr;140(4):318–21. PMID:26288396
159. Cimbaluk D, Kasuganti D, Kluskens L, et al. Malignant biphasic pleural mesothelioma metastatic to the liver diagnosed by fine-needle aspiration. Diagn Cytopathol. 2006 Jan;34(1):33–6. PMID:16355399
160. Cimic A, Rekhtman N. CytoJounal quiz case: Fine-needle aspiration of peripancreatic mass clinically mimicking a lymphoma. Cytojournal. 2019 May 24;16:11. PMID:31367219
161. Clark SB, Alsubait S. Non small cell lung cancer. 2022 Sep 5. In: StatPearls. Treasure Island (FL): StatPearls Publishing; 2022 Jan–. PMID:32965978
162. Clement MJ, Luce JM, Hopewell PC. Diagnosis of pulmonary diseases. Clin Chest Med. 1988 Sep;9(3):497–505. PMID:3044685
163. Coffin CM, Hornick JL, Fletcher CD. Inflammatory myofibroblastic tumor: comparison of clinicopathologic, histologic, and immunohistochemical features including ALK expression in atypical and aggressive cases. Am J Surg Pathol. 2007 Apr;31(4):509–20. PMID:17414097
164. Collins AM, Rylance J, Wootton DG, et al. Bronchoalveolar lavage (BAL) for research; obtaining adequate sample yield. J Vis Exp. 2014 Mar 24;(85):4345. PMID:24686157
165. Collins BT, Cramer HM. Fine needle aspiration cytology of carcinoid tumors. Acta Cytol. 1996 Jul-Aug;40(4):695–707. PMID:8693889
166. Collins KA, Geisinger KR, Wagner PH, et al. The cytologic evaluation of lipid-laden alveolar macrophages as an indicator of aspiration pneumonia in young children. Arch Pathol Lab Med. 1995 Mar;119(3):229–31. PMID:7887776
167. Conde E, Suárez-Gauthier A, Benito A, et al. Accurate identification of ALK positive lung carcinoma patients: novel FDA-cleared automated fluorescence in situ hybridization scanning system and ultrasensitive immunohistochemistry. PLoS One. 2014 Sep 23;9(9):e107200. PMID:25248157
168. Conner JR, Hornick JL. Metastatic carcinoma of unknown primary: diagnostic approach using immunohistochemistry. Adv Anat Pathol. 2015 May;22(3):149–67. PMID:25844674
169. Cook JR, Dehner LP, Collins MH, et al. Anaplastic lymphoma kinase (ALK) expression in the inflammatory myofibroblastic tumor: a comparative immunohistochemical study. Am J Surg Pathol. 2001 Nov;25(11):1364–71. PMID:11684952
170. Cooper JD. Management of the solitary pulmonary nodule: directed resection. Semin Thorac Cardiovasc Surg. 2002 Jul;14(3):286–91. PMID:12232871
171. Córdoba A, de Llano P, Arrechea MA, et al. Partial expectoration of a typical carcinoid: report of a case with diagnosis on sputum cytology. Acta Cytol. 2006 Sep-Oct;50(5):581–3. PMID:17017452
172. Cosgrove MM, Chandrasoma PT, Martin SE. Diagnosis of pulmonary blastoma by fine-needle aspiration biopsy: cytologic and immunocytochemical findings. Diagn Cytopathol. 1991;7(1):83–7. PMID:1709089
173. Cosío BG, Villena V, Echave-Sustaeta J, et al. Endobronchial hamartoma. Chest. 2002 Jul;122(1):202–5. PMID:12114359
174. Crapanzano JP, Heymann JJ, Monaco S, et al. The state of cell block variation and satisfaction in the era of molecular diagnostics and personalized medicine. Cytojournal. 2014 Mar 20;11:7. PMID:24799951
175. Crapanzano JP, Loukeris K, Borczuk AC, et al. Cytological, histological, and immunohistochemical findings of pulmonary carcinomas with basaloid features. Diagn Cytopathol. 2011 Feb;39(2):92–100. PMID:21254456
176. Crapanzano JP, Saqi A. Pitfalls in pulmonary cytopathology. Diagn Cytopathol. 2011 Feb;39(2):144–54. PMID:20607685
177. Creaney J, Dick IM, Meniawy TM, et al. Comparison of fibulin-3 and mesothelin as markers in malignant mesothelioma. Thorax. 2014 Oct;69(10):895–902. PMID:25037982
178. Cree IA, Foss AJ, Luthert PJ. Undefined high-power fields. Lancet. 1996 Jan 27;347(8996):273–4. PMID:8551926
179. Cree IA, Tan PH, Travis WD, et al. Counting mitoses: SI(ze) matters! Mod Pathol. 2021 Sep;34(9):1651–7. PMID:34079071
180. Crombé A, Alberti N, Villard N, et al. Imaging features of SMARCA4-deficient thoracic sarcomas: a multi-centric study of 21 patients. Eur Radiol. 2019 Sep;29(9):4730–41. PMID:30762113
181. Cromwell HA, Papanicolaou GN. Use of the cytologic method in industrial medicine with special reference to tumors of the lung and the bladder. AMA Arch Ind Hyg Occup Med. 1952 Mar;5(3):232–3. PMID:14902140
182. Curtis BV, Calcaterra TC, Coulson WF. Multiple granular cell tumor: a case report and review of the literature. Head Neck. 1997 Oct;19(7):634–7. PMID:9323154
183. Cutlan RT, Eltorky M. Pulmonary granular cell tumor coexisting with bronchogenic carcinoma. Ann Diagn Pathol. 2001 Apr;5(2):74–9. PMID:11294991
184. Cwierzyk TA, Glasberg SS, Virshup MA, et al. Pulmonary oncocytoma. Report of a case with cytologic, histologic and electron microscopic study. Acta Cytol. 1985 Jul-Aug;29(4):620–3. PMID:2992204
185. da Cunha Santos G, Saieg MA, Troncone G, et al. Cytological preparations for molecular analysis: a review of technical procedures, advantages and limitations for referring samples for testing. Cytopathology. 2018 Apr;29(2):125–32. PMID:29575423
186. Dagli AF, Pehlivan S, Cihangiroglu G, et al. Cytology of mixed germ cell tumor with mediastinal metastasis. J Cytol. 2009 Jul;26(3):120–2. PMID:21938171
187. Dagogo-Jack I, Schrock AB, Kem M, et al. Clinicopathologic characteristics of BRG1-deficient NSCLC. J Thorac Oncol. 2020 May;15(5):766–76. PMID:31988001
188. Dahiya N, Patel MD, Young SW. Neck procedures: thyroid and parathyroid. Radiol Clin North Am. 2020 Nov;58(6):1085–98. PMID:33040850
189. Dahl I, Hagmar B, Idvall I. Benign solitary neurilemoma (schwannoma). A correlative cytological and histological study of 28 cases. Acta Pathol Microbiol Immunol Scand A. 1984 Mar;92(2):91–101. PMID:6702462
190. Das S, Das RN, Sen A, et al. Cytological and histological correlation of granular cell tumor in a series of three cases. J Cancer Res Ther. 2018 Jan-Mar;14(2):459–61. PMID:29516941
191. Davidson B. CD24 is highly useful in differentiating high-grade serous carcinoma from benign and malignant mesothelial cells. Hum Pathol. 2016 Dec;58:123–7. PMID:27589896
192. Davidson B, Firat P, Michael CW, editors. Serous effusions: etiology, diagnosis, prognosis and therapy. 2nd ed. Cham (Switzerland): Springer; 2018.
193. Davidson B, Nielsen S, Christensen J, et al. The role of desmin and N-cadherin in effusion cytology: a comparative study using established markers of mesothelial and epithelial cells. Am J Surg Pathol. 2001 Nov;25(11):1405–12. PMID:11684957
194. Davidson B, Stavnes HT, Hellesylt E, et al. MMP-7 is a highly specific negative marker for benign and malignant mesothelial cells in serous effusions. Hum Pathol. 2016 Jan;47(1):104–8. PMID:26520416
195. Davidson B, Tötsch M, Wohlschlaeger J, et al. The diagnostic role of BAP1 in serous effusions. Hum Pathol. 2018 Sep;79:122–6. PMID:29802871
196. Davidson KR, Ha DM, Schwarz MI, et al. Bronchoalveolar lavage as a diagnostic procedure: a review of known cellular and molecular findings in various lung diseases. J Thorac Dis. 2020 Sep;12(9):4991–5019. PMID:33145073
197. Davies KD, Le AT, Theodoro MF, et al. Identifying and targeting ROS1 gene fusions in non-small cell lung cancer. Clin Cancer Res. 2012 Sep 1;18(17):4570–9. PMID:22919003
198. Davis GS. The role of endobronchial ultrasound-guided transbronchial needle aspiration (EBUS TBNA) in the diagnosis of sarcoidosis. Cancer Cytopathol. 2014 Apr;122(4):239–40. PMID:24500810
199. De Giacomi F, Vassallo R, Yi ES, et al. Acute eosinophilic pneumonia. Causes, diagnosis, and management. Am J Respir Crit Care Med. 2018 Mar 15;197(6):728–36. PMID:29206477
200. de Gracia J, Bravo C, Miravitlles M, et al. Diagnostic value of bronchoalveolar lavage in peripheral lung cancer. Am Rev Respir Dis. 1993 Mar;147(3):649–52. PMID:8442600

201. de Gracia J, Curull V, Vidal R, et al. Diagnostic value of bronchoalveolar lavage in suspected pulmonary tuberculosis. Chest. 1988 Feb;93(2):329–32. PMID:3123151

202. De Palma A, Lorusso M, Di Gennaro F, et al. Pulmonary and mediastinal paragangliomas: rare endothoracic malignancies with challenging diagnosis and treatment. J Thorac Dis. 2018 Sep;10(9):5318–27. PMID:30416779

203. Deans ZC, Costa JL, Cree I, et al. Integration of next-generation sequencing in clinical diagnostic molecular pathology laboratories for analysis of solid tumours; an expert opinion on behalf of IQN Path ASBL. Virchows Arch. 2017 Jan;470(1):5–20. PMID:27678269

204. Deavers M, Guinee D, Koss MN, et al. Granular cell tumors of the lung. Clinicopathologic study of 20 cases. Am J Surg Pathol. 1995 Jun;19(6):627–35. PMID:7755149

205. Delattre C, Fournier C, Bouchindhomme B, et al. Endoscopic ultrasound guided transbronchial fine needle aspiration: a French department of pathology's 4-year experience. J Clin Pathol. 2011 Dec;64(12):1117–22. PMID:21965831

206. DellaGiustina D, Falconieri G, Bonifacio-Gori D, et al. Bronchial cytology in pleural mesothelioma. A report of 3 positive cases, including 1 diagnosed initially on bronchial brushings. Acta Cytol. 2003 Nov-Dec;47(6):1017–22. PMID:14674071

207. Denda T, Kamoshida S, Kawamura J, et al. Optimal antigen retrieval for ethanol-fixed cytologic smears. Cancer Cytopathol. 2012 Jun 25;120(3):167–76. PMID:22434540

208. Denda T, Kamoshida S, Kawamura J, et al. Rapid immunocytochemistry with simple heat-induced antigen retrieval technique for improvement in the quality of cytological diagnosis. J Histochem Cytochem. 2013 Dec;61(12):920–30. PMID:24004858

209. Dettrick A, Meikle A, Fong KM. Fine-needle aspiration diagnosis of sclerosing hemangioma (pneumocytoma): report of a case and review of the literature. Diagn Cytopathol. 2014 Mar;42(3):242–6. PMID:22645055

210. Devouassoux-Shisheboran M, Hayashi T, Linnoila RI, et al. A clinicopathologic study of 100 cases of pulmonary sclerosing hemangioma with immunohistochemical studies: TTF-1 is expressed in both round and surface cells, suggesting an origin from primitive respiratory epithelium. Am J Surg Pathol. 2000 Jul;24(7):906–16. PMID:10895813

211. Dewaele B, Floris G, Finalet-Ferreiro J, et al. Coactivated platelet-derived growth factor receptor alpha and epidermal growth factor receptor are potential therapeutic targets in intimal sarcoma. Cancer Res. 2010 Sep 15;70(18):7304–14. PMID:20685895

212. Dhooria S, Sehgal IS, Prasad KT, et al. Diagnostic yield and safety of the ProCore versus the standard EBUS-TBNA needle in subjects with suspected sarcoidosis. Expert Rev Med Devices. 2021 Feb;18(2):211–6. PMID:33435733

213. Di Crescenzo V, Vitale M, Valvano L, et al. Surgical management of cervico-mediastinal goiters: our experience and review of the literature. Int J Surg. 2016 Apr;28 Suppl 1:S47–53. PMID:26721191

214. Di Mari N, Barbagli L, Mourmouras V, et al. Ectopic thyroid of the lung. An additional case. Pathologica. 2010 Jun;102(3):102–3. PMID:21171513

215. Diken ÖE, Karnak D, Çiledağ A, et al. Electromagnetic navigation-guided TBNA vs conventional TBNA in the diagnosis of mediastinal lymphadenopathy. Clin Respir J. 2015 Apr;9(2):214–20. PMID:25849298

216. Domagala-Kulawik J. The relevance of bronchoalveolar lavage fluid analysis for lung cancer patients. Expert Rev Respir Med. 2020 Mar;14(3):329–37. PMID:31865801

217. Domanski HA, Akerman M, Engellau J, et al. Fine-needle aspiration of neurilemoma (schwannoma). A clinicocytopathologic study of 116 patients. Diagn Cytopathol. 2006 Jun;34(6):403–12. PMID:16680779

218. Domanski HA, Akerman M, Rissler P, et al. Fine-needle aspiration of soft tissue leiomyosarcoma: an analysis of the most common cytologic findings and the value of ancillary techniques. Diagn Cytopathol. 2006 Sep;34(9):597–604. PMID:16900474

219. Dômont J, Salas S, Lacroix L, et al. High frequency of beta-catenin heterozygous mutations in extra-abdominal fibromatosis: a potential molecular tool for disease management. Br J Cancer. 2010 Mar 16;102(6):1032–6. PMID:20197769

220. Dotto J, Pelosi G, Rosai J. Expression of p63 in thymomas and normal thymus. Am J Clin Pathol. 2007 Mar;127(3):415–20. PMID:17276940

222. Doxtader EE, Mukhopadhyay S. Insulinoma-associated protein 1 is a sensitive and specific marker of neuroendocrine lung neoplasms in cytology specimens. Cancer Cytopathol. 2018 Apr;126(4):243–52. PMID:29360191

223. Doxtader EE, Shah AA, Zhang Y, et al. Primary salivary gland-type tumors of the tracheobronchial tree diagnosed by transbronchial fine needle aspiration: clinical and cytomorphologic features with histopathologic correlation. Diagn Cytopathol. 2019 Nov;47(11):1168–76. PMID:31343850

224. Drilon A, Cappuzzo F, Ou SI, et al. Targeting MET in lung cancer: Will expectations finally be MET? J Thorac Oncol. 2017 Jan;12(1):15–26. PMID:27794501

225. Drilon A, Laetsch TW, Kummar S, et al. Efficacy of larotrectinib in TRK fusion-positive cancers in adults and children. N Engl J Med. 2018 Feb 22;378(8):731–9. PMID:29466156

226. Drilon A, Oxnard GR, Tan DSW, et al. Efficacy of selpercatinib in RET fusion-positive non-small-cell lung cancer. N Engl J Med. 2020 Aug 27;383(9):813–24. PMID:32846060

227. Driscoll TR, Baker GJ, Daniels S, et al. Clinical aspects of malignant mesothelioma in Australia. Aust N Z J Med. 1993 Feb;23(1):19–25. PMID:8460968

228. Duan K, Mete O. Algorithmic approach to neuroendocrine tumors in targeted biopsies: practical applications of immunohistochemical markers. Cancer Cytopathol. 2016 Dec;124(12):871–84. PMID:27529763

229. Dugan JM. Cytologic diagnosis of basal cell (basaloid) carcinoma of the lung. A report of two cases. Acta Cytol. 1995 May-Jun;39(3):539–42. PMID:7762348

230. Dulmet EM, Macchiarini P, Suc B, et al. Germ cell tumors of the mediastinum. A 30-year experience. Cancer. 1993 Sep 15;72(6):1894–901. PMID:7689921

231. Dumonceau JM, Deprez PH, Jenssen C, et al. Indications, results, and clinical impact of endoscopic ultrasound (EUS)-guided sampling in gastroenterology: European Society of Gastrointestinal Endoscopy (ESGE) Clinical Guideline - Updated January 2017. Endoscopy. 2017 Jul;49(7):695–714. PMID:28511234

232. Dunbar F, Leiman G. The aspiration cytology of pulmonary hamartomas. Diagn Cytopathol. 1989;5(2):174–80. PMID:2776600

233. Dupré MP, Courtade-Saidi M. Immunocytochemistry as an adjunct to diagnostic cytology. Ann Pathol. 2012 Dec;32(6):e47–51, 433–7. PMID:23244485

234. Durieu I, Berger N, Loire R, et al. Contralateral haemorrhagic pulmonary metastases ("choriocarcinoma syndrome") after pneumonectomy for primary pulmonary choriocarcinoma. Thorax. 1994 May;49(5):523–4. PMID:7517072

235. Dutta R, Nambirajan A, Mittal S, et al. Cytomorphology of primary pulmonary NUT carcinoma in different cytology preparations. Cancer Cytopathol. 2021 Jan;129(1):53–61. PMID:32877005

236. El Hallani S, Udager AM, Bell D, et al. Epithelial-myoepithelial carcinoma: frequent morphologic and molecular evidence of preexisting pleomorphic adenoma, common HRAS mutations in PLAG1-intact and HMGA2-intact cases, and occasional TP53, FBXW7, and SMARCB1 alterations in high-grade cases. Am J Surg Pathol. 2018 Jan;42(1):18–27. PMID:29135520

237. Elliott DD, Fanning CV, Caraway NP. The utility of fine-needle aspiration in the diagnosis of gastrointestinal stromal tumors: a cytomorphologic and immunohistochemical analysis with emphasis on malignant tumors. Cancer. 2006 Feb 25;108(1):49–55. PMID:16130141

238. Ellis DW, Srigley J. Does standardised structured reporting contribute to quality in diagnostic pathology? The importance of evidence-based datasets. Virchows Arch. 2016 Jan;468(1):51–9. PMID:26316184

239. Elnayal A, Moran CA, Fox PS, et al. Primary salivary gland-type lung cancer: imaging and clinical predictors of outcome. AJR Am J Roentgenol. 2013 Jul;201(1):W57–63. PMID:23789697

240. Endo C, Nakashima R, Taguchi A, et al. Inter-rater agreement of sputum cytology for lung cancer screening in Japan. Diagn Cytopathol. 2015 Jul;43(7):545–50. PMID:25645403

241. Engelman JA, Jänne PA. Mechanisms of acquired resistance to epidermal growth factor receptor tyrosine kinase inhibitors in non-small cell lung cancer. Clin Cancer Res. 2008 May 15;14(10):2895–9. PMID:18483355

242. Engels F, Oosting RS, Nijkamp FP. Pulmonary macrophages induce deterioration of guinea-pig tracheal beta-adrenergic function through release of oxygen radicals. Eur J Pharmacol. 1985 Apr 23;111(1):143–4. PMID:2990941

243. Engleson J, Soller M, Panagopoulos I, et al. Midline carcinoma with t(15;19) and BRD4-NUT fusion oncogene in a 30-year-old female with response to docetaxel and radiotherapy. BMC Cancer. 2006 Mar 16;6:69. PMID:16542442

244. Erickson LA, Mete O. Immunohistochemistry in diagnostic parathyroid pathology. Endocr Pathol. 2018 Jun;29(2):113–29. PMID:29626276

245. Erkiliç S, Ozsaraç C, Küllü S. Sputum cytology for the diagnosis of lung cancer. Comparison of smear and modified cell block methods. Acta Cytol. 2003 Nov-Dec;47(6):1023–7. PMID:14674072

246. Esterbrook G, Anathhanam S, Plant PK. Adequacy of endobronchial ultrasound transbronchial needle aspiration samples in the subtyping of non-small cell lung cancer. Lung Cancer. 2013 Apr;80(1):30–4. PMID:23312886

247. Esterson YB, Edelman MC, Lipskar AM, et al. A case of bronchial granular cell tumor in a pediatric patient. Clin Imaging. 2017 May-Jun;43:15–8. PMID:28160713

248. Falk N, Weissferdt A, Kalhor N, et al. Primary pulmonary salivary gland-type tumors: a review and update. Adv Anat Pathol. 2016 Jan;23(1):13–23. PMID:26645458

249. Fallet V, Saffroy R, Girard N, et al. High-throughput somatic mutation profiling in pulmonary sarcomatoid carcinomas using the LungCarta™ panel: exploring therapeutic targets. Ann Oncol. 2015 Aug;26(8):1748–53. PMID:25969368

250. Fanburg-Smith JC, Majidi M, Miettinen M. Keratin expression in schwannoma; a study of 115 retroperitoneal and 22 peripheral schwannomas. Mod Pathol. 2006 Jan;19(1):115–21. PMID:16357842

251. Fang HY, Wu CY, Huang HJ, et al. Granular cell tumor of the lung. Lung. 2010 Aug;188(4):355–7. PMID:20066540

252. Feragalli B, Mantini C, Sperandeo M, et al. The lung in systemic vasculitis: radiological patterns and differential diagnosis. Br J Radiol. 2016;89(1061):20150992. PMID:26876879

253. Fernandez-Cuesta L, Peifer M, Lu X, et al. Frequent mutations in chromatin-remodelling genes in pulmonary carcinoids. Nat Commun. 2014 Mar 27;5:3518. PMID:24670920

254. Ferreira-Junior JR, Koenigkam-Santos M, Magalhães Tenório AP, et al. CT-based radiomics for prediction of histologic subtype and metastatic disease in primary malignant lung neoplasms. Int J Comput Assist Radiol Surg. 2020 Jan;15(1):163–72. PMID:31722085

255. Fetsch PA, Fetsch JF, Marincola FM, et al. Comparison of melanoma antigen recognized by T cells (MART-1) to HMB-45: additional evidence to support a common lineage for angiomyolipoma, lymphangiomyomatosis, and clear cell sugar tumor. Mod Pathol. 1998 Aug;11(8):699–703. PMID:9720495

256. Fetsch PA, Simsir A, Brosky K, et al. Comparison of three commonly used cytologic preparations in effusion immunocytochemistry. Diagn Cytopathol. 2002 Jan;26(1):61–6. PMID:11782091

257. Field AS. Cytopathology in low medical infrastructure countries: why and how to integrate to capacitate health care. Clin Lab Med. 2018 Mar;38(1):175–82. PMID:29412881

258. Field AS, Geddie WR. Role of fine needle aspiration biopsy cytology in the diagnosis of infections. Diagn Cytopathol. 2016 Dec;44(12):1024–38. PMID:27555237

259. Fielding D, Dalley AJ, Bashirzadeh F, et al. Diff-Quik cytology smears from endobronchial ultrasound transbronchial needle aspiration lymph node specimens as a source of DNA for next-generation sequencing instead of cell blocks. Respiration. 2019;97(6):525–39. PMID:30731462

260. Fielding D, Oki M. Technologies for targeting the peripheral pulmonary nodule including robotics. Respirology. 2020 Sep;25(9):914–23. PMID:32103596

261. Fijołek J, Wiatr E, Langfort R, et al. [Recurrent pneumothorax as alone manifestation of mesothelioma pleurae]. Pneumonol Alergol Pol. 2005;73(3):281–4. Polish. PMID:16989167

262. Finer EB, Villalba JA, Pitman MB. Granular cell tumor of the lung. Diagn Cytopathol. 2019 Apr;47(4):345–6. PMID:30582298

263. Fischler DF, Hall GS, Gordon S, et al. Aspergillus in cytology specimens: a review of 45 specimens from 36 patients. Diagn Cytopathol. 1997 Jan;16(1):26–30. PMID:9034732

264. Fishback NF, Travis WD, Moran CA, et al. Pleomorphic (spindle/giant cell) carcinoma of the lung. A clinicopathologic correlation of 78 cases. Cancer. 1994 Jun 15;73(12):2936–45. PMID:8199991

265. Fite JJ, Maleki Z. Paraganglioma: cytomorphologic features, radiologic and clinical findings in 12 cases. Diagn Cytopathol. 2018 Jun;46(6):473–81. PMID:29575826

266. Fletcher JA, Pinkus GS, Donovan K, et al. Clonal rearrangement of chromosome band 6p21 in the mesenchymal component of pulmonary chondroid hamartoma. Cancer Res. 1992 Nov 15;52(22):6224–8. PMID:1423265

267. Flieder DB, Koss MN, Nicholson A, et al. Solitary pulmonary papillomas in adults: a clinicopathologic and in situ hybridization study of 14 cases combined with 27 cases in the literature. Am J Surg Pathol. 1998 Nov;22(11):1328–42. PMID:9808125

268. Flieder DB, Travis WD. Clear cell "sugar" tumor of the lung: association with lymphangioleiomyomatosis and multifocal micronodular pneumocyte hyperplasia in a patient with tuberous sclerosis. Am J Surg Pathol. 1997 Oct;21(10):1242–7. PMID:9331299

269. Fowler LJ, Lachar WA. Application of immunohistochemistry to cytology. Arch Pathol Lab Med. 2008 Mar;132(3):373–83. PMID:18318580

270. Francischetti IMB, Cajigas A, Suhrland M, et al. Incidental primary mediastinal choriocarcinoma diagnosed by endobronchial ultrasound-guided fine needle aspiration in a patient presenting with transient ischemic attack and stroke. Diagn Cytopathol. 2017 Aug;45(8):738–43. PMID:28397369

271. Franke KJ, Hein M, Domanski U, et al. Transbronchial catheter aspiration and transbronchial needle aspiration in the diagnostic workup of peripheral lung lesions. Lung. 2015 Oct;193(5):767–72. PMID:26156311

272. Frazier AA, Hossain R. A spectrum of metastatic disease in the chest: insights for the radiologist. Semin Roentgenol. 2020 Jan;55(1):51–9. PMID:31964481

273. Gaffey MJ, Mills SE, Askin FB, et al. Clear cell tumor of the lung. A clinicopathologic, immunohistochemical, and ultrastructural study of eight cases. Am J Surg Pathol. 1990 Mar;14(3):248–59. PMID:1689555

274. Gaffey MJ, Mills SE, Ritter JH. Clear cell tumors of the lower respiratory tract. Semin Diagn Pathol. 1997 Nov;14(4):222–32. PMID:9383822

275. Gaffey MJ, Mills SE, Zarbo RJ, et al. Clear cell tumor of the lung. Immunohistochemical and ultrastructural evidence of melanogenesis. Am J Surg Pathol. 1991 Jul;15(7):644–53. PMID:1711793

276. Gailey MP, Keeney ME, Jensen CS. A cytomorphometric analysis of pulmonary and mediastinal granulomas: differentiating histoplasmosis from sarcoidosis by fine-needle aspiration. Cancer Cytopathol. 2015 Jan;123(1):51–8. PMID:25318988

277. Gailey MP, Klutts JS, Jensen CS. Fine-needle aspiration of histoplasmosis in the era of endoscopic ultrasound and endobronchial ultrasound: cytomorphologic features and correlation with clinical laboratory testing. Cancer Cytopathol. 2013 Sep;121(9):508–17. PMID:23677891

278. Galluccio G, Palazzolo M, Battistoni P, et al. Role of transbronchial needle core biopsy in the diagnosis of mediastinal diseases: experience with an innovative endoscopic technique using a rigid Tru-Cut needle. J Bronchology Interv Pulmonol. 2018 Jul;25(3):239–44. PMID:27261933

279. Gao F, Zang L, He J, et al. A case of solid variant of adenoid cystic carcinoma from trachea: a case report and review of literature. Onco Targets Ther. 2021 Mar 18;14:1997–2002. PMID:33776449

280. García-Escudero A, González-Cámpora R, Villar-Rodríguez JL, et al. Thyroid transcription factor-1 expression in pulmonary blastoma. Histopathology. 2004 May;44(5):507–8. PMID:15140003

281. Garg PK, Sharma G, Rai S, et al. Primary salivary gland-type tumors of the lung: a systematic review and pooled analysis. Lung India. 2019 Mar-Apr;36(2):118–22. PMID:30829245

282. Gaude GS, Patil P, Malur PR, et al. Primary mediastinal choriocarcinoma. South Asian J Cancer. 2013 Apr;2(2):79. PMID:24455559

283. Geller RL, Hookim K, Sullivan HC, et al. Cytologic features of angiosarcoma: a review of 26 cases diagnosed on FNA. Cancer Cytopathol. 2016 Sep;124(9):659–68. PMID:27088896

284. Georgakopoulos B, Al Khalili Y. Anatomy, head and neck, parathyroid, ectopic glands. 2022 Jul 25. In: StatPearls. Treasure Island (FL): StatPearls Publishing; 2022 Jan–. PMID:31082016

285. Geraci G, Pisello F, Sciumè C, et al. [Complication of flexible fiberoptic bronchoscopy. Literature review]. Ann Ital Chir. 2007 May-Jun;78(3):183–92. Italian. PMID:17722491

286. Ghigna MR, Crutu A, Florea V, et al. The role of endobronchial ultrasound-guided fine needle aspiration in the diagnosis of pleural mesothelioma. Cytopathology. 2016 Aug;27(4):284–8. PMID:26315262

287. Ghosh M, Islam N, Saha H, et al. Cytodiagnosis of inflammatory myofibroblastic tumor: a report of three cases in infants. Diagn Cytopathol. 2018 Sep;46(9):776–81. PMID:29673102

288. Girard P, Caliandro R, Seguin-Givelet A, et al. Sensitivity of cytology specimens from bronchial aspirate or washing during bronchoscopy in the diagnosis of lung malignancies: an update. Clin Lung Cancer. 2017 Sep;18(5):512–8. PMID:28007409

289. Giti R, Hosseinzadeh M. Efficacy of bronchial washing and brushing cytology in the diagnosis of non-neoplastic lung diseases. Acta Med Iran. 2017 Oct;55(10):636–41. PMID:29228529

290. Glaser LJ, Montone KT. A practical guide to the role of ancillary techniques in the diagnosis of infectious agents in fine needle aspiration samples. Acta Cytol. 2020;64(1-2):81–91. PMID:30889574

291. Gleason BC, Hornick JL. Inflammatory myofibroblastic tumours: Where are we now? J Clin Pathol. 2008 Apr;61(4):428–37. PMID:17938159

292. Gledhill A, Bates C, Henderson D, et al. Sputum cytology: a limited role. J Clin Pathol. 1997 Jul;50(7):566–8. PMID:9306936

293. Gleeson T, Thiessen R, Hannigan A, et al. Pulmonary hamartomas: CT pixel analysis for fat attenuation using radiologic-pathologic correlation. J Med Imaging Radiat Oncol. 2013 Oct;57(5):534–43. PMID:24119266

294. Gong Y, Sun X, Michael CW, et al. Immunocytochemistry of serous effusion specimens: a comparison of ThinPrep vs cell block. Diagn Cytopathol. 2003 Jan;28(1):1–5. PMID:12508174

295. Gonzalez-Vela JL, Savage PD, Manivel JC, et al. Poor prognosis of mediastinal germ cell cancers containing sarcomatous components. Cancer. 1990 Sep 15;66(6):1114–6. PMID:1698114

296. Gorman BK, Kosarac O, Chakraborty S, et al. Comparison of breast carcinoma prognostic/predictive biomarkers on cell blocks obtained by various methods: Cellient, formalin and thrombin. Acta Cytol. 2012;56(3):289–96. PMID:22555532

297. Gosney JR, Boothman AM, Ratcliffe M, et al. Cytology for PD-L1 testing: a systematic review. Lung Cancer. 2020 Mar;141:101–6. PMID:32007657

298. Goyal G, Heaney ML, Collin M, et al. Erdheim-Chester disease: consensus recommendations for evaluation, diagnosis, and treatment in the molecular era. Blood. 2020 May 28;135(22):1929–45. PMID:32187362

299. Green R, King M, Reid H, et al. Management of pulmonary nodules in head and neck cancer patients - our experience and interpretation of the British Thoracic Society Guidelines. Surgeon. 2017 Aug;15(4):227–30. PMID:27838234

300. Greenberg SD. Recent advances in pulmonary cytopathology. Hum Pathol. 1983 Oct;14(10):901–12. PMID:6352461

301. Groth SS, Whitson BA, D'Cunha J, et al. Endobronchial ultrasound-guided fine-needle aspiration of mediastinal lymph nodes: a single institution's early learning curve. Ann Thorac Surg. 2008 Oct;86(4):1104–9. PMID:18805141

302. Gruchy JR, Barnes PJ, Dakin Haché KA. CytoLyt® fixation and decalcification pretreatments alter antigenicity in normal tissues compared with standard formalin fixation. Appl Immunohistochem Mol Morphol. 2015 Apr;23(4):297–302. PMID:25265430

303. Gu P, Zhao YZ, Jiang LY, et al. Endobronchial ultrasound-guided transbronchial needle aspiration for staging of lung cancer: a systematic review and meta-analysis. Eur J Cancer. 2009 May;45(8):1389–96. PMID:19124238

304. Guan JL, Zhong WZ, An SJ, et al. KRAS mutation in patients with lung cancer: a predictor for poor prognosis but not for EGFR-TKIs or chemotherapy. Ann Surg Oncol. 2013 Apr;20(4):1381–8. PMID:23208128

305. Guillou L, Gloor E, Anani PA, et al. Bronchial granular-cell tumor. Report of a case with preoperative cytologic diagnosis on bronchial brushings and immunohistochemical studies. Acta Cytol. 1991 Jul-Aug;35(4):375–80. PMID:1927169

306. Guo H, Liu S, Guo J, et al. Rapid on-site evaluation during endobronchial ultrasound-guided transbronchial needle aspiration for the diagnosis of hilar and mediastinal lymphadenopathy in patients with lung cancer. Cancer Lett. 2016 Feb 28;371(2):182–6. PMID:26656954

307. Gupta R, Mathur SR, Arora VK, et al. Cytologic features of extragonadal germ cell tumors: a study of 88 cases with aspiration cytology. Cancer. 2008 Dec 25;114(6):504–11. PMID:18980289

308. Gupta RK, Naran S, Lallu S, et al. Fine-needle aspiration cytology in neurilemoma (schwannoma) of the breast: report of two cases in a man and a woman. Diagn Cytopathol. 2001 Jan;24(1):76–7. PMID:11135474

309. Gurbuz AK, Giardiello FM, Petersen GM, et al. Desmoid tumours in familial adenomatous polyposis. Gut. 1994 Mar;35(3):377–81. PMID:8150351

310. Haack H, Johnson LA, Fry CJ, et al. Diagnosis of NUT midline carcinoma using a NUT-specific monoclonal antibody. Am J Surg Pathol. 2009 Jul;33(7):984–91. PMID:19363441

311. Habougit C, Yvorel V, Sulaiman A, et al. Mediastinal mature teratoma with malignant carcinomatous transformation (somatic-type malignancy) with metastatic course. Int J Surg Pathol. 2015 Dec;23(8):682–4. PMID:26113666

312. Haefliger S, Savice Prince S, Rebetez J, et al. Putative malignant pleural mesothelioma in situ (MPMIS) with sequential acquisition of genomic alterations on fluorescence in situ hybridization (FISH) examination. Acta Cytol. 2021;65(1):99–104. PMID:32814330

313. Halperin DM, Shen C, Dasari A, et al. Frequency of carcinoid syndrome at neuroendocrine tumour diagnosis: a population-based study. Lancet Oncol. 2017 Apr;18(4):525–34. PMID:28238592

314. Hamzaoui K, Chelbi H, Kamoun M, et al. Increased endothelin-1 levels of BAL fluid in patients with Behçet's disease. Mediators Inflamm. 2007;2007:93726. PMID:17497041

315. Han X, Zhang J, Fan J, et al. Radiological and clinical features and outcomes of patients with primary pulmonary salivary gland-type tumors. Can Respir J. 2019 Apr 1;2019:1475024. PMID:31065298

316. Hanley KZ, Birdsong GG, Cohen C, et al. Immunohistochemical detection of estrogen receptor, progesterone receptor, and human epidermal growth factor receptor 2 expression in breast carcinomas: comparison on cell block, needle-core, and tissue block preparations. Cancer. 2009 Aug 25;117(4):279–88. PMID:19551847

317. Hanley KZ, Dureau ZJ, Cohen C, et al. Orthopedia homeobox is preferentially expressed in typical carcinoids of the lung. Cancer Cytopathol. 2018 Apr;126(4):236–42. PMID:29316326

318. Hansell DM, Bankier AA, MacMahon H, et al. Fleischner Society: glossary of terms for thoracic imaging. Radiology. 2008 Mar;246(3):697–722. PMID:18195376

319. Hansen T, Pedersen H, Brauner V, et al. Control specimens for immunocytochemistry in liquid-based cytology. Cytopathology. 2011 Aug;22(4):243–6. PMID:20482720

320. Harbhajanka A, Dahoud W, Michael CW, et al. Cytohistological correlation, immunohistochemistry and Murine Double Minute Clone 2 amplification of pulmonary artery intimal sarcoma: a case report with review of literature. Diagn Cytopathol. 2019 May;47(5):494–7. PMID:30552756

321. Haroche J, Charlotte F, Arnaud L, et al. High prevalence of BRAF V600E mutations in Erdheim-Chester disease but not in other non-Langerhans cell histiocytoses. Blood. 2012 Sep 27;120(13):2700–3. PMID:22879539

322. Harris K, Chalhoub M. Tracheal papillomatosis: What do we know so far? Chron Respir Dis. 2011;8(4):233–5. PMID:21971565

323. Healy TM, Borrie J. Lung cancer diagnosis: evaluation of diagnostic techniques. N Z Med J. 1975 May 14;81(539):423–4. PMID:1057739

324. Heerink WJ, de Bock GH, de Jonge GJ, et al. Complication rates of CT-guided transthoracic lung biopsy: meta-analysis. Eur Radiol. 2017 Jan;27(1):138–48. PMID:27108299

325. Henderson DW, Reid G, Kao SC, et al. Challenges and controversies in the diagnosis of mesothelioma: part 1. Cytology-only diagnosis, biopsies, immunohistochemistry, discrimination between mesothelioma and reactive mesothelial hyperplasia, and biomarkers. J Clin Pathol. 2013 Oct;66(10):847–53. PMID:23814259

326. Henke AC, Salomao DR, Hughes JH. Cellular schwannoma mimics a sarcoma: an example of a potential pitfall in aspiration cytodiagnosis. Diagn Cytopathol. 1999 May;20(5):312–6. PMID:10319235

327. Henry M, Landers R, Kealy WF, et al. Solitary columnar bronchial papilloma: a rare endoscopic finding. Respir Med. 1998 Jun;92(6):878–9. PMID:9850375

328. Hermans BCM, de Vos-Geelen J, Derks JL, et al. Unique metastatic patterns in neuroendocrine neoplasms of different primary origin. Neuroendocrinology. 2021;111(11):1111–20. PMID:33227805

329. Hermans BCM, Derks JL, Moonen L, et al. Pulmonary neuroendocrine neoplasms with well differentiated morphology and high proliferative activity: illustrated by a case series and review of the literature. Lung Cancer. 2020 Dec;150:152–8. PMID:33171403

330. Hermans BCM, Derks JL, Thunnissen E, et al. Prevalence and prognostic value of PD-L1 expression in molecular subtypes of metastatic large cell neuroendocrine carcinoma (LCNEC). Lung Cancer. 2019 Apr;130:179–86. PMID:30885341

331. Herpel E, Rieker RJ, Dienemann H, et al. SMARCA4 and SMARCA2 deficiency in non-small cell lung cancer: immunohistochemical survey of 316 consecutive specimens. Ann Diagn Pathol. 2017 Feb;26:47–51. PMID:28038711

332. Hewer E. The oncologist's guide to synoptic reporting: a primer. Oncology. 2020;98(6):396–402. PMID:31177262

333. Hida T, Hamasaki M, Matsumoto S, et al. Immunohistochemical detection of MTAP and BAP1 protein loss for mesothelioma diagnosis: comparison with 9p21 FISH and BAP1 immunohistochemistry. Lung Cancer. 2017 Feb;104:98–105. PMID:28213009

334. Highman WJ, Oliver RT. Diagnosis of metastases from testicular germ cell tumours using fine needle aspiration cytology. J Clin Pathol. 1987 Nov;40(11):1324–33. PMID:3693570

335. Hiroshima K, Dosaka-Akita H, Usuda K, et al. Cytological characteristics of pulmonary pleomorphic and giant cell carcinomas. Acta Cytol. 2011;55(2):173–9. PMID:21325803

336. Hiroshima K, Iyoda A, Shida T, et al. Distinction of pulmonary large cell neuroendocrine carcinoma from small cell lung carcinoma: a morphological, immunohistochemical, and molecular analysis. Mod Pathol. 2006 Oct;19(10):1358–68. PMID:16862075

337. Hiroshima K, Wu D, Hamakawa S, et al. HEG1, BAP1, and MTAP are useful in cytologic diagnosis of malignant mesothelioma with effusion. Diagn Cytopathol. 2021 May;49(5):622–32. PMID:32441895

338. Hiroshima K, Yoshizawa A, Takenaka A, et al. Cytology reporting system for lung cancer from the Japan Lung Cancer Society and Japanese Society of Clinical Cytology: an interobserver reproducibility study and risk of malignancy evaluation on cytology specimens. Acta Cytol. 2020;64(5):452–62. PMID:32222718

339. Hissong E, Rao R. Pneumocytoma (sclerosing hemangioma), a potential pitfall. Diagn Cytopathol. 2017 Aug;45(8):744–9. PMID:28398699

340. Hjerpe A, Abd-Own S, Dobra K. Cytopathologic diagnosis of epithelioid and mixed-type malignant mesothelioma: ten years of clinical experience in relation to international guidelines. Arch Pathol Lab Med. 2018 Aug;142(8):893–901. PMID:30040460

341. Hjerpe A, Ascoli V, Bedrossian CW, et al. Guidelines for the cytopathologic diagnosis of epithelioid and mixed-type malignant mesothelioma: a secondary publication. Cytopathology. 2015 Jun;26(3):142–56. PMID:26052757

342. Horadagoda D, Smith T, Varikatt W. Nuclear protein in testis (NUT) carcinoma diagnosed using only FNA material in the absence of a histological sample. Cytopathology. 2018 Aug;29(4):390–3. PMID:29520920

343. Howlader N, Forjaz G, Mooradian MJ, et al. The effect of advances in lung-cancer treatment on population mortality. N Engl J Med. 2020 Aug 13;383(7):640–9. PMID:32786189

344. Hu J, Ngiam KY, Parameswaran R. Mediastinal parathyroid adenomas and their surgical implications. Ann R Coll Surg Engl. 2015 May;97(4):259–61. PMID:26263931

345. Huang CC, Collins BT, Flint A, et al. Pulmonary neuroendocrine tumors: an entity in search of cytologic criteria. Diagn Cytopathol. 2013 Aug;41(8):689–96. PMID:23166111

346. Huang HC, Zhao L, Cao XH, et al. Primary salivary gland tumors of the lung: two cases date report and literature review. Respir Med Case Rep. 2020 Dec 31;32:101333. PMID:33457200

347. Huang M, Wei S. Overview of molecular testing of cytology specimens. Acta Cytol. 2020;64(1-2):136–46. PMID:30917368

348. Hubers AJ, Prinsen CF, Sozzi G, et al. Molecular sputum analysis for the diagnosis of lung cancer. Br J Cancer. 2013 Aug 6;109(3):530–7. PMID:23868001

349. Hughes JH, Jensen CS, Donnelly AD, et al. The role of fine-needle aspiration cytology in the evaluation of metastatic clear cell tumors. Cancer. 1999 Dec 25;87(6):380–9. PMID:10603192

350. Hughes JH, Young NA, Wilbur DC, et al. Fine-needle aspiration of pulmonary hamartoma: a common source of false-positive diagnoses in the College of American Pathologists Interlaboratory Comparison Program in Nongynecologic Cytology. Arch Pathol Lab Med. 2005 Jan;129(1):19–22. PMID:15628903

351. Hulbert A, Jusue-Torres I, Stark A, et al. Early detection of lung cancer using DNA promoter hypermethylation in plasma and sputum. Clin Cancer Res. 2017 Apr 15;23(8):1998–2005. PMID:27729459

352. Hummel P, Cangiarella JF, Cohen JM, et al. Transthoracic fine-needle aspiration biopsy of pulmonary spindle cell and mesenchymal lesions: a study of 61 cases. Cancer. 2001 Jun 25;93(3):187–98. PMID:11391606

353. Hung YP. Neuroendocrine tumors of the lung: updates and diagnostic pitfalls. Surg Pathol Clin. 2019 Dec;12(4):1055–71. PMID:31672294

354. Hung YP, Chen AL, Taylor MS, et al. Thoracic nuclear protein in testis (NUT) carcinoma: expanded pathological spectrum with expression of thyroid transcription factor-1 and neuroendocrine markers. Histopathology. 2021 May;78(6):896–904. PMID:33231320

355. Huo L, Moran CA, Fuller GN, et al. Pulmonary artery sarcoma: a clinicopathologic and immunohistochemical study of 12 cases. Am J Clin Pathol. 2006 Mar;125(3):419–24. PMID:16613346

356. Huo Z, Wu H, Li J, et al. Primary pulmonary mucoepidermoid carcinoma: histopathological and moleculargenetic studies of 26 cases. PLoS One. 2015 Nov 17;10(11):e0143169. PMID:26575266

357. Hupp M, Najmuddin M, Dincer HE, et al. Cytomorphologic features of malignant solitary fibrous tumor with mediastinal involvement sampled by endoscopic and endobronchial ultrasound-guided fine-needle aspiration: a comparison of two cases. Diagn Cytopathol. 2019 Aug;47(8):821–7. PMID:31016889

358. Hussien A, Lin CT. CT findings of fungal pneumonia with emphasis on aspergillosis. Emerg Radiol. 2018 Dec;25(6):685–9. PMID:29956050

359. Hyun TS, Barnes M, Tabatabai ZL. The diagnostic utility of D2-40, calretinin, CK5/6, desmin and MOC-31 in the differentiation of mesothelioma from adenocarcinoma in pleural effusion cytology. Acta Cytol. 2012;56(5):527–32. PMID:23075894

360. Idowu MO, Powers CN. Lung cancer cytology: potential pitfalls and mimics - a review. Int J Clin Exp Pathol. 2010 Mar 25;3(4):367–85. PMID:20490328

361. Ikeda K, Tate G, Suzuki T, et al. Comparison of immunocytochemical sensitivity between formalin-fixed and alcohol-fixed specimens reveals the diagnostic value of alcohol-fixed cytocentrifuged preparations in malignant effusion cytology. Am J Clin Pathol. 2011 Dec;136(6):934–42. PMID:22095380

362. Ikeda N, Hayashi A, Iwasaki K, et al. Comprehensive diagnostic bronchoscopy of central type early stage lung cancer. Lung Cancer. 2007 Jun;56(3):295–302. PMID:17291623

363. Ilahi A, Muco E, Ilahi TB. Anatomy, head and neck, parathyroid. 2022 Aug 8. In: StatPearls. Treasure Island (FL): StatPearls Publishing; 2022 Jan–. PMID:30725888

364. Illei PB, Rusch VW, Zakowski MF, et al. Homozygous deletion of CDKN2A and codeletion of the methylthioadenosine phosphorylase gene in the majority of pleural mesotheliomas. Clin Cancer Res. 2003 Jun;9(6):2108–13. PMID:12796375

365. Inage T, Nakajima T, Fujiwara T, et al. Pathological diagnosis of pulmonary large cell neuroendocrine carcinoma by endobronchial ultrasound-guided transbronchial needle aspiration. Thorac Cancer. 2018 Feb;9(2):273–7. PMID:29271588

366. Inage T, Nakajima T, Yoshino I. Staging lung cancer: role of endobronchial ultrasound. Lung Cancer (Auckl). 2014 Nov 4;5:67–72. PMID:28210144

367. Incarbone M, Ceresoli GL, Di Tommaso L, et al. Primary pulmonary meningioma: report of a case and review of the literature. Lung Cancer. 2008 Dec;62(3):401–7. PMID:18486986

368. Inoue Y, Oka M, Ishii H, et al. A solitary bronchial papilloma with malignant changes. Intern Med. 2001 Jan;40(1):56–60. PMID:11201373

369. Ismail-Khan R, Robinson LA, Williams CC Jr, et al. Malignant pleural mesothelioma: a comprehensive review. Cancer Control. 2006 Oct;13(4):255–63. PMID:17075562

370. Iwamoto N, Ishida M, Yoshida K, et al. Mediastinal seminoma: a case report with special emphasis on SALL4 as a new immunocytochemical marker. Diagn Cytopathol. 2013 Sep;41(9):821–4. PMID:22298374

372. Jain D, Allen TC, Aisner DL, et al. Rapid on-site evaluation of endobronchial ultrasound-guided transbronchial needle aspirations for the diagnosis of lung cancer: a perspective from members of the Pulmonary Pathology Society. Arch Pathol Lab Med. 2018 Feb;142(2):253–62. PMID:28639854

373. Jain D, Mathur SR, Iyer VK. Cell blocks in cytopathology: a review of preparative methods, utility in diagnosis and role in ancillary studies. Cytopathology. 2014 Dec;25(6):356–71. PMID:25113785

374. Jain D, Nambirajan A, Borczuk A, et al. Immunocytochemistry for predictive biomarker testing in lung cancer cytology. Cancer Cytopathol. 2019 May;127(5):325–39. PMID:31050216

375. Jain D, Nambirajan A, Chen G, et al. NSCLC subtyping in conventional cytology: results of the International Association for the Study of Lung Cancer Cytology Working Group survey to determine specific cytomorphologic criteria for adenocarcinoma and squamous cell carcinoma. J Thorac Oncol. 2022 Jun;17(6):793–805. PMID:35331963

376. Jain D, Roy-Chowdhuri S. Molecular pathology of lung cancer cytology specimens: a concise review. Arch Pathol Lab Med. 2018 Sep;142(9):1127–33. PMID:29547001

377. Jatakanon A, Lim S, Barnes PJ. Changes in sputum eosinophils predict loss of asthma control. Am J Respir Crit Care Med. 2000 Jan;161(1):64–72. PMID:10619799

378. Jeffus SK, Joiner AK, Siegel ER, et al. Rapid on-site evaluation of EBUS-TBNA specimens of lymph nodes: comparative analysis and recommendations for standardization. Cancer Cytopathol. 2015 Jun;123(6):362–72. PMID:25931443

379. Jeung MY, Gasser B, Gangi A, et al. Bronchial carcinoid tumors of the thorax: spectrum of radiologic findings. Radiographics. 2002 Mar-Apr;22(2):351–65. PMID:11896225

380. Jiang G, Zhang M, Tan Q, et al. Identification of the BRAF V600E mutation in a patient with sclerosing pneumocytoma: a case report. Lung Cancer. 2019 Nov;137:52–5. PMID:31546071

381. Jiang M, Anderson T, Nwogu C, et al. Pulmonary malignant granular cell tumor. World J Surg Oncol. 2003 Oct 21;1(1):22. PMID:14613555

382. Jiang X, Liu Y, Chen C, et al. The value of biomarkers in patients with sarcomatoid carcinoma of the lung: molecular analysis of 33 cases. Clin Lung Cancer. 2012 Jul;13(4):288–96. PMID:22169481

383. Jiménez-Heffernan JA, López-Ferrer P, Vicandi B, et al. Cytologic features of malignant peripheral nerve sheath tumor. Acta Cytol. 1999 Mar-Apr;43(2):175–83. PMID:10097706

384. Jimenez-Heffernan JA, Lopez-Ferrer P, Vicandi B, et al. Fine-needle aspiration cytology of large cell neuroendocrine carcinoma of the lung: a cytohistologic correlation study of 11 cases. Cancer. 2008 Jun 25;114(3):180–6. PMID:18433011

385. Jiménez-Heffernan JA, Vicandi B, López-Ferrer P, et al. Cytologic features of pheochromocytoma and retroperitoneal paraganglioma: a morphologic and immunohistochemical study of 13 cases. Acta Cytol. 2006 Jul-Aug;50(4):372–8. PMID:16900997

386. Jin M, Wakely PE Jr. Lymph node cytopathology: essential ancillary studies as applied to lymphoproliferative neoplasms. Cancer Cytopathol. 2018 Aug;126 Suppl 8:615–26. PMID:30156771

387. Jin MS, Ha HJ, Baek HJ, et al. Adenomyomatous hamartoma of lung mimicking benign mucinous tumor in fine needle aspiration biopsy: a case report. Acta Cytol. 2008 May-Jun;52(3):357–60. PMID:18540306

388. Jo VY, Cibas ES, Pinkus GS. Claudin-4 immunohistochemistry is highly effective in distinguishing adenocarcinoma from malignant mesothelioma in effusion cytology. Cancer Cytopathol. 2014 Apr;122(4):299–306. PMID:24421209

389. Jones KD, Churg A, Henderson DW, et al. Data set for reporting of lung carcinomas: recommendations from International Collaboration on Cancer Reporting. Arch Pathol Lab Med. 2013 Aug;137(8):1054–62. PMID:23899061

390. Jouneau S, Ménard C, Lederlin M. Pulmonary alveolar proteinosis. Respirology. 2020 Aug;25(8):816–26. PMID:32363736

391. Kaba S, Tokoro Y, Washiya K, et al. Cytology of pulmonary marginal zone B-cell lymphoma of MALT type: lessons learned for intra-operative diagnosis. Cytopathology. 2011 Oct;22(5):346–9. PMID:21166908

392. Kadota K, Haba R, Katsuki N, et al. Cytological findings of mixed squamous cell and glandular papilloma in the lung. Diagn Cytopathol. 2010 Dec;38(12):913–7. PMID:20301213

393. Kadota K, Suzuki K, Colovos C, et al. A nuclear grading system is a strong predictor of survival in epitheloid diffuse malignant pleural mesothelioma. Mod Pathol. 2012 Feb;25(2):260–71. PMID:21983936

394. Kadota K, Suzuki K, Sima CS, et al. Pleomorphic epithelioid diffuse malignant pleural mesothelioma: a clinicopathological review and conceptual proposal to reclassify as biphasic or sarcomatoid mesothelioma. J Thorac Oncol. 2011 May;6(5):896–904. PMID:21358344

395. Kadota K, Yeh YC, D'Angelo SP, et al. Associations between mutations and histologic patterns of mucin in lung adenocarcinoma: invasive mucinous pattern and extracellular mucin are associated with KRAS mutation. Am J Surg Pathol. 2014 Aug;38(8):1118–27. PMID:25029118

396. Kakinuma H, Mikami T, Iwabuchi K, et al. Diagnostic findings of bronchial brush cytology for pulmonary large cell neuroendocrine carcinomas: comparison with poorly differentiated adenocarcinomas, squamous cell carcinomas, and small cell carcinomas. Cancer. 2003 Aug 25;99(4):247–54. PMID:12925987

397. Kalemkerian GP, Narula N, Kennedy EB, et al. Molecular testing guideline for the selection of patients with lung cancer for treatment with targeted tyrosine kinase inhibitors: American Society of Clinical Oncology endorsement of the College of American Pathologists/International Association for the Study of Lung Cancer/Association for Molecular Pathology clinical practice guideline update. J Clin Oncol. 2018 Mar 20;36(9):911–9. PMID:29401004

398. Kalhor N, Moran CA. Pulmonary mucoepidermoid carcinoma: diagnosis and treatment. Expert Rev Respir Med. 2018 Mar;12(3):249–55. PMID:29338644

399. Kandalaft PL, Gown AM. Practical applications in immunohistochemistry: carcinomas of unknown primary site. Arch Pathol Lab Med. 2016 Jun;140(6):508–23. PMID:26457625

400. Kao CS, Idrees MT, Young RH, et al. Solid pattern yolk sac tumor: a morphologic and immunohistochemical study of 52 cases. Am J Surg Pathol. 2012 Mar;36(3):360–7. PMID:22261704

401. Kaparianos A, Argyropoulou E, Sampsonas F, et al. Indications, results and complications of flexible fiberoptic bronchoscopy: a 5-year experience in a referral population in Greece. Eur Rev Med Pharmacol Sci. 2008 Nov-Dec;12(6):355–63. PMID:19146197

402. Kapatia G, Rajasekaran S, Rohilla M, et al. Fine-needle aspiration cytology of extra-salivary adenoid cystic carcinoma. Cytopathology. 2020 May;31(3):215–22. PMID:31743547

403. Karamchandani JR, Nielsen TO, van de Rijn M, et al. Sox10 and S100 in the diagnosis of soft-tissue neoplasms. Appl Immunohistochem Mol Morphol. 2012 Oct;20(5):445–50. PMID:22495377

404. Karki A, Shah R, Fein A. Multiple pulmonary nodules in malignancy. Curr Opin Pulm Med. 2017 Jul;23(4):285–9. PMID:28463856

405. Karunamurthy A, Cai G, Dacic S, et al. Evaluation of endobronchial ultrasound-guided fine-needle aspirations (EBUS-FNA): correlation with adequacy and histologic follow-up. Cancer Cytopathol. 2014 Jan;122(1):23–32. PMID:24127207

406. Katabi N, Ghossein R, Ho A, et al. Consistent PLAG1 and HMGA2 abnormalities distinguish carcinoma ex-pleomorphic adenoma from its de novo counterparts. Hum Pathol. 2015 Jan;46(1):26–33. PMID:25439740

407. Kathuria S, Jablokow VR. Primary choriocarcinoma of mediastinum with immunohistochemical study and review of the literature. J Surg Oncol. 1987 Jan;34(1):39–42. PMID:2433543

408. Katsumata Y, Terada J, Abe M, et al. An analysis of the clinical benefit of 37 bronchoalveolar lavage procedures in patients with hematologic disease and pulmonary complications. Intern Med. 2019 Apr 15;58(8):1073–80. PMID:30568132

409. Kavunkal AM, Pandiyan MS, Philip MA, et al. Large clear cell tumor of the lung mimicking malignant behavior. Ann Thorac Surg. 2007 Jan;83(1):310–2. PMID:17184693

410. Kawaguchi T, Matumura A, Iuchi K, et al. Solitary squamous papilloma of the bronchus associated with human papilloma virus type 11. Intern Med. 1999 Oct;38(10):817–9. PMID:10526947

411. Kelemen K, Rimsza LM, Craig FE. Primary pulmonary B-cell lymphoma. Semin Diagn Pathol. 2020 Nov;37(6):259–67. PMID:32444246

412. Keppens C, Tack V, Hart N, et al. A stitch in time saves nine: external quality assessment rounds demonstrate improved quality of biomarker analysis in lung cancer. Oncotarget. 2018 Apr 17;9(29):20524–38. PMID:29755669

413. Khajotia RR, Mohn A, Pokieser L, et al. Induced sputum and cytological diagnosis of lung cancer. Lancet. 1991 Oct 19;338(8773):976–7. PMID:1681343

414. Khilnani GC, Hadda V. Lipoid pneumonia: an uncommon entity. Indian J Med Sci. 2009 Oct;63(10):474–80. PMID:19901490

415. Kiffer JD, Sandeman TF. Primary malignant mediastinal germ cell tumours: a literature review and a study of 18 cases. Australas Radiol. 1999 Feb;43(1):58–68. PMID:10901872

416. Kim CH, Jeong JS, Kim SR, et al. Endobronchial epithelial-myoepithelial carcinoma of the lung. Thorax. 2018 Jun;73(6):593–4. PMID:29196470

417. Kim J, Lazar AJ, Davies MA, et al. BRAF, NRAS and KIT sequencing analysis of spindle cell melanoma. J Cutan Pathol. 2012 Sep;39(9):821–5. PMID:22809251

418. Kim MK, Park SH, Cho HD, et al. Fine needle aspiration cytology of primary pulmonary paraganglioma. A case report. Acta Cytol. 2001 May-Jun;45(3):459–64. PMID:11393086

419. Kim S, Kim MY, Koh J, et al. Programmed death-1 ligand 1 and 2 are highly expressed in pleomorphic carcinomas of the lung: comparison of sarcomatous and carcinomatous areas. Eur J Cancer. 2015 Nov;51(17):2698–707. PMID:26329973

420. Kim SR, Park JK, Park SJ, et al. Solitary bronchial squamous papilloma presenting as a plaque-like lesion in a subject with asthma. Am J Respir Crit Care Med. 2011 Feb 15;183(4):555–6. PMID:21325086

421. Kim TH, Kim SJ, Ryu YH, et al. Pleomorphic carcinoma of lung: comparison of CT features and pathologic findings. Radiology. 2004 Aug;232(2):554–9. PMID:15215543

422. Kim TS, Han J, Lee KS, et al. CT findings of surgically resected pleomorphic carcinoma of the lung in 30 patients. AJR Am J Roentgenol. 2005 Jul;185(1):120–5. PMID:15972411

423. Kim WJ, Kim SR, Choe YH, et al. Clear cell "sugar" tumor of the lung: a well-enhanced mass with an early washout pattern on dynamic contrast-enhanced computed tomography. J Korean Med Sci. 2008 Dec;23(6):1121–4. PMID:19119463

424. Kim YW, Kwon BS, Lim SY, et al. Diagnostic value of bronchoalveolar lavage and bronchial washing in sputum-scarce or smear-negative cases with suspected pulmonary tuberculosis: a randomized study. Clin Microbiol Infect. 2020 Jul;26(7):911–6. PMID:31759097

425. Kinoshita Y, Hamasaki M, Matsumoto S, et al. Fluorescence in situ hybridization detection of chromosome 22 monosomy in pleural effusion cytology for the diagnosis of mesothelioma. Cancer Cytopathol. 2021 Jul;129(7):526–36. PMID:33493384

426. Kinoshita Y, Hamasaki M, Yoshimura M, et al. Hemizygous loss of NF2 detected by fluorescence in situ hybridization is useful for the diagnosis of malignant pleural mesothelioma. Mod Pathol. 2020 Feb;33(2):235–44. PMID:31231129

427. Kinoshita Y, Hida T, Hamasaki M, et al. A combination of MTAP and BAP1 immunohistochemistry in pleural effusion cytology for the diagnosis of mesothelioma. Cancer Cytopathol. 2018 Jan;126(1):54–63. PMID:29053210

428. Kinslow CJ, May MS, Saqi A, et al. Large-cell neuroendocrine carcinoma of the lung: a population-based study. Clin Lung Cancer. 2020 Mar;21(2):e99–113. PMID:31601526

429. Kirby JG, Hargreave FE, Gleich GJ, et al. Bronchoalveolar cell profiles of asthmatic and nonasthmatic subjects. Am Rev Respir Dis. 1987 Aug;136(2):379–83. PMID:3304046

430. Klebe S, Nakatani Y, Dobra K, et al. The concept of mesothelioma in situ, with consideration of its potential impact on cytology diagnosis. Pathology. 2021 Jun;53(4):446–53. PMID:33775406

431. Klein O, Kee D, Markman B, et al. Immunotherapy of ipilimumab and nivolumab in patients with advanced neuroendocrine tumors: a subgroup analysis of the CA209-538 clinical trial for rare cancers. Clin Cancer Res. 2020 Sep 1;26(17):4454–9. PMID:32532787

432. Kleinberg L, Holth A, Fridman E, et al. The diagnostic role of claudins in serous effusions. Am J Clin Pathol. 2007 Jun;127(6):928–37. PMID:17509990

433. Klijanienko J, Caillaud JM, Lagacé R, et al. Cytohistologic correlations in angiosarcoma including classic and epithelioid variants: Institut Curie's experience. Diagn Cytopathol. 2003 Sep;29(3):140–5. PMID:12951681

434. Ko HM, Geddie WR, Boerner SL, et al. Cytomorphological and clinicopathological spectrum of pulmonary marginal zone lymphoma: the utility of immunophenotyping, PCR and FISH studies. Cytopathology. 2014 Aug;25(4):250–8. PMID:24261323

435. Kobayashi N, Koizumi T, Eguchi T, et al. A mediastinal somatic-type germ cell tumor with hepatic metastasis successfully treated by multiple modalities. Anticancer Res. 2010 Dec;30(12):5117–20. PMID:21187499

436. Kobayashi T, Man-I M, Shin E, et al. Hyperfunctioning intrathyroid parathyroid adenoma: report of two cases. Surg Today. 1999;29(8):766–8. PMID:10483753

437. König D, Savic Prince S, Rothschild SI. Targeted therapy in advanced and metastatic non-small cell lung cancer. An update on treatment of the most important actionable oncogenic driver alterations. Cancers (Basel). 2021 Feb 15;13(4):804. PMID:33671873

438. Koss MN, Hochholzer L, O'Leary T. Pulmonary blastomas. Cancer. 1991 May 1;67(9):2368–81. PMID:1849449

439. Krause A, Roma L, Lorber T, et al. Deciphering the clonal relationship between glandular and squamous components in adenosquamous carcinoma of the lung using whole exome sequencing. Lung Cancer. 2020 Dec;150:132–8. PMID:33137577

440. Kriegsmann K, Zgorzelski C, Kazdal D, et al. Insulinoma-associated protein 1 (INSM1) in thoracic tumors is less sensitive but more specific compared with synaptophysin, chromogranin A, and CD56. Appl Immunohistochem Mol Morphol. 2020 Mar;28(3):237–42. PMID:30358615

441. Krishnamurthy SC, Naresh KN, Soni M, et al. Sclerosing hemangioma of the lung: a potential source of error in fine needle aspiration cytology. Acta Cytol. 1994 Jan-Feb;38(1):111–2. PMID:8291347

441A. Krogerus L, Kholová I. Cell block in cytological diagnostics: review of preparatory techniques. Acta Cytol. 2018;62(4):237–43. PMID:29909418

442. Krüger S, Buck AK, Blumstein NM, et al. Use of integrated FDG PET/CT imaging in pulmonary carcinoid tumours. J Intern Med. 2006 Dec;260(6):545–50. PMID:17116005

443. Krupar R, Kümpers C, Haenel A, et al. [Cryptogenic organizing pneumonia versus secondary organizing pneumonia]. Pathologe. 2021 Feb;42(1):55–63. German. PMID:33462627

444. Kubik MJ, Bovbel A, Goli H, et al. Diagnostic value and accuracy of imprint cytology evaluation during image-guided core needle biopsies: review of our experience at a large academic center. Diagn Cytopathol. 2015 Oct;43(10):773–9. PMID:26119885

445. Kuhajda I, Zarogoulidis K, Tsirgogianni K, et al. Lung abscess-etiology, diagnostic and treatment options. Ann Transl Med. 2015 Aug;3(13):183. PMID:26366400

446. Kumar V, Soni P, Garg M, et al. A comparative study of primary adenoid cystic and mucoepidermoid carcinoma of lung. Front Oncol. 2018 May 15;8:153. PMID:29868475

447. Kuroda S, Suzuki S, Kurita A, et al. Cytological features of a variant NUT midline carcinoma of the lung harboring the NSD3-NUT fusion gene: a case report and literature review. Case Rep Pathol. 2015;2015:572951. PMID:25685583

448. Kurtin PJ, Myers JL, Adlakha H, et al. Pathologic and clinical features of primary pulmonary extranodal marginal zone B-cell lymphoma of MALT type. Am J Surg Pathol. 2001 Aug;25(8):997–1008. PMID:11474283

449. Kurtycz DF, Logrono R, Leopando M, et al. Immunocytochemistry controls using cell culture. Diagn Cytopathol. 1997 Jul;17(1):74–9. PMID:9218910

450. Kwak EL, Bang YJ, Camidge DR, et al. Anaplastic lymphoma kinase inhibition in non-small-cell lung cancer. N Engl J Med. 2010 Oct 28;363(18):1693–703. PMID:20979469

451. Kwon D, Koh J, Kim S, et al. MET exon 14 skipping mutation in triple-negative pulmonary adenocarcinomas and pleomorphic carcinomas: an analysis of intratumoral MET status heterogeneity and clinicopathological characteristics. Lung Cancer. 2017 Apr;106:131–7. PMID:28285687

452. Kwon YS, Koh WJ. Diagnosis and treatment of nontuberculous mycobacterial lung disease. J Korean Med Sci. 2016 May;31(5):649–59. PMID:27134484

454. Lang TU, Khalbuss WE, Monaco SE, et al. Solitary tracheobronchial papilloma: cytomorphology and ancillary studies with histologic correlation. Cytojournal. 2011 Mar 3;8:6. PMID:21383960

455. Lankshear S, Srigley J, McGowan T, et al. Standardized synoptic cancer pathology reports - so what and who cares? A population-based satisfaction survey of 970 pathologists, surgeons, and oncologists. Arch Pathol Lab Med. 2013 Nov;137(11):1599–602. PMID:23432456

456. Lantuejoul S, Rouquette I, Brambilla E, et al. [New WHO classification of lung adenocarcinoma and preneoplasia]. Ann Pathol. 2016 Jan;36(1):5–14. French. PMID:26791238

457. Lapkus O, Elsheikh TM, Ujevich BA, et al. Pitfalls in the diagnosis of herpes simplex infection in respiratory cytology. Acta Cytol. 2006 Nov-Dec;50(6):617–20. PMID:17152271

458. LaRocque RC, Katz JT, Perruzzi P, et al. The utility of sputum induction for diagnosis of Pneumocystis pneumonia in immunocompromised patients without human immunodeficiency virus. Clin Infect Dis. 2003 Nov 15;37(10):1380–3. PMID:14583873

459. Larone DH. Medically important fungi: a guide to identification. 2nd ed. Washington, DC: American Society for Microbiology; 1993.

460. Latimer KM. Lung cancer: clinical presentation and diagnosis. FP Essent. 2018 Jan;464:23–6. PMID:29313654

461. Law MR, Hodson ME, Turner-Warwick M. Malignant mesothelioma of the pleura: clinical aspects and symptomatic treatment. Eur J Respir Dis. 1984 Apr;65(3):162–8. PMID:6202538

463. Layfield LJ. The Papanicolaou Society of Cytopathology classification for pulmonary specimens: an overview. Cytopathology. 2016 Jun;27(3):149–52. PMID:27221749

464. Layfield LJ, Baloch Z, editors. The Papanicolaou Society of Cytopathology System for Reporting Respiratory Cytology: definitions, criteria, explanatory notes, and recommendations for ancillary testing. Cham (Switzerland): Springer; 2019.

465. Layfield LJ, Baloch Z, Elsheikh T, et al. Standardized terminology and nomenclature for respiratory cytology: the Papanicolaou Society of Cytopathology guidelines. Diagn Cytopathol. 2016 May;44(5):399–409. PMID:26990836

466. Layfield LJ, Dodd L, Witt B. Malignancy risk for the categories: non-diagnostic, benign, atypical, suspicious, and malignant used in the categorization of endobronchial ultrasound guided-fine needle aspirates of pulmonary nodules. Diagn Cytopathol. 2015 Nov;43(11):892–6. PMID:26331778

467. Layfield LJ, Esebua M. A modified Papanicolaou Society of Cytopathology system for reporting respiratory cytology specimens: implications for estimates of malignancy risk and diagnostic accuracy. Diagn Cytopathol. 2021 Nov;49(11):1167–72. PMID:34319004

468. Layfield LJ, Esebua M, Dodd L, et al. The Papanicolaou Society of Cytopathology guidelines for respiratory cytology: reproducibility of categories among observers. Cytojournal. 2018 Sep 21;15:22. PMID:30294354

469. Layfield LJ, Esebua M, Schmidt RL, et al. Malignancy risk associated with the EBUS-FNA diagnostic categories nondiagnostic, benign, atypical, suspicious for malignancy, and malignant for mediastinal lymph node aspirate specimens. J Am Soc Cytopathol. 2015 Sep-Oct;4(5):276–81. PMID:31051765
470. Layfield LJ, Pearson L, Walker BS, et al. Diagnostic accuracy of fine-needle aspiration cytology for discrimination of squamous cell carcinoma from adenocarcinoma in non-small cell lung cancer: a systematic review and meta-analysis. Acta Cytol. 2018;62(5-6):318–26. PMID:30380531
471. Layfield LJ, Roy-Chowdhuri S, Baloch Z, et al. Utilization of ancillary studies in the cytologic diagnosis of respiratory lesions: the Papanicolaou Society of Cytopathology consensus recommendations for respiratory cytology. Diagn Cytopathol. 2016 Dec;44(12):1000–9. PMID:27561242
472. Layfield LJ, Wallander ML. Diagnosis of gastrointestinal stromal tumors from minute specimens: cytomorphology, immunohistochemistry, and molecular diagnostic findings. Diagn Cytopathol. 2012 Jun;40(6):484–90. PMID:22351482
473. Lazar AJ, Tuvin D, Hajibashi S, et al. Specific mutations in the beta-catenin gene (CTNNB1) correlate with local recurrence in sporadic desmoid tumors. Am J Pathol. 2008 Nov;173(5):1518–27. PMID:18832571
474. Le BH, Boyer PJ, Lewis JE, et al. Granular cell tumor: immunohistochemical assessment of inhibin-alpha, protein gene product 9.5, S100 protein, CD68, and Ki-67 proliferative index with clinical correlation. Arch Pathol Lab Med. 2004 Jul;128(7):771–5. PMID:15214825
475. Le Loarer F, Watson S, Pierron G, et al. SMARCA4 inactivation defines a group of undifferentiated thoracic malignancies transcriptionally related to BAF-deficient sarcomas. Nat Genet. 2015 Oct;47(10):1200–5. PMID:26343384
476. Le Stang N, Burke L, Blaizot G, et al. Differential diagnosis of epithelioid malignant mesothelioma with lung and breast pleural metastasis: a systematic review compared with a standardized panel of antibodies-a new proposal that may influence pathologic practice. Arch Pathol Lab Med. 2020 Apr;144(4):446–56. PMID:31389715
477. Le X, Desai NV, Majid A, et al. De novo pulmonary small cell carcinomas and large cell neuroendocrine carcinomas harboring EGFR mutations: lack of response to EGFR inhibitors. Lung Cancer. 2015 Apr;88(1):70–3. PMID:25700797
478. Lee AC, Kwong YI, Fu KH, et al. Disseminated mediastinal carcinoma with chromosomal translocation (15;19). A distinctive clinicopathologic syndrome. Cancer. 1993 Oct 1;72(7):2273–6. PMID:8374886
479. Lee KH, Lim KY, Suh YJ, et al. Nondiagnostic percutaneous transthoracic needle biopsy of lung lesions: a multicenter study of malignancy risk. Radiology. 2019 Mar;290(3):814–23. PMID:30561276
480. Lee KW, Lee Y, Oh SW, et al. Large cell neuroendocrine carcinoma of the lung: CT and FDG PET findings. Eur J Radiol. 2015 Nov;84(11):2332–8. PMID:26279139
481. Lee W, Chung WS, Hong KS, et al. Clinical usefulness of bronchoalveolar lavage cellular analysis and lymphocyte subsets in diffuse interstitial lung diseases. Ann Lab Med. 2015 Mar;35(2):220–5. PMID:25729724
483. Leung SW, Bédard YC. Immunocytochemical staining on ThinPrep processed smears. Mod Pathol. 1996 Mar;9(3):304–6. PMID:8685232
484. Levy EB, Fiel MI, Hamilton SR, et al. State of the art: toward improving outcomes of lung and liver tumor biopsies in clinical trials-a multidisciplinary approach. J Clin Oncol. 2020 May 10;38(14):1633–40. PMID:32134701
485. Li C, Lu H. Adenosquamous carcinoma of the lung. Onco Targets Ther. 2018 Aug 14;11:4829–35. PMID:30147334
486. Li F, He M, Li F, et al. Histologic characteristics and prognosis of lung mixed squamous cell and glandular papilloma: six case reports. Int J Clin Exp Pathol. 2019 Sep 1;12(9):3542–8. PMID:31934202
487. Lichtenberger JP 3rd, Biko DM, Carter BW, et al. Primary lung tumors in children: radiologic-pathologic correlation from the Radiologic Pathology Archives. Radiographics. 2018 Nov-Dec;38(7):2151–72. PMID:30422774
488. Lim JH, Kim MJ, Jeon SH, et al. The optimal sequence of bronchial brushing and washing for diagnosing peripheral lung cancer using non-guided flexible bronchoscopy. Sci Rep. 2020 Jan 23;10(1):1036. PMID:31974454
489. Lim SM, Chang H, Cha YJ, et al. Validation of ALK/ROS1 dual break apart FISH probe probe in non-small-cell lung cancer. Lung Cancer. 2017 Sep;111:79–83. PMID:28838404
490. Lin F, Liu H. Immunohistochemistry in undifferentiated neoplasm/tumor of uncertain origin. Arch Pathol Lab Med. 2014 Dec;138(12):1583–610. PMID:25427040
491. Lin O. Telecytology for rapid on-site evaluation: current status. J Am Soc Cytopathol. 2018 Jan-Feb;7(1):1–6. PMID:29546032
492. Lin O, Olgac S, Green I, et al. Immunohistochemical staining of cytologic smears with MIB-1 helps distinguish low-grade from high-grade neuroendocrine neoplasms. Am J Clin Pathol. 2003 Aug;120(2):209–16. PMID:12931551
493. Lindeman NI, Cagle PT, Aisner DL, et al. Updated molecular testing guideline for the selection of lung cancer patients for treatment with targeted tyrosine kinase inhibitors: guideline from the College of American Pathologists, the International Association for the Study of Lung Cancer, and the Association for Molecular Pathology. Arch Pathol Lab Med. 2018 Mar;142(3):321–46. PMID:29355391
494. Lindeman NI, Cagle PT, Aisner DL, et al. Updated molecular testing guideline for the selection of lung cancer patients for treatment with targeted tyrosine kinase inhibitors: guideline from the College of American Pathologists, the International Association for the Study of Lung Cancer, and the Association for Molecular Pathology. J Mol Diagn. 2018 Mar;20(2):129–59. PMID:29398453
495. Lindeman NI, Cagle PT, Aisner DL, et al. Updated molecular testing guideline for the selection of lung cancer patients for treatment with targeted tyrosine kinase inhibitors: guideline from the College of American Pathologists, the International Association for the Study of Lung Cancer, and the Association for Molecular Pathology. J Thorac Oncol. 2018 Mar;13(3):323–58. PMID:29396253
496. Lindeman NI, Cagle PT, Beasley MB, et al. Molecular testing guideline for selection of lung cancer patients for EGFR and ALK tyrosine kinase inhibitors: guideline from the College of American Pathologists, International Association for the Study of Lung Cancer, and Association for Molecular Pathology. Arch Pathol Lab Med. 2013 Jun;137(6):828–60. PMID:23551194
497. Littooij AS, McHugh K, McCarville MB, et al. Yolk sac tumour: a rare cause of raised serum alpha-foetoprotein in a young child with a large liver mass. Pediatr Radiol. 2014 Jan;44(1):18–22. PMID:23982265
498. Liu A, Cheng L, Du J, et al. Diagnostic utility of novel stem cell markers SALL4, OCT4, NANOG, SOX2, UTF1, and TCL1 in primary mediastinal germ cell tumors. Am J Surg Pathol. 2010 May;34(5):697–706. PMID:20410807
499. Liu QH, Arias S, Wang KP. International Association for the Study of Lung Cancer map, Wang lymph node map and rapid on-site evaluation in transbronchial needle aspiration. J Thorac Dis. 2016 Sep;8(9):E869–74. PMID:27747023
500. Liu RB, Zhou DL, Xu BH, et al. Comparison of the diagnostic performances of US-guided fine needle aspiration cytology and thyroglobulin measurement for lymph node metastases in patients with differentiated thyroid carcinoma: a meta-analysis. Eur Radiol. 2021 May;31(5):2903–14. PMID:33125564
501. Liu X, Huang Z, Zhang J. [Analysis of clinical characteristics of 35 cases of pulmonary sclerosing pneumocytoma]. Zhongguo Fei Ai Za Zhi. 2020 Dec 20;23(12):1049–58. Chinese. PMID:33357311
502. Liu X, Jia Y, Stoopler MB, et al. Next-generation sequencing of pulmonary sarcomatoid carcinoma reveals high frequency of actionable MET gene mutations. J Clin Oncol. 2016 Mar 10;34(8):794–802. PMID:26215952
503. Lococo F, Torricelli F, Rossi G, et al. Inter-relationship between PD-L1 expression and clinic-pathological features and driver gene mutations in pulmonary sarcomatoid carcinomas. Lung Cancer. 2017 Nov;113:93–101. PMID:29110857
504. Long B, Long D, Koyfman A. Emergency medicine evaluation of community-acquired pneumonia: history, examination, imaging and laboratory assessment, and risk scores. J Emerg Med. 2017 Nov;53(5):642–52. PMID:28941558
505. Loo PS, Thomas SC, Nicolson MC, et al. Subtyping of undifferentiated non-small cell carcinomas in bronchial biopsy specimens. J Thorac Oncol. 2010 Apr;5(4):442–7. PMID:20195168
506. Lopes CV, Rigon P, Zettler CG, et al. Differential diagnosis of mesenchymal neoplasms of the digestive tract by cell block and immunohistochemistry. Cytopathology. 2018 Dec;29(6):531–6. PMID:30218589
507. Lou F, Sarkaria I, Pietanza C, et al. Recurrence of pulmonary carcinoid tumors after resection: implications for postoperative surveillance. Ann Thorac Surg. 2013 Oct;96(4):1156–62. PMID:23915584
508. Louw M, Brundyn K, Schubert PT, et al. Comparison of the quality of smears in transbronchial fine-needle aspirates using two staining methods for rapid on-site evaluation. Diagn Cytopathol. 2012 Sep;40(9):777–81. PMID:21322124
509. Lozano MD, Abengozar-Muela M, Echeveste JI, et al. Programmed death-ligand 1 expression on direct Pap-stained cytology smears from non-small cell lung cancer: comparison with cell blocks and surgical resection specimens. Cancer Cytopathol. 2019 Jul;127(7):470–80. PMID:31245924
510. Lozano MD, Echeveste JI, Abengozar M, et al. Cytology smears in the era of molecular biomarkers in non-small cell lung cancer: doing more with less. Arch Pathol Lab Med. 2018 Mar;142(3):291–8. PMID:29494220
511. Lozowski W, Hajdu SI, Melamed MR. Cytomorphology of carcinoid tumors. Acta Cytol. 1979 Sep-Oct;23(5):360–5. PMID:230682
512. Lukáš J, Drábek J, Lukáš D, et al. Ectopic thyroid with benign and malignant findings: a case series. Int J Surg Case Rep. 2020;66:33–8. PMID:31790949
513. Lynch TJ, Bell DW, Sordella R, et al. Activating mutations in the epidermal growth factor receptor underlying responsiveness of non-small-cell lung cancer to gefitinib. N Engl J Med. 2004 May 20;350(21):2129–39. PMID:15118073
514. Maan MSA, Waleed M, Sohail AH, et al. Solitary endobronchial papilloma: a rare entity. J Coll Physicians Surg Pak. 2019 Dec;29(12):S120–2. PMID:31779763
515. MacMahon H, Naidich DP, Goo JM, et al. Guidelines for management of incidental pulmonary nodules detected on CT images: from the Fleischner Society 2017. Radiology. 2017 Jul;284(1):228–43. PMID:28240562
516. MacMillan M, Roy B, McLaren S, et al. Widespread pulmonary invasion by malignant pleural mesothelioma: an important diagnostic consideration. Respirol Case Rep. 2020 Oct 26;8(9):e00675. PMID:33133607
517. Maddock SD, Cirulis MM, Callahan SJ, et al. Pulmonary lipid-laden macrophages and vaping. N Engl J Med. 2019 Oct 10;381(15):1488–9. PMID:31491073
518. Magers MJ, Kao CS, Cole CD, et al. "Somatic-type" malignancies arising from testicular germ cell tumors: a clinicopathologic study of 124 cases with emphasis on glandular tumors supporting frequent yolk sac tumor origin. Am J Surg Pathol. 2014 Oct;38(10):1396–409. PMID:24921638
519. Mahon BM, Placido JB, Gattuso P. Fine-needle aspiration of classic biphasic pulmonary blastoma. Diagn Cytopathol. 2010 Jun;38(6):427–9. PMID:19937760
520. Makris D, Scherpereel A, Leroy S, et al. Electromagnetic navigation diagnostic bronchoscopy for small peripheral lung lesions. Eur Respir J. 2007 Jun;29(6):1187–92. PMID:17360724
521. Malapelle U, Mayo-de-Las-Casas C, Molina-Vila MA, et al. Consistency and reproducibility of next-generation sequencing and other multigene mutational assays: a worldwide ring trial study on quantitative cytological molecular reference specimens. Cancer Cytopathol. 2017 Aug;125(8):615–26. PMID:28475299
522. Maleki S, Dorokhova O, Sunkara J, et al. Estrogen, progesterone, and HER-2 receptor immunostaining in cytology: the effect of varied fixation on human breast cancer cells. Diagn Cytopathol. 2013 Oct;41(10):864–70. PMID:23447357
523. Maleki Z. Diagnostic issues with cytopathologic interpretation of lung neoplasms displaying high-grade basaloid or neuroendocrine morphology. Diagn Cytopathol. 2011 Mar;39(3):159–67. PMID:21319315
524. Maleki Z, Muller S, Layfield L, et al. Pulmonary sclerosing pneumocytoma: cytomorphology and immunoprofile. Cancer Cytopathol. 2020 Jun;128(6):414–23. PMID:32022435
525. Malpica A, Euscher ED, Marques-Piubelli ML, et al. Malignant mesothelioma of the peritoneum in women: a clinicopathologic study of 164 cases. Am J Surg Pathol. 2021 Jan;45(1):45–58. PMID:32769428
526. Mancini R, Giarnieri E, De Vitis C, et al. Spheres derived from lung adenocarcinoma pleural effusions: molecular characterization and tumor engraftment. PLoS One. 2011;6(7):e21320. PMID:21789168
527. Maneenil K, Xue Z, Liu M, et al. Sarcomatoid carcinoma of the lung: the Mayo Clinic experience in 127 patients. Clin Lung Cancer. 2018 May;19(3):e323–33. PMID:29454534
528. Manhire A, Charig M, Clelland C, et al. Guidelines for radiologically guided lung biopsy. Thorax. 2003 Nov;58(11):920–36. PMID:14586042
529. Manukyan I, Sidawy M, DeBrito P. Spindle cell lesion on fine needle aspiration as an initial step for diagnosis of lymphangioleiomyomatosis: report of a rare case. Diagn Cytopathol. 2021 Sep;49(9):E352–5. PMID:34000096
530. Manzotti G, Torricelli F, Benedetta D, et al. An epithelial-to-mesenchymal transcriptional switch triggers evolution of pulmonary sarcomatoid

carcinoma (PSC) and identifies dasatinib as new therapeutic option. Clin Cancer Res. 2019 Apr 1;25(7):2348–60. PMID:30587547
531. Marchetti A, Barberis M, Papotti M, et al. ALK rearrangement testing by FISH analysis in non-small-cell lung cancer patients: results of the first Italian external quality assurance scheme. J Thorac Oncol. 2014 Oct;9(10):1470–6. PMID:25170637
532. Marchetti A, Felicioni L, Buttitta F. Assessing EGFR mutations. N Engl J Med. 2006 Feb 2;354(5):526–8. PMID:16452569
533. Marchevsky AM, LeStang N, Hiroshima K, et al. The differential diagnosis between pleural sarcomatoid mesothelioma and spindle cell/pleomorphic (sarcomatoid) carcinomas of the lung: evidence-based guidelines from the International Mesothelioma Panel and the MESOPATH National Reference Center. Hum Pathol. 2017 Sep;67:160–8. PMID:28782639
534. Marchiò C, Scaltriti M, Ladanyi M, et al. ESMO recommendations on the standard methods to detect NTRK fusions in daily practice and clinical research. Ann Oncol. 2019 Sep 1;30(9):1417–27. PMID:31268127
535. Mariño-Enríquez A, Fletcher CD. Round cell sarcomas - biologically important refinements in subclassification. Int J Biochem Cell Biol. 2014 Aug;53:493–504. PMID:24801613
536. Marks RA, Cramer HM, Wu HH. Fine-needle aspiration cytology of basaloid squamous cell carcinoma and small cell carcinoma-a comparison study. Diagn Cytopathol. 2013 Jan;41(1):81–4. PMID:22102491
537. Marmor S, Koren R, Halpern M, et al. Transthoracic needle biopsy in the diagnosis of large-cell neuroendocrine carcinoma of the lung. Diagn Cytopathol. 2005 Oct;33(4):238–43. PMID:16138368
538. Marotti JD, Rao KP, Brister KJ, et al. Cytologic rapid on-site evaluation of transthoracic computed tomography-guided lung needle biopsies: Who should perform ROSE? A cross-institutional analysis of procedural and diagnostic outcomes. J Am Soc Cytopathol. 2015 May-Jun;4(3):160–9. PMID:31051697
539. Martínez-Giron R, Doganci L, Ribas A. From the 19th century to the 21st, an old dilemma: ciliocytophthoria, multiflagellated protozoa, or both? Diagn Cytopathol. 2008 Aug;36(8):609–11. PMID:18618722
540. Martini K, Eberhard M, Frauenfelder T. [Pulmonary nodules - an overview]. Ther Umsch. 2020;77(2):75–80. German. PMID:32633224
541. Martinu T, Koutsokera A, Benden C, et al. International Society for Heart and Lung Transplantation consensus statement for the standardization of bronchoalveolar lavage in lung transplantation. J Heart Lung Transplant. 2020 Nov;39(11):1171–90. PMID:32773322
542. Matsubara D, Kishaba Y, Ishikawa S, et al. Lung cancer with loss of BRG1/BRM, shows epithelial mesenchymal transition phenotype and distinct histologic and genetic features. Cancer Sci. 2013 Feb;104(2):266–73. PMID:23163725
543. Matsubayashi H, Yamashita R, Sasaki K, et al. Retroperitoneal choriocarcinoma diagnosed by endoscopic ultrasonography-guided fine needle aspiration biopsy. Arab J Gastroenterol. 2018 Sep;19(3):130–3. PMID:30262237
544. Matsuda K, Kashima J, Yatabe Y. The isoform matters in NUT carcinoma: a diagnostic pitfall of p40 immunohistochemistry. J Thorac Oncol. 2020 Oct;15(10):e176–8. PMID:32981612
545. Matsuda KM, Nóbrega R, Quezado M, et al. Melanocytic bronchopulmonary carcinoid tumor in a patient with multiple endocrine neoplasia syndrome type 1: a case report with emphasis on intraoperative cytological findings. Diagn Cytopathol. 2010 Sep;38(9):669–74. PMID:20196165
546. Matsuguma H, Nakahara R, Kondo T, et al. Risk of pleural recurrence after needle biopsy in patients with resected early stage lung cancer. Ann Thorac Surg. 2005 Dec;80(6):2026–31. PMID:16305838
547. Matsushita M, Kuwamoto S. Cytologic features of SMARCA4-deficient thoracic sarcoma: a case report and comparison with other SWI/SNF complex-deficient tumors. Acta Cytol. 2018;62(5-6):456–62. PMID:30286456
548. Matter MS, Chijioke O, Savic S, et al. Narrative review of molecular pathways of kinase fusions and diagnostic approaches for their detection in non-small cell lung carcinomas. Transl Lung Cancer Res. 2020 Dec;9(6):2645–55. PMID:33489824
549. Mazza E, Maddau C, Ricciardi A, et al. On-site evaluation of percutaneous CT-guided fine needle aspiration of pulmonary lesions. A study of 321 cases. Radiol Med. 2005 Sep;110(3):141–8. PMID:16200036
550. McCarthy MJ, Rosado-de-Christenson ML. Tumors of the trachea. J Thorac Imaging. 1995 Summer;10(3):180–98. PMID:7674431
551. McCaughan BC, Martini N, Bains MS. Bronchial carcinoids. Review of 124 cases. J Thorac Cardiovasc Surg. 1985 Jan;89(1):8–17. PMID:2981373
552. McHugh KE, Sturgis CD, Procop GW, et al. The cytopathology of Actinomyces, Nocardia, and their mimickers. Diagn Cytopathol. 2017 Dec;45(12):1105–15. PMID:28888064
553. Medalie NS, Vallejo CE, Wasserman P. Metastatic pulmonary artery sarcoma. Report of a case with diagnosis by fine needle aspiration. Acta Cytol. 1998 Jul-Aug;42(4):968–72. PMID:9684587
554. Mehnert JM, Bergsland E, O'Neil BH, et al. Pembrolizumab for the treatment of programmed death-ligand 1-positive advanced carcinoid or pancreatic neuroendocrine tumors: results from the KEYNOTE-028 study. Cancer. 2020 Jul 1;126(13):3021–30. PMID:32320048
555. Mehrad M, Roy S, Bittar HT, et al. Next-generation sequencing approach to non-small cell lung carcinoma yields more actionable alterations. Arch Pathol Lab Med. 2018 Mar;142(3):353–7. PMID:29219616
556. Mei K, Liu A, Allan RW, et al. Diagnostic utility of SALL4 in primary germ cell tumors of the central nervous system: a study of 77 cases. Mod Pathol. 2009 Dec;22(12):1628–36. PMID:19820689
557. Mei L, Alikhan M, Mujacic I, et al. Genomic alterations in undifferentiated malignant tumors with rhabdoid phenotype and loss of BRG1 immunoexpression identified by fine needle aspirates. Acta Cytol. 2019;63(5):438–44. PMID:31230044
558. Meisinger QC, Klein JS, Butnor KJ, et al. CT features of peripheral pulmonary carcinoid tumors. AJR Am J Roentgenol. 2011 Nov;197(5):1073–80. PMID:22021498
559. Meng Q, Dong Y, Tao H, et al. ALK-rearranged squamous cell carcinoma of the lung. Thorac Cancer. 2021 Apr;12(7):1106–14. PMID:33565277
560. Metintaş M, Ozdemir N, Işiksoy S, et al. CT-guided pleural needle biopsy in the diagnosis of malignant mesothelioma. J Comput Assist Tomogr. 1995 May-Jun;19(3):370–4. PMID:7790544
561. Metintaş S, Batırel HF, Bayram H, et al. Turkey National Mesothelioma Surveillance and Environmental Asbestos Exposure Control Program. Int J Environ Res Public Health. 2017 Oct 25;14(11):1293. PMID:29068368
562. Metovic J, Barella M, Bianchi F, et al. Morphologic and molecular classification of lung neuroendocrine neoplasms. Virchows Arch. 2021 Jan;478(1):5–19. PMID:33474631
563. Metovic J, Righi L, Delsedime L, et al. Role of immunocytochemistry in the cytological diagnosis of pulmonary tumors. Acta Cytol. 2020;64(1-2):16–29. PMID:30878997
564. Mettler TN, Andrade RS, Pambuccian SE. Spindle cell typical carcinoid tumor (well-differentiated neuroendocrine carcinoma) diagnosed by electromagnetic navigation bronchoscopy with cytologic rapid on-site evaluation. Diagn Cytopathol. 2012 Oct;40(10):898–902. PMID:21987437
565. Meyer KC, Raghu G, Baughman RP, et al. An official American Thoracic Society clinical practice guideline: the clinical utility of bronchoalveolar lavage cellular analysis in interstitial lung disease. Am J Respir Crit Care Med. 2012 May 1;185(9):1004–14. PMID:22550210
566. Micello D, Bossi A, Marando A, et al. Expression of calretinin in high-grade hormone receptor-negative invasive breast carcinomas: correlation with histological and molecular subtypes. Virchows Arch. 2017 Jul;471(1):13–21. PMID:28550498
567. Michael CW, Bedrossian CC. The implementation of liquid-based cytology for lung and pleural-based diseases. Acta Cytol. 2014;58(6):563–73. PMID:25427721
568. Michael CW, Faquin W, Jing X, et al. Committee II: Guidelines for cytologic sampling techniques of lung and mediastinal lymph nodes. Diagn Cytopathol. 2018 Oct;46(10):815–25. PMID:30195266
569. Michael CW, Hoda RS, Saqi A, et al. Committee I: Indications for pulmonary cytology sampling methods. Diagn Cytopathol. 2016 Dec;44(12):1010–23. PMID:27753244
570. Michelow P, Omar T, Field A, et al. The cytopathology of mycobacterial infection. Diagn Cytopathol. 2016 Mar;44(3):255–62. PMID:26800030
571. Miettinen M, McCue PA, Sarlomo-Rikala M, et al. GATA3: a multispecific but potentially useful marker in surgical pathology: a systematic analysis of 2500 epithelial and nonepithelial tumors. Am J Surg Pathol. 2014 Jan;38(1):13–22. PMID:24145643
572. Miettinen M, McCue PA, Sarlomo-Rikala M, et al. Sox10–a marker for not only schwannian and melanocytic neoplasms but also myoepithelial cell tumors of soft tissue: a systematic analysis of 5134 tumors. Am J Surg Pathol. 2015 Jun;39(6):826–35. PMID:25724000
573. Milano MT, Zhang H. Malignant pleural mesothelioma: a population-based study of survival. J Thorac Oncol. 2010 Nov;5(11):1841–8. PMID:20975379
574. Milman N, Faurschou P, Grode G. Diagnostic yield of transthoracic needle aspiration biopsy following negative fiberoptic bronchoscopy in 103 patients with peripheral circumscribed pulmonary lesions. Respiration. 1995;62(1):1–3. PMID:7716347
575. Mimica X, McGill M, Hay A, et al. Distant metastasis of salivary gland cancer: incidence, management, and outcomes. Cancer. 2020 May 15;126(10):2153–62. PMID:32097509
576. Mitchell ML, Parker FP. Capillaries. A cytologic feature of pulmonary carcinoid tumors. Acta Cytol. 1991 Mar-Apr;35(2):183–5. PMID:2028691
577. Miyoshi T, Umemura S, Matsumura Y, et al. Genomic profiling of large-cell neuroendocrine carcinoma of the lung. Clin Cancer Res. 2017 Feb 1;23(3):757–65. PMID:27507618
578. Mizuguchi K, Minato H, Onishi H, et al. Cytopathological findings of primary pulmonary Ewing family of tumors with EWSR1 translocation: a case report. Thorac Cancer. 2016 Sep;7(5):602–6. PMID:27766786
579. Mokhtari M, Kumar PV. Intranuclear pseudo-inclusions and grooves in fine needle aspiration cytology of pulmonary carcinoid tumor. Arch Iran Med. 2016 Feb;19(2):150–2. PMID:26838088
580. Molina JR, Aubry MC, Lewis JE, et al. Primary salivary gland-type lung cancer: spectrum of clinical presentation, histopathologic and prognostic factors. Cancer. 2007 Nov 15;110(10):2253–9. PMID:17918258
581. Monaco SE, Khalbuss WE, Ustinova E, et al. The cytomorphologic spectrum of salivary gland type tumors in the lung and mediastinum: a report of 16 patients. Diagn Cytopathol. 2012 Dec;40(12):1062–70. PMID:21591276
582. Montezuma D, Azevedo R, Lopes P, et al. A panel of four immunohistochemical markers (CK7, CK20, TTF-1, and p63) allows accurate diagnosis of primary and metastatic lung carcinoma on biopsy specimens. Virchows Arch. 2013 Dec;463(6):749–54. PMID:24126803
583. Mooney EE, Layfield LJ, Dodd LG. Fine-needle aspiration of neural lesions. Diagn Cytopathol. 1999 Jan;20(1):1–5. PMID:9884818
584. Moran CA. Primary salivary gland-type tumors of the lung. Semin Diagn Pathol. 1995 May;12(2):106–22. PMID:7638445
585. Moran CA, Hochholzer L, Rush W, et al. Primary intrapulmonary meningiomas. A clinicopathologic and immunohistochemical study of ten cases. Cancer. 1996 Dec 1;78(11):2328–33. PMID:8941002
586. Moran CA, Lindholm KE, Brunnström H, et al. Typical and atypical carcinoid tumors of the lung: a clinicopathological correlation of 783 cases with emphasis on histological features. Hum Pathol. 2020 Apr;98:98–109. PMID:32145220
587. Moran CA, Suster S. Primary germ cell tumors of the mediastinum: I. Analysis of 322 cases with special emphasis on teratomatous lesions and a proposal for histopathologic classification and clinical staging. Cancer. 1997 Aug 15;80(4):681–90. PMID:9264351
588. Moran CA, Suster S. Primary mediastinal choriocarcinomas: a clinicopathologic and immunohistochemical study of eight cases. Am J Surg Pathol. 1997 Sep;21(9):1007–12. PMID:9298876
589. Moran CA, Suster S, Koss MN. Primary germ cell tumors of the mediastinum: III. Yolk sac tumor, embryonal carcinoma, choriocarcinoma, and combined nonteratomatous germ cell tumors of the mediastinum–a clinicopathologic and immunohistochemical study of 64 cases. Cancer. 1997 Aug 15;80(4):699–707. PMID:9264353
590. Moran CA, Suster S, Przygodzki RM, et al. Primary germ cell tumors of the mediastinum: II. Mediastinal seminomas–a clinicopathologic and immunohistochemical study of 120 cases. Cancer. 1997 Aug 15;80(4):691–8. PMID:9264352
591. Moreira AL. Evolution of guidelines for respiratory cytology by the Papanicolaou Society of Cytopathology. Diagn Cytopathol. 2020 Oct;48(10):867–9. PMID:32359109
592. Morikawa K, Misumi S, Fukuda T, et al. Pulmonary sclerosing pneumocytoma presenting as slow-growing multiple nodules over a long period. Radiol Case Rep. 2019 Mar 7;14(5):602–7. PMID:30891111
593. Mukhopadhyay S, Dermawan JK, Lanigan CP, et al. Insulinoma-associated protein 1 (INSM1) is a sensitive and highly specific marker of neuroendocrine differentiation in primary lung neoplasms: an immunohistochemical study of 345 cases, including 292 whole-tissue sections. Mod Pathol. 2019 Jan;32(1):100–9. PMID:30154579
594. Mukhopadhyay S, Mehta AC. Utility of core needle biopsies and transbronchial biopsies for diagnosing nonneoplastic lung diseases. Arch Pathol Lab Med. 2018 Sep;142(9):1054–68. PMID:30141992
595. Mullerpattan JB, Udwadia ZF, Udwadia FE. Tropical pulmonary eosinophilia–a review. Indian J Med Res. 2013 Sep;138(3):295–302. PMID:24135173

596. Mundt F, Johansson HJ, Forshed J, et al. Proteome screening of pleural effusions identifies galectin 1 as a diagnostic biomarker and highlights several prognostic biomarkers for malignant mesothelioma. Mol Cell Proteomics. 2014 Mar;13(3):701–15. PMID:24361865
597. Mundt F, Nilsonne G, Arslan S, et al. Hyaluronan and N-ERC/mesothelin as key biomarkers in a specific two-step model to predict pleural malignant mesothelioma. PLoS One. 2013 Aug 21;8(8):e72030. PMID:23991032
598. Murgu SD. Robotic assisted-bronchoscopy: technical tips and lessons learned from the initial experience with sampling peripheral lung lesions. BMC Pulm Med. 2019 May 9;19(1):89. PMID:31072355
599. Murray KL, Duvall E, Salter DM, et al. Efficacy and pattern of use of sputum cytology as a diagnostic test. Cytopathology. 2002 Dec;13(6):350–4. PMID:12485170
600. Naidoo J, Santos-Zabala ML, Iyriboz T, et al. Large cell neuroendocrine carcinoma of the lung: clinico-pathologic features, treatment, and outcomes. Clin Lung Cancer. 2016 Sep;17(5):e121–9. PMID:26898325
601. Najafi N, Demanet C, Dab I, et al. Differential cytology of bronchoalveolar lavage fluid in asthmatic children. Pediatr Pulmonol. 2003 Apr;35(4):302–8. PMID:12629629
602. Nakagiri T, Nakayama T, Tokunaga T, et al. intraoperative diagnosis and surgical procedure with imprint cytology for small pulmonary adenocarcinoma. J Cancer. 2020 Feb 20;11(10):2724–9. PMID:32226490
603. Nakagiri T, Nakayama T, Tokunaga T, et al. Novel imprint cytological classification for small pulmonary adenocarcinoma using surgical specimens: comparison with the 8th Lung Cancer Staging System and Histopathological Classification. J Cancer. 2020 Feb 21;11(10):2845–51. PMID:32226502
604. Nakaguro M, Nagao T. Epithelial-myoepithelial carcinoma. Surg Pathol Clin. 2021 Mar;14(1):97–109. PMID:33526226
605. Nakanishi K, Sakakura N, Matsui T, et al. Clinicopathological features, surgical outcomes, oncogenic status and PD-L1 expression of pulmonary pleomorphic carcinoma. Anticancer Res. 2019 Oct;39(10):5789–95. PMID:31570483
606. Nakashima K, Demura Y, Oi M, et al. Utility of endoscopic ultrasound with bronchoscope-guided fine-needle aspiration for detecting driver oncogenes in non-small-cell lung cancer during emergency situations: case series. Intern Med. 2021 Apr 1;60(7):1061–5. PMID:33132332
607. Nakatani Y, Miyagi Y, Takemura T, et al. Aberrant nuclear/cytoplasmic localization and gene mutation of beta-catenin in classic pulmonary blastoma: beta-catenin immunostaining is useful for distinguishing between classic pulmonary blastoma and a blastomatoid variant of carcinosarcoma. Am J Surg Pathol. 2004 Jul;28(7):921–7. PMID:15223963
608. Nakayama T, Ohtsuka T, Kazama A, et al. Classic pulmonary blastoma: a subtype of biphasic pulmonary blastoma. Ann Thorac Cardiovasc Surg. 2012;18(2):125–7. PMID:22001215
609. Nambirajan A, Dutta R, Malik PS, et al. Cytology of SMARCA4-deficient thoracic neoplasms: comparative analysis of SMARCA4-deficient non-small cell lung carcinomas and SMARCA4-deficient thoracic sarcomas. Acta Cytol. 2021;65(1):67–74. PMID:32854100
610. Nambirajan A, Jain D. Cell blocks in cytopathology: an update. Cytopathology. 2018 Dec;29(6):505–24. PMID:30153355
611. Nambirajan A, Kaur H, Jangra K, et al. Adenocarcinoma predominant pattern subtyping and nuclear grading in cytology: Is there a role in prognostication of advanced pulmonary adenocarcinomas? Cytopathology. 2018 Apr;29(2):163–71. PMID:29388266
613. Nambirajan A, Singh V, Bhardwaj N, et al. SMARCA4/BRG1-deficient non-small cell lung carcinomas: a case series and review of the literature. Arch Pathol Lab Med. 2021 Jan 1;145(1):90–8. PMID:33367658
614. Naryshkin S, Bedrossian CW. Selected mimics of malignancy in sputum and bronchoscopic cytology specimens. Diagn Cytopathol. 1995 Dec;13(5):443–7. PMID:8834319
615. Naryshkin S, Young NA. Respiratory cytology: a review of non-neoplastic mimics of malignancy. Diagn Cytopathol. 1993;9(1):89–97. PMID:8384547
616. Nath D, Arava S, Joshi P, et al. Primary pulmonary leiomyosarcoma of lung: an unusual entity with brief review. Indian J Pathol Microbiol. 2015 Jul-Sep;58(3):338–40. PMID:26275258
617. National Comprehensive Cancer Network (NCCN) [Internet]. Fort Washington (PA): NCCN; 2021 [accessed 2021 Feb 23]. Available from: https://www.nccn.org.
618. National Comprehensive Cancer Network (NCCN) [Internet]. Fort Washington (PA): NCCN; 2021 [accessed 2021 Nov 16]. Available from: https://www.nccn.org.
619. National Comprehensive Cancer Network (NCCN). NCCN clinical practice guidelines in oncology (NCCN guidelines): Non-small cell lung cancer. Version 3.2022. Fort Washington (PA): NCCN; 2022 [accessed 2021 Mar 2]. Available from: https://www.nccn.org/professionals/physician_gls/default.aspx.
620. National Comprehensive Cancer Network (NCCN). NCCN clinical practice guidelines in oncology (NCCN guidelines): Non-small cell lung cancer. Version 3.2022. Fort Washington (PA): NCCN; 2022 [accessed 2022 Apr 30]. Available from: https://www.nccn.org/professionals/physician_gls/default.aspx.
621. Natu S, Hoffman J, Siddiqui M, et al. The role of endobronchial ultrasound guided transbronchial needle aspiration cytology in the investigation of mediastinal lymphadenopathy and masses, the North Tees experience. J Clin Pathol. 2010 May;63(5):445–51. PMID:20299387
622. Nayak A, Sugrue C, Koenig S, et al. Endobronchial ultrasound-guided transbronchial needle aspirate (EBUS-TBNA): a proposal for on-site adequacy criteria. Diagn Cytopathol. 2012 Feb;40(2):128–37. PMID:22246929
623. Nelson BA, Lee EY, French CA, et al. BRD4-NUT carcinoma of the mediastinum in a pediatric patient: multidetector computed tomography imaging findings. J Thorac Imaging. 2010 Aug;25(3):W93–6. PMID:20395873
624. Neumann T, Meyer M, Patten FW, et al. Premalignant and malignant cells in sputum from lung cancer patients. Cancer. 2009 Dec 25;117(6):473–81. PMID:19852034
625. Neumann V, Müller KM, Fischer M. [Peritoneal mesothelioma–incidence and etiology]. Pathologe. 1999 May;20(3):169–76. German. PMID:10412176
626. Ng AB, Horak GC. Factors significant in the diagnostic accuracy of lung cytology in bronchial washing and sputum samples. II. Sputum samples. Acta Cytol. 1983 Jul-Aug;27(4):397–402. PMID:6308932
627. Nguyen GK. Cytopathology of pulmonary carcinoid tumors in sputum and bronchial brushings. Acta Cytol. 1995 Nov-Dec;39(6):1152–60. PMID:7483991
628. Nguyen P, Bashirzadeh F, Hundloe J, et al. Grey scale texture analysis of endobronchial ultrasound mini probe images for prediction of benign or malignant aetiology. Respirology. 2015 Aug;20(6):960–6. PMID:26113224
629. Nguyen Y, Guillevin L. Eosinophilic granulomatosis with polyangiitis (Churg-Strauss). Semin Respir Crit Care Med. 2018 Aug;39(4):471–81. PMID:30404114
630. Nicholson AG, Sauter JL, Nowak AK, et al. EURACAN/IASLC proposals for updating the histologic classification of pleural mesothelioma: towards a more multidisciplinary approach. J Thorac Oncol. 2020 Jan;15(1):29–49. PMID:31546041
631. Nicholson DW, Neupert W. Import of cytochrome c into mitochondria: reduction of heme, mediated by NADH and flavin nucleotides, is obligatory for its covalent linkage to apocytochrome c. Proc Natl Acad Sci U S A. 1989 Jun;86(12):4340–4. PMID:2543970
632. Nicholson SA, Beasley MB, Brambilla E, et al. Small cell lung carcinoma (SCLC): a clinicopathologic study of 100 cases with surgical specimens. Am J Surg Pathol. 2002 Sep;26(9):1184–97. PMID:12218575
633. Niederkohr RD, Cameron MJ, French CA. FDG PET/CT imaging of NUT midline carcinoma. Clin Nucl Med. 2011 Sep;36(9):e124–6. PMID:21825839
634. Nishii Y, Nakamura Y, Fujiwara K, et al. Use of ultrathin bronchoscope on a need basis improves diagnostic yield of difficult-to-approach pulmonary lesions. Front Med (Lausanne). 2020 Dec 15;7:588048. PMID:33385003
635. Nishino M, Hoang MP, Della Pelle P, et al. Napsin A/p40 antibody cocktail for subtyping non-small cell lung carcinoma on cytology and small biopsy specimens. Cancer Cytopathol. 2016 Jul;124(7):472–84. PMID:27412420
636. Nizzoli R, Tiseo M, Gelsomino F, et al. Accuracy of fine needle aspiration cytology in the pathological typing of non-small cell lung cancer. J Thorac Oncol. 2011 Mar;6(3):489–93. PMID:21258246
637. Noll B, Wang WL, Gong Y, et al. Programmed death ligand 1 testing in non-small cell lung carcinoma cytology cell block and aspirate smear preparations. Cancer Cytopathol. 2018 May;126(5):342–52. PMID:29499101
638. Nonaka D, Chiriboga L, Rubin BP. Sox10: a pan-schwannian and melanocytic marker. Am J Surg Pathol. 2008 Sep;32(9):1291–8. PMID:18636017
639. Noussios G, Anagnostis P, Natsis K. Ectopic parathyroid glands and their anatomical, clinical and surgical implications. Exp Clin Endocrinol Diabetes. 2012 Nov;120(10):604–10. PMID:23174995
640. Ntanasis-Stathopoulos I, Tsilimigras DI, Klapsinou E, et al. Challenging differential diagnosis of an extra-adrenal paraganglioma; the role of fine needle aspiration cytology. Diagn Cytopathol. 2017 Jun;45(6):565–8. PMID:28261927
641. Nunes H, Brillet PY, Valeyre D, et al. Imaging in sarcoidosis. Semin Respir Crit Care Med. 2007 Feb;28(1):102–20. PMID:17330195
642. Oda T, Ogata S, Kawaguchi S, et al. Immunocytochemical utility of claudin-4 versus those of Ber-EP4 and MOC-31 in effusion cytology. Diagn Cytopathol. 2016 Jun;44(6):499–504. PMID:27015745
643. Ogino S, al-Kaisi N, Abdul-Karim FW. Cytopathology of oncocytic carcinoid tumor of the lung mimicking granular cell tumor. A case report. Acta Cytol. 2000 Mar-Apr;44(2):247–50. PMID:10740615
644. Ohashi-Nakatani K, Shibuki Y, Fujima M, et al. Primary pulmonary meningioma: a rare case report of aspiration cytological features and immunohistochemical assessment. Diagn Cytopathol. 2019 Apr;47(4):330–3. PMID:30548187
645. Ohshimo S, Guzman J, Costabel U, et al. Differential diagnosis of granulomatous lung disease: clues and pitfalls: Number 4 in the Series "Pathology for the clinician" Edited by Peter Dorfmüller and Alberto Cavazza. Eur Respir Rev. 2017 Aug 9;26(145):170012. PMID:28794143
646. Oike T, Ogiwara H, Tominaga Y, et al. A synthetic lethality-based strategy to treat cancers harboring a genetic deficiency in the chromatin remodeling factor BRG1. Cancer Res. 2013 Sep 1;73(17):5508–18. PMID:23872584
647. Oki M, Saka H, Ando M, et al. How many passes are needed for endobronchial ultrasound-guided transbronchial needle aspiration for sarcoidosis? A prospective multicenter study. Respiration. 2018;95(4):251–7. PMID:29320774
648. Onofre FB, Onofre AS, Pomjanski N, et al. 9p21 deletion in the diagnosis of malignant mesothelioma in serous effusions additional to immunocytochemistry, DNA-ICM, and AgNOR analysis. Cancer. 2008 Jun 25;114(3):204–15. PMID:18306350
649. Ordóñez NG. Mesothelioma with rhabdoid features: an ultrastructural and immunohistochemical study of 10 cases. Mod Pathol. 2006 Mar;19(3):373–83. PMID:16400322
650. Ordóñez NG. Napsin A expression in lung and kidney neoplasia: a review and update. Adv Anat Pathol. 2012 Jan;19(1):66–73. PMID:22156835
651. Ordóñez NG. Pleomorphic mesothelioma: report of 10 cases. Mod Pathol. 2012 Jul;25(7):1011–22. PMID:22388762
652. Ordóñez NG. The diagnostic utility of immunohistochemistry and electron microscopy in distinguishing between peritoneal mesotheliomas and serous carcinomas: a comparative study. Mod Pathol. 2006 Jan;19(1):34–48. PMID:16056246
653. Ordóñez NG. The diagnostic utility of immunohistochemistry in distinguishing between epithelioid mesotheliomas and squamous carcinomas of the lung: a comparative study. Mod Pathol. 2006 Mar;19(3):417–28. PMID:16415794
654. Ordóñez NG. What are the current best immunohistochemical markers for the diagnosis of epithelioid mesothelioma? A review and update. Hum Pathol. 2007 Jan;38(1):1–16. PMID:17056092
655. Oshiro Y, Kusumoto M, Matsuno Y, et al. CT findings of surgically resected large cell neuroendocrine carcinoma of the lung in 38 patients. AJR Am J Roentgenol. 2004 Jan;182(1):87–91. PMID:14684518
656. Ost DE, Ernst A, Lei X, et al. Diagnostic yield and complications of bronchoscopy for peripheral lung lesions. Results of the AQuIRE registry. Am J Respir Crit Care Med. 2016 Jan 1;193(1):68–77. PMID:26367186
657. Ou SH, Kawaguchi T, Soo RA, et al. Rare subtypes of adenocarcinoma of the lung. Expert Rev Anticancer Ther. 2011 Oct;11(10):1535–42. PMID:21999127
658. Owens CL, Sharma R, Ali SZ. Deep fibromatosis (desmoid tumor): cytopathologic characteristics, clinicoradiologic features, and immunohistochemical findings on fine-needle aspiration. Cancer. 2007 Jun 25;111(3):166–72. PMID:17477374
659. Oxnard GR, Lo PC, Nishino M, et al. Natural history and molecular characteristics of lung cancers harboring EGFR exon 20 insertions. J Thorac Oncol. 2013 Feb;8(2):179–84. PMID:23328547
660. Ozan E, Oztekin O, Alacacioğlu A, et al. Esophageal gastrointestinal stromal tumor with pulmonary and bone metastases. Diagn Interv Radiol. 2010 Sep;16(3):217–20. PMID:19838991
661. Oz Atalay F, Aytac Vuruskan B, Vuruskan H. CDX2 immunostaining in primary and metastatic germ cell tumours of the testis.

J Int Med Res. 2016 Dec;44(6):1323–30. PMID:28322096
662. Ozturk A, Cicek T, Aktas Z, et al. Mediastinal ectopic thyroid diagnosed by endobronchial ultrasound-guided transbronchial needle aspiration: report of three cases. J Clin Ultrasound. 2018 May;46(4):299–301. PMID:28940588
663. Paez JG, Jänne PA, Lee JC, et al. EGFR mutations in lung cancer: correlation with clinical response to gefitinib therapy. Science. 2004 Jun 4;304(5676):1497–500. PMID:15118125
664. Pal P, Chetty R. Multiple sclerosing pneumocytomas: a review. J Clin Pathol. 2020 Sep;73(9):531–4. PMID:32317291
665. Paliouras D, Gogakos A, Rallis T, et al. Coexistence of squamous cell tracheal papilloma and carcinoma treated with chemotherapy and radiotherapy: a case report. Ther Clin Risk Manag. 2015 Dec 21;12:1–4. PMID:26730195
667. Pambuccian SE. The COVID-19 pandemic: implications for the cytology laboratory. J Am Soc Cytopathol. 2020 May-Jun;9(3):202–11. PMID:32284276
668. Panigrahi MK, Pradhan G, Sahoo N, et al. Primary pulmonary synovial sarcoma: a reappraisal. J Cancer Res Ther. 2018 Apr-Jun;14(3):481–9. PMID:29893303
669. Panizo-Santos A, Sola I, de Alava E, et al. Angiomyolipoma and PEComa are immunoreactive for MyoD1 in cell cytoplasmic staining pattern. Appl Immunohistochem Mol Morphol. 2003 Jun;11(2):156–60. PMID:12778001
670. Pao W, Miller V, Zakowski M, et al. EGF receptor gene mutations are common in lung cancers from "never smokers" and are associated with sensitivity of tumors to gefitinib and erlotinib. Proc Natl Acad Sci U S A. 2004 Sep 7;101(36):13306–11. PMID:15329413
671. Pao W, Miller VA, Politi KA, et al. Acquired resistance of lung adenocarcinomas to gefitinib or erlotinib is associated with a second mutation in the EGFR kinase domain. PLoS Med. 2005 Mar;2(3):e73. PMID:15737014
672. Papanicolaou GN. Diagnostic value of exfoliated cells from cancerous tissues. J Am Med Assoc. 1946 Jun 1;131:372–8. PMID:20983696
673. Papanicolaou GN, Cromwell HA. Diagnosis of cancer of the lung by the cytologic method. Dis Chest. 1949 Apr;15(4):412–21. PMID:18114650
674. Papanicolaou GN, Koprowska I. Carcinoma in situ of the right lower bronchus; a case report. Cancer. 1951 Jan;4(1):141–6. PMID:14801781
675. Papanicolaou Society of Cytopathology Task Force on Standards of Practice. Guidelines of the Papanicolaou Society of Cytopathology for fine-needle aspiration procedure and reporting. Diagn Cytopathol. 1997 Oct;17(4):239–47. PMID:9316777
676. Papanicolaou Society of Cytopathology Task Force on Standards of Practice. Guidelines of the Papanicolaou Society of Cytopathology for the examination of cytologic specimens obtained from the respiratory tract. Diagn Cytopathol. 1999 Jul;21(1):61–9. PMID:10405813
677. Papaxoinis G, Lamarca A, Quinn AM, et al. Clinical and pathologic characteristics of pulmonary carcinoid tumors in central and peripheral locations. Endocr Pathol. 2018 Sep;29(3):259–68. PMID:29770932
678. Park JS, Chung JH, Jheon S, et al. EBUS-TBNA in the differential diagnosis of pulmonary artery sarcoma and thromboembolism. Eur Respir J. 2011 Dec;38(6):1480–2. PMID:22130766
679. Patel A, Borczuk AC, Siddiqui MT. Utility of claudin-4 versus BerEP4 and B72.3 in pleural fluids with metastatic lung adenocarcinoma. J Am Soc Cytopathol. 2020 May-Jun;9(3):146–51. PMID:32184064
680. Patel TS, Shah MG, Gandhi JS, et al. Accuracy of cytology in sub typing non small cell lung carcinomas. Diagn Cytopathol. 2017 Jul;45(7):598–603. PMID:28429425
681. Pearson L, Factor RE, White SK, et al. Rapid on-site evaluation of fine-needle aspiration by non-cytopathologists: a systematic review and meta-analysis of diagnostic accuracy studies for adequacy assessment. Acta Cytol. 2018;62(4):244–52. PMID:29874653
682. Pei J, Flieder DB, Patchefsky A, et al. Detecting MYB and MYBL1 fusion genes in tracheobronchial adenoid cystic carcinoma by targeted RNA-sequencing. Mod Pathol. 2019 Oct;32(10):1416–20. PMID:31028361
683. Pelosi G, Fabbri A, Cossa M, et al. What clinicians are asking pathologists when dealing with lung neuroendocrine neoplasms? Semin Diagn Pathol. 2015 Nov;32(6):469–79. PMID:26561395
684. Pelosi G, Fraggetta F, Maffini F, et al. Pulmonary epithelial-myoepithelial tumor of unproven malignant potential: report of a case and review of the literature. Mod Pathol. 2001 May;14(5):521–6. PMID:11353064
685. Pelosi G, Fraggetta F, Nappi O, et al. Pleomorphic carcinomas of the lung show a selective distribution of gene products involved in cell differentiation, cell cycle control, tumor growth, and tumor cell motility: a clinicopathologic and immunohistochemical study of 31 cases. Am J Surg Pathol. 2003 Sep;27(9):1203–15. PMID:12960804
686. Pelosi G, Massa F, Gatti G, et al. Ki-67 evaluation for clinical decision in metastatic lung carcinoids: a proof of concept. Clin Pathol. 2019 Feb 19;12:X19829259. PMID:31041430
687. Pelosi G, Rodriguez J, Viale G, et al. Typical and atypical pulmonary carcinoid tumor overdiagnosed as small-cell carcinoma on biopsy specimens: a major pitfall in the management of lung cancer patients. Am J Surg Pathol. 2005 Feb;29(2):179–87. PMID:15644774
688. Pelosi G, Rossi G, Cavazza A, et al. ΔNp63 (p40) distribution inside lung cancer: a driver biomarker approach to tumor characterization. Int J Surg Pathol. 2013 Jun;21(3):229–39. PMID:23486764
689. Pelosi G, Sonzogni A, De Pas T, et al. Review article: pulmonary sarcomatoid carcinomas: a practical overview. Int J Surg Pathol. 2010 Apr;18(2):103–20. PMID:19124452
690. Perret R, Chalabreysse L, Watson S, et al. SMARCA4-deficient thoracic sarcomas: clinicopathologic study of 30 cases with an emphasis on their nosology and differential diagnoses. Am J Surg Pathol. 2019 Apr;43(4):455–65. PMID:30451731
691. Petri N, Holten I. Parathyroid cyst: report of case in the mediastinum. J Laryngol Otol. 1990 Jan;104(1):56–7. PMID:2313181
692. Petscavage JM, Richardson ML, Nett M, et al. Primary chordoid meningioma of the lung. J Thorac Imaging. 2011 Feb;26(1):W14-6. PMID:20634760
693. Petursdottir A, Sigurdardottir J, Fridriksson BM, et al. Pulmonary carcinoid tumours: incidence, histology, and surgical outcome. A population-based study. Gen Thorac Cardiovasc Surg. 2020 May;68(5):523–9. PMID:31782060
694. Pezzuto F, Fortarezza F, Mammana M, et al. Immunohistochemical neuroendocrine marker expression in primary pulmonary NUT carcinoma: a diagnostic pitfall. Histopathology. 2020 Sep;77(3):508–10. PMID:32502287
695. Piao Y, Guo M, Gong Y. Diagnostic challenges of metastatic spindle cell melanoma on fine-needle aspiration specimens. Cancer. 2008 Apr 25;114(2):94–101. PMID:18260089
696. Piña-Oviedo S, Weissferdt A, Kalhor N, et al. Primary pulmonary lymphomas. Adv Anat Pathol. 2015 Nov;22(6):355–75. PMID:26452211
697. Pisani RJ, Colby TV, Williams DE. Malignant mesothelioma of the pleura. Mayo Clin Proc. 1988 Dec;63(12):1234–44. PMID:3059081
698. Pisapia P, Lozano MD, Vigliar E, et al. ALK and ROS1 testing on lung cancer cytologic samples: perspectives. Cancer Cytopathol. 2017 Nov;125(11):817–30. PMID:28743163
699. Pisapia P, Malapelle U, Roma G, et al. Consistency and reproducibility of next-generation sequencing in cytopathology: a second worldwide ring trial study on improved cytological molecular reference specimens. Cancer Cytopathol. 2019 May;127(5):285–96. PMID:31021538
700. Planchard D, Besse B, Groen HJM, et al. Dabrafenib plus trametinib in patients with previously treated BRAF(V600E)-mutant metastatic non-small cell lung cancer: an open-label, multicentre phase 2 trial. Lancet Oncol. 2016 Jul;17(7):984–93. PMID:27283860
701. Planchard D, Popat S, Kerr K, et al. Metastatic non-small cell lung cancer: ESMO Clinical Practice Guidelines for diagnosis, treatment and follow-up. Ann Oncol. 2018 Oct 1;29(Suppl 4):iv192–237. PMID:30285222
702. Poletti V, Ravaglia C, Tomassetti S, et al. Lymphoproliferative lung disorders: clinicopathological aspects. Eur Respir Rev. 2013 Dec;22(130):427–36. PMID:24293460
703. Policarpio-Nicolas ML, Covell J, Bregman S, et al. Fine needle aspiration cytology of clear cell "sugar" tumor (PEComa) of the lung: report of a case. Diagn Cytopathol. 2008 Feb;36(2):89–93. PMID:18181192
704. Policarpio-Nicolas ML, Wick MR. False-positive interpretations in respiratory cytopathology: exemplary cases and literature review. Diagn Cytopathol. 2008 Jan;36(1):13–9. PMID:18064688
705. Polsani A, Braithwaite KA, Alazraki AL, et al. NUT midline carcinoma: an imaging case series and review of literature. Pediatr Radiol. 2012 Feb;42(2):205–10. PMID:22033856
706. Ponti G, Manfredini M, Tomasi A. Non-blood sources of cell-free DNA for cancer molecular profiling in clinical pathology and oncology. Crit Rev Oncol Hematol. 2019 Sep;141:36–42. PMID:31212145
707. Popp W, Merkle M, Schreiber B, et al. How much brushing is enough for the diagnosis of lung tumors? Cancer. 1992 Nov 1;70(9):2278–80. PMID:1394056
708. Popper HH, el-Shabrawi Y, Wöckel W, et al. Prognostic importance of human papilloma virus typing in squamous cell papilloma of the bronchus: comparison of in situ hybridization and the polymerase chain reaction. Hum Pathol. 1994 Nov;25(11):1191–7. PMID:7959664
709. Postmus PE, Kerr KM, Oudkerk M, et al. Early and locally advanced non-small-cell lung cancer (NSCLC): ESMO Clinical Practice Guidelines for diagnosis, treatment and follow-up. Ann Oncol. 2017 Jul 1;28(suppl_4):iv1–21. PMID:28881918
710. Powers CN. Diagnosis of infectious diseases: a cytopathologist's perspective. Clin Microbiol Rev. 1998 Apr;11(2):341–65. PMID:9564567
711. Prayson RA, Farver CF. Primary pulmonary malignant meningioma. Am J Surg Pathol. 1999 Jun;23(6):722–6. PMID:10366156
712. Pritt BS, Aubry MC. Histopathology of viral infections of the lung. Semin Diagn Pathol. 2017 Nov;34(6):510–7. PMID:28693907
713. Proietti A, Alì G, Pelliccioni S, et al. Anaplastic lymphoma kinase gene rearrangements in cytological samples of non-small cell lung cancer: comparison with histological assessment. Cancer Cytopathol. 2014 Jun;122(6):445–53. PMID:24648382
714. Pu RT, Pang Y, Michael CW. Utility of WT-1, p63, MOC31, mesothelin, and cytokeratin (K903 and CK5/6) immunostains in differentiating adenocarcinoma, squamous cell carcinoma, and malignant mesothelioma in effusions. Diagn Cytopathol. 2008 Jan;36(1):20–5. PMID:18064689
715. Pulford E, Huilgol K, Moffat D, et al. Malignant mesothelioma, BAP1 immunohistochemistry, and VEGFA: Does BAP1 have potential for early diagnosis and assessment of prognosis? Dis Markers. 2017;2017:1310478. PMID:29085180
716. Puliyel MM, Mascarenhas L, Zhou S, et al. Nuclear protein in testis midline carcinoma misdiagnosed as adamantinoma. J Clin Oncol. 2014 May 20;32(15):e57–60. PMID:24470009
717. Qin BD, Jiao XD, Liu K, et al. Clinical, pathological and treatment factors associated with the survival of patients with primary pulmonary salivary gland-type tumors. Lung Cancer. 2018 Dec;126:174–81. PMID:30527184
718. Qiu S, Nampoothiri MM, Zaharopoulos P, et al. Primary pulmonary adenoid cystic carcinoma: report of a case diagnosed by fine-needle aspiration cytology. Diagn Cytopathol. 2004 Jan;30(1):51–6. PMID:14696146
719. Quinn AM, Chaturvedi A, Nonaka D. High-grade neuroendocrine carcinoma of the lung with carcinoid morphology: a study of 12 cases. Am J Surg Pathol. 2017 Feb;41(2):263–70. PMID:27879513
720. Quintanal-Villalonga Á, Chan JM, Yu HA, et al. Lineage plasticity in cancer: a shared pathway of therapeutic resistance. Nat Rev Clin Oncol. 2020 Jun;17(6):360–71. PMID:32152485
721. Raab SS, Silverman JF, McLeod DL, et al. Fine needle aspiration biopsy of fibromatoses. Acta Cytol. 1993 May-Jun;37(3):323–8. PMID:8498134
722. Radzikowska E. Update on pulmonary Langerhans cell histiocytosis. Front Med (Lausanne). 2021 Mar 8;7:582581. PMID:33763431
723. Rakich PM, Latimer KS. Cytology of the respiratory tract. Vet Clin North Am Small Anim Pract. 1989 Sep;19(5):823–50. PMID:2678710
724. Ramalingam P, Teague D, Reid-Nicholson M. Imprint cytology of high-grade immature ovarian teratoma: a case report, literature review, and distinction from other ovarian small round cell tumors. Diagn Cytopathol. 2008 Aug;36(8):595–9. PMID:18618728
725. Ramani NS, Chen H, Broaddus RR, et al. Utilization of cytology smears improves success rates of RNA-based next-generation sequencing gene fusion assays for clinically relevant predictive biomarkers. Cancer Cytopathol. 2021 May;129(5):374–82. PMID:33119213
726. Ramos SG, Rezende GG, Faccio AA. A rare presentation of biphasic pulmonary blastoma. Arch Pathol Lab Med. 2002 Jul;126(7):875–6. PMID:12125652
727. Randall MB, Geisinger KR. Angiosarcoma of the heart: pericardial fluid cytology. Diagn Cytopathol. 1990;6(1):58–62. PMID:2323298
728. Rao N. Adenosquamous carcinoma. Semin Diagn Pathol. 2014 Jul;31(4):271–7. PMID:25002356
729. Rao S, Rao S, Lal A, et al. Bronchial wash cytology: a study on morphology and morphometry. J Cytol. 2014 Apr;31(2):63–7. PMID:25210231
730. Rapicetta C, Lococo F, Stefani A, et al. Primary sarcomatoid carcinoma of the lung: radiometabolic ((18)F-FDG PET/CT) findings and correlation with clinico-pathological and survival results. Lung. 2016 Aug;194(4):653–7. PMID:27300448
731. Raso MG, Bota-Rabassedas N, Wistuba II. Pathology and classification of SCLC. Cancers (Basel). 2021 Feb 16;13(4):820. PMID:33669241

732. Ravaioli S, Bravaccini S, Tumedei MM, et al. Easily detectable cytomorphological features to evaluate during ROSE for rapid lung cancer diagnosis: from cytology to histology. Oncotarget. 2017 Feb 14;8(7):11199–205. PMID:27833073

733. Reck M, Rodríguez-Abreu D, Robinson AG, et al. Pembrolizumab versus chemotherapy for PD-L1-positive non-small-cell lung cancer. N Engl J Med. 2016 Nov 10;375(19):1823–33. PMID:27718847

734. Rekhtman N. Neuroendocrine tumors of the lung: an update. Arch Pathol Lab Med. 2010 Nov;134(11):1628–38. PMID:21043816

735. Rekhtman N, Ang DC, Sima CS, et al. Immunohistochemical algorithm for differentiation of lung adenocarcinoma and squamous cell carcinoma based on large series of whole-tissue sections with validation in small specimens. Mod Pathol. 2011 Oct;24(10):1348–59. PMID:21623384

736. Rekhtman N, Brandt SM, Sigel CS, et al. Suitability of thoracic cytology for new therapeutic paradigms in non-small cell lung carcinoma: high accuracy of tumor subtyping and feasibility of EGFR and KRAS molecular testing. J Thorac Oncol. 2011 Mar;6(3):451–8. PMID:21266922

737. Rekhtman N, Desmeules P, Litvak AM, et al. Stage IV lung carcinoids: spectrum and evolution of proliferation rate, focusing on variants with elevated proliferation indices. Mod Pathol. 2019 Jul;32(8):1106–22. PMID:30923345

738. Rekhtman N, Montecalvo J, Chang JC, et al. SMARCA4-deficient thoracic sarcomatoid tumors represent primarily smoking-related undifferentiated carcinomas rather than primary thoracic sarcomas. J Thorac Oncol. 2020 Feb;15(2):231–47. PMID:31751681

739. Rekhtman N, Paik PK, Arcila ME, et al. Clarifying the spectrum of driver oncogene mutations in biomarker-verified squamous carcinoma of lung: lack of EGFR/KRAS and presence of PIK3CA/AKT1 mutations. Clin Cancer Res. 2012 Feb 15;18(4):1167–76. PMID:22228640

740. Rekhtman N, Pietanza CM, Sabari J, et al. Pulmonary large cell neuroendocrine carcinoma with adenocarcinoma-like features: napsin A expression and genomic alterations. Mod Pathol. 2018 Jan;31(1):111–21. PMID:28884744

741. Rekhtman N, Pietanza MC, Hellmann MD, et al. Next-generation sequencing of pulmonary large cell neuroendocrine carcinoma reveals small cell carcinoma-like and non-small cell carcinoma-like subsets. Clin Cancer Res. 2016 Jul 15;22(14):3618–29. PMID:26960398

741A. Rekhtman N, Roy-Chowdhuri S. Cytology specimens: a goldmine for molecular testing. Arch Pathol Lab Med. 2016 Nov;140(11):1189–90. PMID:27788046

742. Ren WH, Zou SM, Zhang YM, et al. The role of cytology in endobronchial ultrasound-guided transbronchial needle aspiration: a study of 813 cases focusing on diagnostic yield, an analysis of misdiagnosed cases and diagnostic accordance rate of cytological subtyping. Diagn Cytopathol. 2021 Jan;49(1):119–26. PMID:32894657

743. Renshaw AA, Haja J, Lozano RL, et al. Distinguishing carcinoid tumor from small cell carcinoma of the lung: correlating cytologic features and performance in the College of American Pathologists Non-Gynecologic Cytology Program. Arch Pathol Lab Med. 2005 May;129(5):614–8. PMID:15859631

744. Resio BJ, Chiu AS, Hoag J, et al. Primary salivary type lung cancers in the National Cancer Database. Ann Thorac Surg. 2018 Jun;105(6):1633–9. PMID:29486180

745. Reynolds JH, McDonald G, Alton H, et al. Pneumonia in the immunocompetent patient. Br J Radiol. 2010 Dec;83(996):998–1009. PMID:21088086

746. Richardson SO, Huibers MMH, de Weger RA, et al. One-fits-all pretreatment protocol facilitating fluorescence in situ hybridization on formalin-fixed paraffin-embedded, fresh frozen and cytological slides. Mol Cytogenet. 2019 Jun 17;12:27. PMID:31236139

747. Righi I, Rosso L, Grisorio G, et al. Fine needle aspiration wash out for thyroglobulin determination in the differential diagnosis of lung lesions. Endocrine. 2021 Jan;71(1):253–5. PMID:32506193

748. Righi L, Gatti G, Volante M, et al. Lung neuroendocrine tumors: pathological characteristics. J Thorac Dis. 2017 Nov;9(Suppl 15):S1442–7. PMID:29201447

749. Righi L, Graziano P, Fornari A, et al. Immunohistochemical subtyping of nonsmall cell lung cancer not otherwise specified in fine-needle aspiration cytology: a retrospective study of 103 cases with surgical correlation. Cancer. 2011 Aug 1;117(15):3416–23. PMID:21246522

750. Righi L, Vavalà T, Rapa I, et al. Impact of non-small-cell lung cancer-not otherwise specified immunophenotyping on treatment outcome. J Thorac Oncol. 2014 Oct;9(10):1540–6. PMID:25521399

751. Rindi G, Klimstra DS, Abedi-Ardekani B, et al. A common classification framework for neuroendocrine neoplasms: an International Agency for Research on Cancer (IARC) and World Health Organization (WHO) expert consensus proposal. Mod Pathol. 2018 Dec;31(12):1770–86. PMID:30140036

752. Risse EK, van't Hof MA, Laurini RN, et al. Sputum cytology by the Saccomanno method in diagnosing lung malignancy. Diagn Cytopathol. 1985 Oct-Dec;1(4):286–91. PMID:3915250

753. Rivera MP, Mehta AC, American College of Chest Physicians. Initial diagnosis of lung cancer: ACCP evidence-based clinical practice guidelines (2nd edition). Chest. 2007 Sep;132(3 Suppl):131S–48S. PMID:17873165

754. Rivera MP, Mehta AC, Wahidi MM. Establishing the diagnosis of lung cancer: diagnosis and management of lung cancer, 3rd ed: American College of Chest Physicians evidence-based clinical practice guidelines. Chest. 2013 May;143(5 Suppl):e142S–65S. PMID:23649436

756. Robinson DR, Wu YM, Kalyana-Sundaram S, et al. Identification of recurrent NAB2-STAT6 gene fusions in solitary fibrous tumor by integrative sequencing. Nat Genet. 2013 Feb;45(2):180–5. PMID:23313952

757. Roden AC, Garcia JJ, Wehrs RN, et al. Histopathologic, immunophenotypic and cytogenetic features of pulmonary mucoepidermoid carcinoma. Mod Pathol. 2014 Nov;27(11):1479–88. PMID:24743219

758. Rodriguez FJ, Aubry MC, Tazelaar HD, et al. Pulmonary chondroma: a tumor associated with Carney triad and different from pulmonary hamartoma. Am J Surg Pathol. 2007 Dec;31(12):1844–53. PMID:18043038

759. Røge R, Simonsen C, Petersen AC. Primary mediastinal choriocarcinoma in an elderly patient with concurrent goserelin-treated prostate adenocarcinoma. Case Rep Pathol. 2019 May 6;2019:2734815. PMID:31198613

760. Roglić M, Jukić S, Damjanov I. Cytology of the solitary papilloma of the bronchus. Acta Cytol. 1975 Jan-Feb;19(1):11–3. PMID:1054203

761. Roh MH. The utilization of cytologic and small biopsy samples for ancillary molecular testing. Mod Pathol. 2019 Jan;32(Suppl 1):77–85. PMID:30600323

762. Rolfo C, Mack PC, Scagliotti GV, et al. Liquid biopsy for advanced non-small cell lung cancer (NSCLC): a statement paper from the IASLC. J Thorac Oncol. 2018 Sep;13(9):1248–68. PMID:29885479

763. Ronchi A, Cozzolino I, Montella M, et al. Extragonadal germ cell tumors: not just a matter of location. A review about clinical, molecular and pathological features. Cancer Med. 2019 Nov;8(16):6832–40. PMID:31568647

764. Rooper LM, Sharma R, Li QK, et al. INSM1 demonstrates superior performance to the individual and combined use of synaptophysin, chromogranin and CD56 for diagnosing neuroendocrine tumors of the thoracic cavity. Am J Surg Pathol. 2017 Nov;41(11):1561–9. PMID:28719469

765. Rosado-de-Christenson ML, Templeton PA, Moran CA. From the archives of the AFIP. Mediastinal germ cell tumors: radiologic and pathologic correlation. Radiographics. 1992 Sep;12(5):1013–30. PMID:1326777

766. Roscilli G, De Vitis C, Ferrara FF, et al. Human lung adenocarcinoma cell cultures derived from malignant pleural effusions as model system to predict patients chemosensitivity. J Transl Med. 2016 Feb 29;14:61. PMID:26928703

767. Rosen LE, Karrison T, Ananthanarayanan V, et al. Nuclear grade and necrosis predict prognosis in malignant epithelioid pleural mesothelioma: a multi-institutional study. Mod Pathol. 2018 Apr;31(4):598–606. PMID:29327706

768. Rosen RD, Bordoni B. Embryology, parathyroid. 2022 May 8. In: StatPearls. Treasure Island (FL): StatPearls Publishing; 2022 Jan–. PMID:32119467

769. Rosenbaum DG, Teruya-Feldstein J, Price AP, et al. Radiologic features of NUT midline carcinoma in an adolescent. Pediatr Radiol. 2012 Feb;42(2):249–52. PMID:22057302

770. Rossi G, Cavazza A, Comin C, et al. Mucinous adenomyomatous pulmonary hamartoma: clinicopathologic, immunohistochemical, and molecular features of 6 cases. Int J Surg Pathol. 2021 May;29(3):273–80. PMID:32715806

771. Rossi G, Cavazza A, Spagnolo P, et al. The role of macrophages in interstitial lung diseases: Number 3 in the Series "Pathology for the clinician" Edited by Peter Dorfmüller and Alberto Cavazza. Eur Respir Rev. 2017 Jul 19;26(145):170009. PMID:28724562

772. Rossi G, Cavazza A, Sturm N, et al. Pulmonary carcinomas with pleomorphic, sarcomatoid, or sarcomatous elements: a clinicopathologic and immunohistochemical study of 75 cases. Am J Surg Pathol. 2003 Mar;27(3):311–24. PMID:12604887

773. Rossi G, Pelosi G, Barbareschi M, et al. Subtyping non-small cell lung cancer: relevant issues and operative recommendations for the best pathology practice. Int J Surg Pathol. 2013 Aug;21(4):326–36. PMID:23740564

774. Rougemont AL, Tille JC. Role of HNF1β in the differential diagnosis of yolk sac tumor from other germ cell tumors. Hum Pathol. 2018 Nov;81:26–36. PMID:29753846

775. Rowsell C, Sirbovan J, Rosenblum MK, et al. Primary chordoid meningioma of lung. Virchows Arch. 2005 Mar;446(3):333–7. PMID:15714337

776. Roy-Chowdhuri S, Chen H, Singh RR, et al. Concurrent fine needle aspirations and core needle biopsies: a comparative study of substrates for next-generation sequencing in solid organ malignancies. Mod Pathol. 2017 Apr;30(4):499–508. PMID:28084342

777. Roy-Chowdhuri S, Chow CW, Kane MK, et al. Optimizing the DNA yield for molecular analysis from cytologic preparations. Cancer Cytopathol. 2016 Apr;124(4):254–60. PMID:26630358

778. Roy-Chowdhuri S, Dacic S, Ghofrani M, et al. Collection and handling of thoracic small biopsy and cytology specimens for ancillary studies: guideline from the College of American Pathologists in collaboration with the American College of Chest Physicians, Association for Molecular Pathology, American Society of Cytopathology, American Thoracic Society, Pulmonary Pathology Society, Papanicolaou Society of Cytopathology, Society of Interventional Radiology, and Society of Thoracic Radiology. Arch Pathol Lab Med. 2020 May 13. PMID:32401054

779. Roy-Chowdhuri S, Pisapia P, Salto-Tellez M, et al. Invited review-next-generation sequencing: a modern tool in cytopathology. Virchows Arch. 2019 Jul;475(1):3–11. PMID:30877381

780. Roy-Chowdhuri S, Stewart J. Preanalytic variables in cytology: lessons learned from next-generation sequencing-the MD Anderson experience. Arch Pathol Lab Med. 2016 Nov;140(11):1191–9. PMID:27333361

781. Rubino M, Scoazec JY, Pisa E, et al. Lung carcinoids with high proliferative activity: further support for the identification of a new tumor category in the classification of lung neuroendocrine neoplasms. Lung Cancer. 2020 Oct;148:149–58. PMID:32916569

782. Rudin CM, Brambilla E, Faivre-Finn C, et al. Small-cell lung cancer. Nat Rev Dis Primers. 2021 Jan 14;7(1):3. PMID:33446664

783. Ruiz C, Kustermann S, Pietilae E, et al. Culture and drug profiling of patient derived malignant pleural effusions for personalized cancer medicine. PLoS One. 2016 Aug 22;11(8):e0160807. PMID:27548442

784. Russell DK, Jain D. Cytopreparatory techniques. In: Chandra A, Crothers BA, Kurtycz DFI, et al., editors. The International System for Serous Fluid Cytopathology. Cham (Switzerland): Springer 2020. pp. 239–65.

785. Saad RS, Silverman JF. Respiratory cytology: differential diagnosis and pitfalls. Diagn Cytopathol. 2010 Apr;38(4):297–307. PMID:19856422

786. Saccomanno G, Archer VE, Auerbach O, et al. Development of carcinoma of the lung as reflected in exfoliated cells. Cancer. 1974 Jan;33(1):256–70. PMID:4810100

787. Saccomanno G, Saunders RP, Ellis H, et al. Concentration of carcinoma or atypical cells in sputum. Acta Cytol. 1963 Sep-Oct;7:305–10. PMID:14063649

788. Saeed OAM, Cramer H, Wang X, et al. Fine needle aspiration cytology of hepatic metastases of neuroendocrine tumors: a 20-year retrospective, single institutional study. Diagn Cytopathol. 2018 Jan;46(1):35–9. PMID:29076658

789. Saglietti C, Volante M, La Rosa S, et al. Cytology of primary salivary gland-type tumors of the lower respiratory tract: report of 15 cases and review of the literature. Front Med (Lausanne). 2017 Apr 24;4:43. PMID:28484699

790. Saha K, Sit NK, Jash D, et al. Diagnosis of sclerosing hemangioma of lung: don't rely on fine-needle aspiration cytology diagnosis alone. J Cancer Res Ther. 2013 Oct-Dec;9(4):748–50. PMID:24518736

791. Saito Y, Nagamoto N, Ota S, et al. Results of surgical treatment for roentgenographically occult bronchogenic squamous cell carcinoma. J Thorac Cardiovasc Surg. 1992 Aug;104(2):401–7. PMID:1495303

792. Salem A, Bell D, Sepesi B, et al. Clinicopathologic and genetic features of primary bronchopulmonary mucoepidermoid carcinoma: the MD Anderson Cancer Center experience and comprehensive review of the literature. Virchows Arch. 2017 Jun;470(6):619–26. PMID:28343305

793. Sanati S, Lu DW, Schmidt E, et al. Cytologic diagnosis of Ewing sarcoma/peripheral neuroectodermal tumor with paired prospective molecular genetic analysis. Cancer. 2007 Jun 25;111(3):192–9. PMID:17487851
794. Sanguedolce F, Zanelli M, Zizzo M, et al. Primary pulmonary B-cell lymphoma: a review and update. Cancers (Basel). 2021 Jan 22;13(3):415. PMID:33499258
795. Santagata S, Ligon KL, Hornick JL. Embryonic stem cell transcription factor signatures in the diagnosis of primary and metastatic germ cell tumors. Am J Surg Pathol. 2007 Jun;31(6):836–45. PMID:17527070
796. Santana AN, Nunes FS, Ho N, et al. A rare cause of hemoptysis: benign sugar (clear) cell tumor of the lung. Eur J Cardiothorac Surg. 2004 Apr;25(4):652–4. PMID:15037292
797. Sanz-Santos J, Serra P, Andreo F, et al. Contribution of cell blocks obtained through endobronchial ultrasound-guided transbronchial needle aspiration to the diagnosis of lung cancer. BMC Cancer. 2012 Jan 21;12:34. PMID:22264305
798. Saqi A, Shaham D, Scognamiglio T, et al. Incidence and cytological features of pulmonary hamartomas indeterminate on CT scan. Cytopathology. 2008 Jun;19(3):185–91. PMID:17388933
799. Saraswathy Veena V, Sara George P, Jayasree K, et al. Comparative analysis of cell morphology in sputum samples homogenized with dithiothreitol, N-acetyl-L cysteine, Cytorich(®) red preservative and in cellblock preparations to enhance the sensitivity of sputum cytology for the diagnosis of lung cancer. Diagn Cytopathol. 2015 Jul;43(7):551–8. PMID:25881088
800. Sareen R, Pandey CL. Lung malignancy: diagnostic accuracies of bronchoalveolar lavage, bronchial brushing, and fine needle aspiration cytology. Lung India. 2016 Nov-Dec;33(6):635–41. PMID:27890992
801. Satoh Y, Ishikawa Y. Primary pulmonary meningioma: ten-year follow-up findings for a multiple case, implying a benign biological nature. J Thorac Cardiovasc Surg. 2010 Mar;139(3):e39–40. PMID:19660266
802. Satturwar SP, Rossi ED, Maleki Z, et al. Thyroid paraganglioma: a diagnostic pitfall in thyroid FNA. Cancer Cytopathol. 2021 Jun;129(6):439–49. PMID:33232572
803. Sauter JL, Graham RP, Larsen BT, et al. SMARCA4-deficient thoracic sarcoma: a distinctive clinicopathological entity with undifferentiated rhabdoid morphology and aggressive behavior. Mod Pathol. 2017 Oct;30(10):1422–32. PMID:28643792
804. Sauter JL, Grogg KL, Vrana JA, et al. Young investigator challenge: validation and optimization of immunohistochemistry protocols for use on Cellient cell block specimens. Cancer Cytopathol. 2016 Feb;124(2):89–100. PMID:26882197
805. Savic S, Bode B, Diebold J, et al. Detection of ALK-positive non-small-cell lung cancers on cytological specimens: high accuracy of immunocytochemistry with the 5A4 clone. J Thorac Oncol. 2013 Aug;8(8):1004–11. PMID:23689429
806. Savic S, Bubendorf L. Common fluorescence in situ hybridization applications in cytology. Arch Pathol Lab Med. 2016 Dec;140(12):1323–30. PMID:27479335
807. Savic S, Bubendorf L. Role of fluorescence in situ hybridization in lung cancer cytology. Acta Cytol. 2012;56(6):611–21. PMID:23207439
808. Savic S, Franco N, Grilli B, et al. Fluorescence in situ hybridization in the definitive diagnosis of malignant mesothelioma in effusion cytology. Chest. 2010 Jul;138(1):137–44. PMID:20139227
809. Savic S, Glatz K, Schoenegg R, et al. Multitarget fluorescence in situ hybridization elucidates equivocal lung cytology. Chest. 2006 Jun;129(6):1629–35. PMID:16778285
810. Schaefer IM, Zardo P, Freermann S, et al. Neuroendocrine carcinoma in a mediastinal teratoma as a rare variant of somatic-type malignancy. Virchows Arch. 2013 Nov;463(5):731–5. PMID:23979407
811. Schildhaus HU, Deml KF, Schmitz K, et al. Chromogenic in situ hybridization is a reliable assay for detection of ALK rearrangements in adenocarcinomas of the lung. Mod Pathol. 2013 Nov;26(11):1468–77. PMID:23743932
812. Schmidt RL, Witt BL, Lopez-Calderon LE, et al. The influence of rapid onsite evaluation on the adequacy rate of fine-needle aspiration cytology: a systematic review and meta-analysis. Am J Clin Pathol. 2013 Mar;139(3):300–8. PMID:23429365
813. Schmitt F, Cochand-Priollet B, Toetsch M, et al. Immunocytochemistry in Europe: results of the European Federation of Cytology Societies (EFCS) inquiry. Cytopathology. 2011 Aug;22(4):238–42. PMID:21771093
814. Schmoll HJ. Extragonadal germ cell tumors. Ann Oncol. 2002;13 Suppl 4:265–72. PMID:12401700
815. Schreiber G, McCrory DC. Performance characteristics of different modalities for diagnosis of suspected lung cancer: summary of published evidence. Chest. 2003 Jan;123(1 Suppl):115S–28S. PMID:12527571
816. Schrijver WA, van der Groep P, Hoefnagel LD, et al. Influence of decalcification procedures on immunohistochemistry and molecular pathology in breast cancer. Mod Pathol. 2016 Dec;29(12):1460–70. PMID:27562496
817. Schrock AB, Li SD, Frampton GM, et al. Pulmonary sarcomatoid carcinomas commonly harbor either potentially targetable genomic alterations or high tumor mutational burden as observed by comprehensive genomic profiling. J Thorac Oncol. 2017 Jun;12(6):932–42. PMID:28315738
817A. Schubert P, Wright CA, Louw M, et al. Ultrasound-assisted transthoracic biopsy: cells or sections? Diagn Cytopathol. 2005 Oct;33(4):233–7. PMID:16138366
818. Schulte JJ, Pease G, Taxy JB, et al. Distinguishing parathyromatosis, atypical parathyroid adenomas, and parathyroid carcinomas utilizing histologic and clinical features. Head Neck Pathol. 2021 Sep;15(3):727–36. PMID:33394375
819. Schumann GB, Roby TJ, Swan GE, et al. Quantitative sputum cytologic findings in 109 nonsmokers. Am Rev Respir Dis. 1989 Mar;139(3):601–3. PMID:2923357
820. Schwartz BE, Hofer MD, Lemieux ME, et al. Differentiation of NUT midline carcinoma by epigenomic reprogramming. Cancer Res. 2011 Apr 1;71(7):2686–96. PMID:21447744
821. Segal A, Sterrett GF, Frost FA, et al. A diagnosis of malignant pleural mesothelioma can be made by effusion cytology: results of a 20 year audit. Pathology. 2013 Jan;45(1):44–8. PMID:23222247
822. Segletes LA, Steffee CH, Geisinger KR. Cytology of primary pulmonary mucoepidermoid and adenoid cystic carcinoma. A report of four cases. Acta Cytol. 1999 Nov-Dec;43(6):1091–7. PMID:10578983
823. Selman M, Pardo A, King TE Jr. Hypersensitivity pneumonitis: insights in diagnosis and pathobiology. Am J Respir Crit Care Med. 2012 Aug 15;186(4):314–24. PMID:22679012
824. Selvaggi SM, Guidos BJ. Immature teratoma of the ovary on fluid cytology. Diagn Cytopathol. 2001 Dec;25(6):411–4. PMID:11747240
825. Selves J, Long-Mira E, Mathieu MC, et al. Immunohistochemistry for diagnosis of metastatic carcinomas of unknown primary site. Cancers (Basel). 2018 Apr 5;10(4):108. PMID:29621151
826. Sen S, Senturk E, Kuman NK, et al. PEComa (clear cell "sugar" tumor) of the lung: a benign tumor that presented with thrombocytosis. Ann Thorac Surg. 2009 Dec;88(6):2013–5. PMID:19932282
827. Sequist LV, Waltman BA, Dias-Santagata D, et al. Genotypic and histological evolution of lung cancers acquiring resistance to EGFR inhibitors. Sci Transl Med. 2011 Mar 23;3(75):75ra26. PMID:21430269
828. Shah H, Garbe L, Nussbaum E, et al. Benign tumors of the tracheobronchial tree. Endoscopic characteristics and role of laser resection. Chest. 1995 Jun;107(6):1744–51. PMID:7781378
829. Sharma S, Gupta N, Rajwanshi A, et al. Inflammatory myofibroblastic tumour: a diagnostic challenge on fine needle aspiration cytology. Cytopathology. 2016 Dec;27(6):512–6. PMID:27087029
830. Shatavi S, Fawole A, Haberichter K, et al. Nuclear protein in testis (NUT) midline carcinoma with a novel three-way translocation (4;15;19)(q13;q14;p13.1). Pathology. 2016 Oct;48(6):620–3. PMID:27590195
831. Shaw B, Borchers M, Zander D, et al. Pulmonary Langerhans cell histiocytosis. Semin Respir Crit Care Med. 2020 Apr;41(2):269–79. PMID:32279297
832. Shehata BM, Steelman CK, Abramowsky CR, et al. NUT midline carcinoma in a newborn with multiorgan disseminated tumor and a 2-year-old with a pancreatic/hepatic primary. Pediatr Dev Pathol. 2010 Nov-Dec;13(6):481–5. PMID:20017639
833. Shell R, Nicol K. Pediatric bronchoalveolar lavage: practical considerations and future prospects. Pediatr Dev Pathol. 2010 Jul-Aug;13(4):255–64. PMID:19824821
834. Shelton DA, Rana DN, Holbrook M, et al. Adenosquamous carcinoma of the lung diagnosed by cytology?: A diagnostic dilemma. Diagn Cytopathol. 2012 Sep;40(9):830–3. PMID:21416646
835. Shen C, Wang X, Che G. A rare case of primary peripheral epithelial myoepithelial carcinoma of lung: case report and literature review. Medicine (Baltimore). 2016 Aug;95(35):e4371. PMID:27583848
836. Shen L, Lin J, Ren Z, et al. Clear cell tumor of the lung could be aggressive: a case report and review of the literature. J Cardiothorac Surg. 2020 Jul 20;15(1):177. PMID:32690041
837. Shibahara J, Goto A, Niki T, et al. Primary pulmonary paraganglioma: report of a functioning case with immunohistochemical and ultrastructural study. Am J Surg Pathol. 2004 Jun;28(6):825–9. PMID:15166677
838. Shibuya K, Nakajima T, Fujiwara T, et al. Narrow band imaging with high-resolution bronchovideoscopy: a new approach for visualizing angiogenesis in squamous cell carcinoma of the lung. Lung Cancer. 2010 Aug;69(2):194–202. PMID:20541831
839. Shidham VB. CellBlockistry: chemistry and art of cell-block making - a detailed review of various historical options with recent advances. Cytojournal. 2019 Jun 28;16:12. PMID:31367220
840. Shidham VB, Chang CC, Rao RN, et al. Immunostaining of cytology smears: a comparative study to identify the most suitable method of smear preparation and fixation with reference to commonly used immunomarkers. Diagn Cytopathol. 2003 Oct;29(4):217–21. PMID:14506675
841. Shih IM, Kurman RJ. Immunohistochemical localization of inhibin-alpha in the placenta and gestational trophoblastic lesions. Int J Gynecol Pathol. 1999 Apr;18(2):144–50. PMID:10202672
842. Shin SY, Kim MY, Oh SY, et al. Pulmonary sclerosing pneumocytoma of the lung: CT characteristics in a large series of a tertiary referral center. Medicine (Baltimore). 2015 Jan;94(4):e498. PMID:25634202
843. Shinoda K, Taki H, Tsuda T, et al. Primary pulmonary lymphoma presenting with multiple lung nodules. Am J Respir Crit Care Med. 2014 Nov 1;190(9):e30–1. PMID:25360736
844. Shojaei H, Hong H, Redline RW. High-level expression of divergent endodermal lineage markers in gonadal and extra-gonadal yolk sac tumors. Mod Pathol. 2016 Oct;29(10):1278–88. PMID:27443515
845. Sholl LM, Aisner DL, Varella-Garcia M, et al. Multi-institutional oncogenic driver mutation analysis in lung adenocarcinoma: the Lung Cancer Mutation Consortium experience. J Thorac Oncol. 2015 May;10(5):768–77. PMID:25738220
846. Sholl LM, Nishino M, Pokharel S, et al. Primary pulmonary NUT midline carcinoma: clinical, radiographic, and pathologic characterizations. J Thorac Oncol. 2015 Jun;10(6):951–9. PMID:26001144
847. Sickles EA, Belliveau RE, Wiernik PH. Primary mediastinal choriocarcinoma in the male. Cancer. 1974 Apr;33(4):1196–203. PMID:4856444
848. Siegel RL, Miller KD, Fuchs HE, et al. Cancer statistics, 2021. CA Cancer J Clin. 2021 Jan;71(1):7–33. PMID:33433946
849. Siegel RL, Miller KD, Jemal A. Cancer statistics, 2019. CA Cancer J Clin. 2019 Jan;69(1):7–34. PMID:30620402
850. Sigel CS, Moreira AL, Travis WD, et al. Subtyping of non-small cell lung carcinoma: a comparison of small biopsy and cytology specimens. J Thorac Oncol. 2011 Nov;6(11):1849–56. PMID:21841504
851. Sigel CS, Rudomina DE, Sima CS, et al. Predicting pulmonary adenocarcinoma outcome based on a cytology grading system. Cancer Cytopathol. 2012 Feb 25;120(1):35–43. PMID:22083932
852. Silverman JF. Inflammatory and neoplastic processes of the lung: differential diagnosis and pitfalls in FNA biopsies. Diagn Cytopathol. 1995 Dec;13(5):448–62. PMID:8834320
853. Silverman JF, Johnsrude IS. Fine needle aspiration cytology of granulomatous cryptococcosis of the lung. Acta Cytol. 1985 Mar-Apr;29(2):157–61. PMID:2580411
854. Sing A, Freudenberg N, Kortsik C, et al. Comparison of the sensitivity of sputum and brush cytology in the diagnosis of lung carcinomas. Acta Cytol. 1997 Mar-Apr;41(2):399–408. PMID:9100773
855. Skoog L, Tani E. Immunocytochemistry: an indispensable technique in routine cytology. Cytopathology. 2011 Aug;22(4):215–29. PMID:21771092
856. Slagel DD, Powers CN, Melaragno MJ, et al. Spindle-cell lesions of the mediastinum: diagnosis by fine-needle aspiration biopsy. Diagn Cytopathol. 1997 Sep;17(3):167–76. PMID:9285187
857. Smith ML, Gotway MB, Crotty Alexander LE, et al. Vaping-related lung injury. Virchows Arch. 2021 Jan;478(1):81–8. PMID:33106908
858. Solé Violán J, Rodríguez de Castro F, Caminero Luna J, et al. Comparative efficacy of bronchoalveolar lavage and telescoping plugged catheter in the diagnosis of pneumonia in mechanically ventilated patients. Chest. 1993 Feb;103(2):386–90. PMID:8432124
859. Srinivasan R, Gautam U, Gupta R, et al. Synovial sarcoma: diagnosis on fine-needle aspiration by morphology and molecular analysis. Cancer. 2009 Apr 25;117(2):128–36. PMID:19267417

860. Staaf J, Tran L, Söderlund L, et al. Diagnostic value of insulinoma-associated protein 1 (INSM1) and comparison with established neuroendocrine markers in pulmonary cancers. Arch Pathol Lab Med. 2020 Sep 1;144(9):1075–85. PMID:31913660

861. Stanek J, Busseniers AE. Fine-needle aspiration diagnosis of ectopic thyroid: report of one case. Diagn Cytopathol. 1993;9(1):59–62. PMID:8458284

862. Stanley MW, Powers CN, Pitman MB, et al. Cytology of germ cell tumors: extragonadal, extracranial masses and intraoperative problems. Cancer. 1997 Aug 25;81(4):220–7. PMID:9292737

863. Stelow EB, Debol SM, Stanley MW, et al. Sampling of the adrenal glands by endoscopic ultrasound-guided fine-needle aspiration. Diagn Cytopathol. 2005 Jul;33(1):26–30. PMID:15945088

864. Stelow EB, French CA. Carcinomas of the upper aerodigestive tract with rearrangement of the nuclear protein of the testis (NUT) gene (NUT midline carcinomas). Adv Anat Pathol. 2009 Mar;16(2):92–6. PMID:19550370

865. Stelow EB, Yaziji H. Immunohistochemistry, carcinomas of unknown primary, and incidence rates. Semin Diagn Pathol. 2018 Mar;35(2):143–52. PMID:29224972

866. Sterrett GF, Whitaker D, Shilkin KB, et al. Fine needle aspiration cytology of malignant mesothelioma. Acta Cytol. 1987 Mar-Apr;31(2):185–93. PMID:3469852

867. Stevens TM, Morlote D, Xiu J, et al. NUTM1-rearranged neoplasia: a multi-institution experience yields novel fusion partners and expands the histologic spectrum. Mod Pathol. 2019 Jun;32(6):764–73. PMID:30723300

868. Stewart BD, VandenBussche CJ, Leon ME. Benign lesions of the mediastinum: a review with emphasis on cytology and small biopsy specimens. Semin Diagn Pathol. 2020 Jul;37(4):199–210. PMID:32534865

869. Stichelbout M, Devisme L, Franquet-Ansart H, et al. SALL4 expression in gestational trophoblastic tumors: a useful tool to distinguish choriocarcinoma from placental site trophoblastic tumor and epithelioid trophoblastic tumor. Hum Pathol. 2016 Aug;54:121–6. PMID:27068524

870. Stoll LM, Johnson MW, Burroughs F, et al. Cytologic diagnosis and differential diagnosis of lung carcinoid tumors a retrospective study of 63 cases with histologic correlation. Cancer Cytopathol. 2010 Dec 25;118(6):457–67. PMID:21240996

872. Stoll LM, Li QK. Cytology of fine-needle aspiration of inflammatory myofibroblastic tumor. Diagn Cytopathol. 2011 Sep;39(9):663–72. PMID:20730898

873. Strollo DC, Rosado-de-Christenson ML. Primary mediastinal malignant germ cell neoplasms: imaging features. Chest Surg Clin N Am. 2002 Nov;12(4):645–58. PMID:12471868

874. Strong JW, Worsham GF, Baker AS, et al. Fine-needle aspiration cytology of an endometrioid-like variant of yolk sac tumor. Diagn Cytopathol. 1992;8(6):600–4. PMID:1281767

875. Sturgis CD, Nassar DL, D'Antonio JA, et al. Cytologic features useful for distinguishing small cell from non-small cell carcinoma in bronchial brush and wash specimens. Am J Clin Pathol. 2000 Aug;114(2):197–202. PMID:10941334

876. Sturm N, Rossi G, Lantuéjoul S, et al. 34BetaE12 expression along the whole spectrum of neuroendocrine proliferations of the lung, from neuroendocrine cell hyperplasia to small cell carcinoma. Histopathology. 2003 Feb;42(2):156–66. PMID:12558748

877. Su W, Tian XD, Liu P, et al. Accuracy of endoscopic ultrasound-guided needle aspiration specimens for molecular diagnosis of non-small-cell lung carcinoma. World J Clin Cases. 2020 Nov 6;8(21):5139–48. PMID:33269250

878. Sun W, Song K, Zervos M, et al. The diagnostic value of endobronchial ultrasound-guided needle biopsy in lung cancer and mediastinal adenopathy. Diagn Cytopathol. 2010 May;38(5):337–42. PMID:19890836

879. Sung S, Shirazi M, Shu CA, et al. Pulmonary small cell carcinoma: review, common and uncommon differentials, genomics and management. Diagn Cytopathol. 2020 Aug;48(8):790–803. PMID:32348027

880. Sung S, Tazelaar HD, Crapanzano JP, et al. Adult exogenous lipoid pneumonia: a rare and underrecognized entity in cytology - a case series. Cytojournal. 2018 Jul 13;15:17. PMID:30112015

881. Suri HS, Yi ES, Nowakowski GS, et al. Pulmonary Langerhans cell histiocytosis. Orphanet J Rare Dis. 2012 Mar 19;7:16. PMID:22429393

882. Suster S, Moran CA, Dominguez-Malagon H, et al. Germ cell tumors of the mediastinum and testis: a comparative immunohistochemical study of 120 cases. Hum Pathol. 1998 Jul;29(7):737–42. PMID:9670832

883. Suthipintawong C, Leong AS, Vinyuvat S. Immunostaining of cell preparations: a comparative evaluation of common fixatives and protocols. Diagn Cytopathol. 1996 Aug;15(2):167–74. PMID:8872443

884. Syrjänen K, Syrjänen S. Solitary bronchial squamous cell papilloma - another human papillomavirus (HPV)-associated benign tumor: systematic review and meta-analysis. Contemp Oncol (Pozn). 2013;17(5):427–34. PMID:24596531

885. Syrjänen KJ. HPV infections and lung cancer. J Clin Pathol. 2002 Dec;55(12):885–91. PMID:12461047

886. Szulkin A, Otvös R, Hillerdal CO, et al. Characterization and drug sensitivity profiling of primary malignant mesothelioma cells from pleural effusions. BMC Cancer. 2014 Sep 24;14:709. PMID:25253633

887. Tabbara SO, Sidawy MK, Frost AR, et al. The stability of estrogen and progesterone receptor expression on breast carcinoma cells stored as PreservCyt suspensions and as ThinPrep slides. Cancer. 1998 Dec 25;84(6):355–60. PMID:9915137

888. Takeda M, Tani Y, Saijo N, et al. Cytopathological features of SMARCA4-deficient thoracic sarcoma: report of 2 cases and review of the literature. Int J Surg Pathol. 2020 Feb;28(1):109–14. PMID:31448657

889. Takeda S, Miyoshi S, Ohta M, et al. Primary germ cell tumors in the mediastinum: a 50-year experience at a single Japanese institution. Cancer. 2003 Jan 15;97(2):367–76. PMID:12518361

890. Takeshima Y, Amatya VJ, Kushitani K, et al. Value of immunohistochemistry in the differential diagnosis of pleural sarcomatoid mesothelioma from lung sarcomatoid carcinoma. Histopathology. 2009 May;54(6):667–76. PMID:19438742

891. Tanaka M, Kato K, Gomi K, et al. NUT midline carcinoma: report of 2 cases suggestive of pulmonary origin. Am J Surg Pathol. 2012 Mar;36(3):381–8. PMID:22301500

892. Tane S, Nishio W, Ogawa H, et al. Clinical significance of the 'not otherwise specified' subtype in candidates for resectable non-small cell lung cancer. Oncol Lett. 2014 Sep;8(3):1017–24. PMID:25120650

893. Tani E, Wejde J, Åström K, et al. FNA cytology of solitary fibrous tumors and the diagnostic value of STAT6 immunocytochemistry. Cancer Cytopathol. 2018 Jan;126(1):36–43. PMID:28914981

894. Tao LC. Aspiration biopsy cytology of mesothelioma. Diagn Cytopathol. 1989;5(1):14–21. PMID:2656144

895. Tattevin P, Casalino E, Fleury L, et al. The validity of medical history, classic symptoms, and chest radiographs in predicting pulmonary tuberculosis: derivation of a pulmonary tuberculosis prediction model. Chest. 1999 May;115(5):1248–53. PMID:10334135

896. Tavora F, Miettinen M, Fanburg-Smith J, et al. Pulmonary artery sarcoma: a histologic and follow-up study with emphasis on a subset of low-grade myofibroblastic sarcomas with a good long-term follow-up. Am J Surg Pathol. 2008 Dec;32(12):1751–61. PMID:18779732

897. Teo M, Crotty P, O'Sullivan M, et al. NUT midline carcinoma in a young woman. J Clin Oncol. 2011 Apr 20;29(12):e336–9. PMID:21263084

898. Terra SB, Jang JS, Bi L, et al. Molecular characterization of pulmonary sarcomatoid carcinoma: analysis of 33 cases. Mod Pathol. 2016 Aug;29(8):824–31. PMID:27174587

899. Thakur SK, Singh DP, Choudhary J. Lung cancer identification: a review on detection and classification. Cancer Metastasis Rev. 2020 Sep;39(3):989–98. PMID:32519151

900. Theurer S, Siebolts U, Lorenz K, et al. [Ectopic tissue of the thyroid gland and the parathyroid glands]. Pathologe. 2018 Sep;39(5):379–89. German. PMID:30105609

901. Thivolet-Béjui F. Cytological pitfalls in bronchopulmonary tumors. Diagn Cytopathol. 1997 Dec;17(6):412–6. PMID:9407200

902. Thompson-Wicking K, Francis RW, Stirnweiss A, et al. Novel BRD4-NUT fusion isoforms increase the pathogenic complexity in NUT midline carcinoma. Oncogene. 2013 Sep 26;32(39):4664–74. PMID:23128391

903. Thunnissen E, Borczuk AC, Flieder DB, et al. The use of immunohistochemistry improves the diagnosis of small cell lung cancer and its differential diagnosis. an international reproducibility study in a demanding set of cases. J Thorac Oncol. 2017 Feb;12(2):334–46. PMID:27998793

904. Tobón A, Velásquez M, Pérez B, et al. Pathologic features and clinical course of a non-functioning primary pulmonary paraganglioma: a case report. Ann Med Surg (Lond). 2020 May 27;55:185–9. PMID:32514340

905. Tochigi N, Dacic S, Ohori NP. Bronchoscopic and transthoracic cytology and biopsy for pulmonary nonsmall cell carcinomas: performance characteristics by procedure and tumor type. Diagn Cytopathol. 2012 Aug;40(8):659–63. PMID:21319328

906. Tong JH, Yeung SF, Chan AW, et al. MET amplification and exon 14 splice site mutation define unique molecular subgroups of non-small cell lung carcinoma with poor prognosis. Clin Cancer Res. 2016 Jun 15;22(12):3048–56. PMID:26847053

907. Tongbai T, McDermott S, Kiranantawat N, et al. Non-diagnostic CT-guided percutaneous needle biopsy of the lung: predictive factors and final diagnoses. Korean J Radiol. 2019 Nov;20(11):1515–26. PMID:31606956

908. Torous VF, Brackett D, Brown P, et al. Oil Red O staining for lipid-laden macrophage index of bronchoalveolar lavage: interobserver agreement and challenges to interpretation. J Am Soc Cytopathol. 2020 Nov-Dec;9(6):563–9. PMID:32674937

909. Tosi D, Mendogni P, Carrinola R, et al. CT-guided fine-needle aspiration biopsy of solitary pulmonary nodules under 15 mm in diameter: time for an afterthought? J Thorac Dis. 2019 Mar;11(3):724–31. PMID:31019760

910. Travis WD. Pathology and diagnosis of neuroendocrine tumors: lung neuroendocrine. Thorac Surg Clin. 2014 Aug;24(3):257–66. PMID:25065926

911. Travis WD. Pathology of lung cancer. Clin Chest Med. 2011 Dec;32(4):669–92. PMID:22054879

912. Travis WD. Pathology of pulmonary vasculitis. Semin Respir Crit Care Med. 2004 Oct;25(5):475–82. PMID:16088493

913. Travis WD. Sarcomatoid neoplasms of the lung and pleura. Arch Pathol Lab Med. 2010 Nov;134(11):1645–58. PMID:21043818

914. Travis WD. Update on small cell carcinoma and its differentiation from squamous cell carcinoma and other non-small cell carcinomas. Mod Pathol. 2012 Jan;25 Suppl 1:S18–30. PMID:22214967

915. Travis WD, Brambilla E, Nicholson AG, et al. The 2015 World Health Organization Classification of Lung Tumors: impact of genetic, clinical and radiologic advances since the 2004 classification. J Thorac Oncol. 2015 Sep;10(9):1243–60. PMID:26291008

916. Travis WD, Brambilla E, Noguchi M, et al. International Association for the Study of Lung Cancer/American Thoracic Society/European Respiratory Society international multidisciplinary classification of lung adenocarcinoma. J Thorac Oncol. 2011 Feb;6(2):244–85. PMID:21252716

917. Travis WD, Linnoila RI, Tsokos MG, et al. Neuroendocrine tumors of the lung with proposed criteria for large-cell neuroendocrine carcinoma. An ultrastructural, immunohistochemical, and flow cytometric study of 35 cases. Am J Surg Pathol. 1991 Jun;15(6):529–53. PMID:1709558

918. Travis WD, Rekhtman N. Pathological diagnosis and classification of lung cancer in small biopsies and cytology: strategic management of tissue for molecular testing. Semin Respir Crit Care Med. 2011 Feb;32(1):22–31. PMID:21500121

919. Travis WD, Rush W, Flieder DB, et al. Survival analysis of 200 pulmonary neuroendocrine tumors with clarification of criteria for atypical carcinoid and its separation from typical carcinoid. Am J Surg Pathol. 1998 Aug;22(8):934–44. PMID:9706973

920. Tsao AS, Scagliotti GV, Bunn PA Jr, et al. Scientific advances in lung cancer 2015. J Thorac Oncol. 2016 May;11(5):613–38. PMID:27013409

921. Tsao MS, Hirsch FR, Yatabe Y, editors. IASLC atlas of ALK and ROS1 testing in lung cancer. 2nd ed. Denver (CO): International Association for the Study of Lung Cancer; 2016.

922. Tsilimigras DI, Bakopoulos A, Ntanasis-Stathopoulos I, et al. Clear cell "sugar tumor" of the lung: diagnostic features of a rare pulmonary tumor. Respir Med Case Rep. 2017 Dec 5;23:52–4. PMID:29276673

923. Tsuta K, Kalhor N, Wistuba II, et al. Clinicopathological and immunohistochemical analysis of spindle-cell carcinoid tumour of the lung. Histopathology. 2011 Sep;59(3):526–36. PMID:22034892

924. Turner SR, Buonocore D, Desmeules P, et al. Feasibility of endobronchial ultrasound transbronchial needle aspiration for massively parallel next-generation sequencing in thoracic cancer patients. Lung Cancer. 2018 May;119:85–90. PMID:29656758

925. Ueki S, Hebisawa A, Kitani M, et al. Allergic bronchopulmonary aspergillosis-a luminal hypereosinophilic disease with extracellular trap cell death. Front Immunol. 2018 Oct 11;9:2346. PMID:30364279

926. Ueno M, Fujiyama J, Yamazaki I, et al. Cytology of primary pulmonary meningioma. Report of the first multiple case. Acta Cytol. 1998 Nov-Dec;42(6):1424–30. PMID:9850654

927. Uke MS, Pathuthara S, Shaikh A, et al. Is the morning sputum sample superior to the fresh sputum sample for the detection of malignant cells? Acta Cytol. 2017;61(3):223–9. PMID:28535501

928. Ulbright TM. Pitfalls in the interpretation of specimens from patients with testicular tumours, with an emphasis on variant morphologies. Pathology. 2018 Jan;50(1):88–99. PMID:29129333

929. Ulbright TM, Young RH. Seminoma with tubular, microcystic, and related patterns: a study of 28 cases of unusual morphologic variants that often cause confusion with yolk sac tumor. Am J Surg Pathol. 2005 Apr;29(4):500–5. PMID:15767805

930. Umeda Y, Otsuka M, Nishikiori H, et al. Feasibility of rapid on-site cytological evaluation of lung cancer by a trained pulmonologist during bronchoscopy examination. Cytopathology. 2019 Nov;30(6):628–33. PMID:31479551

931. Urano M, Nakaguro M, Yamamoto Y, et al. Diagnostic significance of HRAS mutations in epithelial-myoepithelial carcinomas exhibiting a broad histopathologic spectrum. Am J Surg Pathol. 2019 Jul;43(7):984–94. PMID:30994537

932. Usman Ali M, Miller J, Peirson L, et al. Screening for lung cancer: a systematic review and meta-analysis. Prev Med. 2016 Aug;89:301–14. PMID:27130532

933. Uzaslan E, Ebsen M, Freudenberg N, et al. Reactive alveolar epithelium in chondroid hamartoma of the lung. Acta Cytol. 2005 Mar-Apr;49(2):154–6. PMID:15839619

934. Vaideeswar P, Chaudhari J. Primary pulmonary meningioma. Indian J Pathol Microbiol. 2019 Jul-Sep;62(3):486–7. PMID:31361249

935. Vaidya A, Gouri M, Sudha HM, et al. Ectopic parathyroid adenoma presenting as a mediastinal mass. J Clin Diagn Res. 2017 May;11(5):ED40–2. PMID:28658791

936. Vaidya PJ, Saha A, Kate AH, et al. Diagnostic value of core biopsy histology and cytology sampling of mediastinal lymph nodes using 21-gauge EBUS-TBNA needle. J Cancer Res Ther. 2016 Jul-Sep;12(3):1172–7. PMID:28054531

937. van den Bosch JM, Wagenaar SS, Corrin B, et al. Mesenchymoma of the lung (so called hamartoma): a review of 154 parenchymal and endobronchial cases. Thorax. 1987 Oct;42(10):790–3. PMID:3321538

938. van der Drift MA, van der Wilt GJ, Thunnissen FB, et al. A prospective study of the timing and cost-effectiveness of bronchial washing during bronchoscopy for pulmonary malignant tumors. Chest. 2005 Jul;128(1):394–400. PMID:16002962

939. VandenBussche CJ, Wakely PE Jr, Siddiqui MT, et al. Cytopathologic characteristics of epithelioid vascular malignancies. Acta Cytol. 2014;58(4):356–66. PMID:25195738

940. VanderLaan PA. Collection and handling of thoracic small biopsy and cytology specimens for ancillary studies guideline from the College of American Pathologists (CAP): implications for the cytology community. J Am Soc Cytopathol. 2020 Jul-Aug;9(4):286–90. PMID:32439185

941. VanderLaan PA, Wang HH, Majid A, et al. Endobronchial ultrasound-guided transbronchial needle aspiration (EBUS-TBNA): an overview and update for the cytopathologist. Cancer Cytopathol. 2014 Aug;122(8):561–76. PMID:24760496

942. VanKoevering KK, Marchiano E, Walline HM, et al. An algorithm to evaluate suspected lung metastases in patients with HPV-associated oropharyngeal cancer. Otolaryngol Head Neck Surg. 2018 Jan;158(1):118–21. PMID:28949800

943. van Meerbeeck JP, Fennell DA, De Ruysscher DK. Small-cell lung cancer. Lancet. 2011 Nov 12;378(9804):1741–55. PMID:21565397

944. Vargas SO, French CA, Faul PN, et al. Upper respiratory tract carcinoma with chromosomal translocation 15;19: evidence for a distinct disease entity of young patients with a rapidly fatal course. Cancer. 2001 Sep 1;92(5):1195–203. PMID:11571733

945. Vidarsdottir H, Tran L, Nodin B, et al. Immunohistochemical profiles in primary lung cancers and epithelial pulmonary metastases. Hum Pathol. 2019 Feb;84:221–30. PMID:30389437

946. Vignaud JM. [Squamous cell carcinoma, basaloid squamous cell carcinoma and adenosquamous carcinoma in the lung]. Ann Pathol. 2016 Jan;36(1):15–23. French. PMID:26746368

947. Vijayabhaskar R, Mehta SS, Deodhar KK, et al. PEComa of the lung. J Cancer Res Ther. 2010 Jan-Mar;6(1):109–11. PMID:20479562

948. Vilmann P, Frost Clementsen P, Colella S, et al. Combined endobronchial and esophageal endosonography for the diagnosis and staging of lung cancer: European Society of Gastrointestinal Endoscopy (ESGE) Guideline, in cooperation with the European Respiratory Society (ERS) and the European Society of Thoracic Surgeons (ESTS). Eur J Cardiothorac Surg. 2015 Jul;48(1):1–15. PMID:26034060

949. Virani N, Pang J, Lew M. Cytologic and immunohistochemical evaluation of low-grade spindle cell lesions of the gastrointestinal tract. Arch Pathol Lab Med. 2016 Oct;140(10):1038–44. PMID:27684974

950. Viswanathan K, Siddiqui MT, Borczuk AC. Insulinoma-associated protein 1 is a sensitive and specific marker for lung neuroendocrine tumors in cytologic and surgical specimens. J Am Soc Cytopathol. 2019 Nov-Dec;8(6):299–308. PMID:31345782

951. Vlajnic T, Savic S, Barascud A, et al. Detection of ROS1-positive non-small cell lung cancer on cytological specimens using immunocytochemistry. Cancer Cytopathol. 2018 Jun;126(6):421–9. PMID:29451745

952. Wagner DG, Russell DK, Benson JM, et al. Cellient™ automated cell block versus traditional cell block preparation: a comparison of morphologic features and immunohistochemical staining. Diagn Cytopathol. 2011 Oct;39(10):730–6. PMID:20949469

953. Wakely P Jr. Pulmonary spindle cell lesions: correlation of aspiration cytopathology and histopathology. Ann Diagn Pathol. 2001 Aug;5(4):216–28. PMID:11510004

954. Wakely PE Jr. Fine needle aspiration in the diagnosis of thymic epithelial neoplasms. Hematol Oncol Clin North Am. 2008 Jun;22(3):433–42. PMID:18514125

955. Wakely PE Jr, Ali SZ, Bishop JA. The cytopathology of malignant peripheral nerve sheath tumor: a report of 55 fine-needle aspiration cases. Cancer Cytopathol. 2012 Oct 25;120(5):334–41. PMID:22434579

956. Walia R, Jain D, Madan K, et al. p40 & thyroid transcription factor-1 immunohistochemistry: a useful panel to characterize non-small cell lung carcinoma-not otherwise specified (NSCLC-NOS) category. Indian J Med Res. 2017 Jul;146(1):42–8. PMID:29168459

957. Walia R, Jain D, Mathur SR, et al. Spindle cell melanoma: a comparison of the cytomorphological features with the epithelioid variant. Acta Cytol. 2013;57(6):557–61. PMID:24107480

958. Wang B, Wu A, Fan Y, et al. [Diagnostic value of computed tomography-guided percutaneous lung biopsy for malignant lung tumors]. Zhonghua Yi Xue Za Zhi. 2013 Oct 15;93(38):3023–6. Chinese. PMID:24417920

959. Wang CY, Chang TC. Preoperative thyroid ultrasonography and fine-needle aspiration cytology in ectopic thyroid. Am Surg. 1995 Dec;61(12):1029–31. PMID:7486437

960. Wang H, Sun Y, Jia J. [Analyzing for 198 cases of ectopic thyroid glands]. Lin Chung Er Bi Yan Hou Tou Jing Wai Ke Za Zhi. 2012 Sep;26(18):814–6. Chinese. PMID:23259300

961. Wang W, Tang Y, Li J, et al. Detection of ALK rearrangements in malignant pleural effusion cell blocks from patients with advanced non-small cell lung cancer: a comparison of Ventana immunohistochemistry and fluorescence in situ hybridization. Cancer Cytopathol. 2015 Feb;123(2):117–22. PMID:25529354

962. Warth A, Muley T, Herpel E, et al. Large-scale comparative analyses of immunomarkers for diagnostic subtyping of non-small-cell lung cancer biopsies. Histopathology. 2012 Dec;61(6):1017–25. PMID:22882703

963. Watanabe K, Ono N, Hoshi T, et al. Fine-needle aspiration cytology of bronchial acinic cell carcinoma: a case report. Diagn Cytopathol. 2004 May;30(5):359–61. PMID:15108238

964. Watanabe Y, Tsuta K, Kusumoto M, et al. Clinicopathologic features and computed tomographic findings of 52 surgically resected adenosquamous carcinomas of the lung. Ann Thorac Surg. 2014 Jan;97(1):245–51. PMID:24206962

965. Weatherhead JE, Gazzinelli-Guimaraes P, Knight JM, et al. Host immunity and inflammation to pulmonary helminth infections. Front Immunol. 2020 Oct 20;11:594520. PMID:33193446

966. Weber C, Pautex S, Zulian GB, et al. Primary pulmonary malignant meningioma with lymph node and liver metastasis in a centenary woman, an autopsy case. Virchows Arch. 2013 Apr;462(4):481–5. PMID:23443940

967. Wee A, Nilsson B. pCEA canalicular immunostaining in fine needle aspiration biopsy diagnosis of hepatocellular carcinoma. Acta Cytol. 1997 Jul-Aug;41(4):1147–55. PMID:9250313

968. Wegman SJ, Parwani AV, Zynger DL. Cytokeratin 7, inhibin, and p63 in testicular germ cell tumor: superior markers of choriocarcinoma compared to β-human chorionic gonadotropin. Hum Pathol. 2019 Feb;84:254–61. PMID:30359635

969. Weissferdt A, Kalhor N, Correa AM, et al. "Sarcomatoid" carcinomas of the lung: a clinicopathological study of 86 cases with a new perspective on tumor classification. Hum Pathol. 2017 May;63:14–26. PMID:27993578

970. Weissferdt A, Kalhor N, Rodriguez Canales J, et al. Primary mediastinal yolk sac tumors: an immunohistochemical analysis of 14 cases. Appl Immunohistochem Mol Morphol. 2019 Feb;27(2):125–33. PMID:27643524

971. Weissferdt A, Rodriguez-Canales J, Liu H, et al. Primary mediastinal seminomas: a comprehensive immunohistochemical study with a focus on novel markers. Hum Pathol. 2015 Mar;46(3):376–83. PMID:25576290

972. Weissferdt A, Tang X, Suster S, et al. Pleuropulmonary meningothelial proliferations: evidence for a common histogenesis. Am J Surg Pathol. 2015 Dec;39(12):1673–8. PMID:26291511

973. Weldon CB, Shamberger RC. Pediatric pulmonary tumors: primary and metastatic. Semin Pediatr Surg. 2008 Feb;17(1):17–29. PMID:18158138

974. Weng X, Zhi L, An X, et al. Diagnostic value of rapid on-site evaluation in interventional pulmonology: a protocol for systematic review and meta analysis. Medicine (Baltimore). 2020 Jul 17;99(29):e21168. PMID:32702873

975. Whitaker D, Sterrett G, Shilkin K, et al. Malignant mesothelioma cells in sputum. Diagn Cytopathol. 1986 Jan-Mar;2(1):21–4. PMID:3720479

976. WHO Classification of Tumours Editorial Board. Thoracic tumours. Lyon (France): International Agency for Research on Cancer; 2021. (WHO classification of tumours series, 5th ed.; vol. 5). https://publications.iarc.fr/595.

977. Wiatrowska BA, Krol J, Zakowski MF. Large-cell neuroendocrine carcinoma of the lung: proposed criteria for cytologic diagnosis. Diagn Cytopathol. 2001 Jan;24(1):58–64. PMID:11135471

978. Wiatrowska BA, Yazdi HM, Matzinger FR, et al. Fine needle aspiration biopsy of pulmonary hamartomas. Radiologic, cytologic and immunocytochemical study of 15 cases. Acta Cytol. 1995 Nov-Dec;39(6):1167–74. PMID:7483993

979. Wick MR. Hamartomas and other tumor-like malformations of the lungs and heart. Semin Diagn Pathol. 2019 Jan;36(1):2–10. PMID:30473462

980. Wick MR, Ritter JH, Nappi O. Inflammatory sarcomatoid carcinoma of the lung: report of three cases and clinicopathologic comparison with inflammatory pseudotumors in adult patients. Hum Pathol. 1995 Sep;26(9):1014–21. PMID:7672783

981. Wile AG, Evans HL, Romsdahl MM. Leiomyosarcoma of soft tissue: a clinicopathologic study. Cancer. 1981 Aug 15;48(4):1022–32. PMID:7272926

982. Witt BL, Wallander ML, Layfield LJ, et al. Respiratory cytology in the era of molecular diagnostics: a review. Diagn Cytopathol. 2012 Jun;40(6):556–63. PMID:22619130

983. Wolf J, Seto T, Han JY, et al. Capmatinib in MET exon 14-mutated or MET-amplified non-small-cell lung cancer. N Engl J Med. 2020 Sep 3;383(10):944–57. PMID:32877583

984. Wood B, Swarbrick N, Frost F. Diagnosis of pulmonary hamartoma by fine needle biopsy. Acta Cytol. 2008 Jul-Aug;52(4):412–7. PMID:18702357

985. Wu CE, Tzen CY, Wang SY, et al. Clinical diagnosis of gastrointestinal stromal tumor (gist): from the molecular genetic point of view. Cancers (Basel). 2019 May 16;11(5):679. PMID:31100836

986. Wu CG, Chiovaro F, Curioni-Fontecedro A, et al. In vitro cell culture of patient derived malignant pleural and peritoneal effusions for personalised drug screening. J Transl Med. 2020 Apr 10;18(1):163. PMID:32276643

987. Wu CW, Yang CY, Chang YL, et al. Successful management of a ROS1-rearranged pulmonary pleomorphic carcinoma using serial tyrosine kinase inhibitors. Onco Targets Ther. 2020 Oct 9;13:10123–7. PMID:33116594

988. Wu X, Huang Y, Li Y, et al. 18F-FDG PET/CT imaging in pulmonary sarcomatoid carcinoma and correlation with clinical and genetic findings. Ann Nucl Med. 2019 Sep;33(9):647–56. PMID:31165974

989. Xiao GQ, Li F, Unger PD, et al. ZBTB16: a novel sensitive and specific biomarker for yolk sac tumor. Mod Pathol. 2016 Jun;29(6):591–8. PMID:26916077

990. Xing D, Banet N, Sharma R, et al. Aberrant Pax-8 expression in well-differentiated papillary mesothelioma and malignant mesothelioma of the peritoneum: a clinicopathologic study. Hum Pathol. 2018 Feb;72:160–6. PMID:29241740

991. Xing L, Todd NW, Yu L, et al. Early detection of squamous cell lung cancer in sputum by a panel of microRNA markers. Mod Pathol. 2010 Aug;23(8):1157–64. PMID:20526284

992. Xu D, Lin X, Qiu X. The epithelioid gastrointestinal stromal tumor with pulmonary metastasis: a rare case report and literature review. Medicine (Baltimore). 2020 Feb;99(9):e19346. PMID:32118771

993. Yamamoto Y, Kodama K, Maniwa T, et al. Anaplastic lymphoma kinase-positive squamous cell carcinoma of the lung: a case report. Mol Clin Oncol. 2016 Jul;5(1):61–3. PMID:27330767

994. Yang GC. Cytohistology of papillary carcinoid and emerging concept of pulmonary neuroendocrine neoplasms. Diagn Cytopathol. 2016 Jan;44(1):52–60. PMID:26457802

995. Yang GC, Hwang SJ, Yee HT. Fine-needle aspiration cytology of unusual germ cell tumors of the mediastinum: atypical seminoma and parietal yolk sac tumor. Diagn Cytopathol. 2002 Aug;27(2):69–74. PMID:12203871

996. Yang SR, Mooney KL, Libiran P, et al. Targeted deep sequencing of cell-free DNA in serous body cavity fluids with malignant, suspicious, and benign cytology. Cancer Cytopathol. 2020 Jan;128(1):43–56. PMID:31751001

997. Yang YJ, Steele CT, Ou XL, et al. Diagnosis of high-grade pulmonary neuroendocrine carcinoma by fine-needle aspiration biopsy: nonsmall-cell or small-cell type? Diagn Cytopathol. 2001 Nov;25(5):292–300. PMID:11747218

998. Yao X, Gomes MM, Tsao MS, et al. Fine-needle aspiration biopsy versus core-needle biopsy in diagnosing lung cancer: a systematic review. Curr Oncol. 2012 Feb;19(1):e16–27. PMID:22328844

999. Yatabe Y, Borczuk AC, Cooper WA, et al., editors. IASLC atlas of diagnostic immunohistochemistry. Denver (CO): International Association for the Study of Lung Cancer; 2020.

1000. Yatabe Y, Dacic S, Borczuk AC, et al. Best practices recommendations for diagnostic immunohistochemistry in lung cancer. J Thorac Oncol. 2019 Mar;14(3):377–407. PMID:30572031

1001. Yates DH, Corrin B, Stidolph PN, et al. Malignant mesothelioma in south east England: clinicopathological experience of 272 cases. Thorax. 1997 Jun;52(6):507–12. PMID:9227715

1002. Yin W, Cheng J, Tang Z, et al. MET amplification (MET/CEP7 ratio ≥ 1.8) is an independent poor prognostic marker in patients with treatment-naive non-small-cell lung cancer. Clin Lung Cancer. 2021 Jul;22(4):e512–8. PMID:33288441

1004. Yoshida A, Kobayashi E, Kubo T, et al. Clinicopathological and molecular characterization of SMARCA4-deficient thoracic sarcomas with comparison to potentially related entities. Mod Pathol. 2017 Jun;30(6):797–809. PMID:28256572

1005. Yoshimoto T, Matsubara D, Nakano T, et al. Frequent loss of the expression of multiple subunits of the SWI/SNF complex in large cell carcinoma and pleomorphic carcinoma of the lung. Pathol Int. 2015 Nov;65(11):595–602. PMID:26345631

1006. Yoshimura M, Kinoshita Y, Hamasaki M, et al. Highly expressed EZH2 in combination with BAP1 and MTAP loss, as detected by immunohistochemistry, is useful for differentiating malignant pleural mesothelioma from reactive mesothelial hyperplasia. Lung Cancer. 2019 Apr;130:187–93. PMID:30885343

1007. Young JA. ACP Broadsheet No 140: July 1993. Techniques in pulmonary cytopathology. J Clin Pathol. 1993 Jul;46(7):589–95. PMID:8157740

1008. Young RH. The yolk sac tumor: reflections on a remarkable neoplasm and two of the many intrigued by it-Gunnar Teilum and Aleksander Talerman-and the bond it formed between them. Int J Surg Pathol. 2014 Dec;22(8):677–87. PMID:25395492

1009. Yousem SA, Wick MR, Randhawa P, et al. Pulmonary blastoma. An immunohistochemical analysis with comparison with fetal lung in its pseudoglandular stage. Am J Clin Pathol. 1990 Feb;93(2):167–75. PMID:2301281

1010. Yu DC, Grabowski MJ, Kozakewich HP, et al. Primary lung tumors in children and adolescents: a 90-year experience. J Pediatr Surg. 2010 Jun;45(6):1090–5. PMID:20620301

1011. Yu HA, Arcila ME, Rekhtman N, et al. Analysis of tumor specimens at the time of acquired resistance to EGFR-TKI therapy in 155 patients with EGFR-mutant lung cancers. Clin Cancer Res. 2013 Apr 15;19(8):2240–7. PMID:23470965

1012. Yuan Y, Nymoen DA, Stavnes HT, et al. Tenascin-X is a novel diagnostic marker of malignant mesothelioma. Am J Surg Pathol. 2009 Nov;33(11):1673–82. PMID:19738457

1013. Yung RC. Tissue diagnosis of suspected lung cancer: selecting between bronchoscopy, transthoracic needle aspiration, and resectional biopsy. Respir Care Clin N Am. 2003 Mar;9(1):51–76. PMID:12820712

1015. Zarbo RJ, Fenoglio-Preiser CM. Interinstitutional database for comparison of performance in lung fine-needle aspiration cytology. A College of American Pathologists Q-Probe Study of 5264 cases with histologic correlation. Arch Pathol Lab Med. 1992 May;116(5):463–70. PMID:1580748

1016. Zarogoulidis P, Tryfon S, Sapalidis K, et al. Bronchial HPV; the good the bad and the unknown. Respir Med Case Rep. 2020 Apr 7;30:101053. PMID:32309132

1017. Zeng J, Zhou F, Wei XJ, et al. Sclerosing hemangioma: a diagnostic dilemma in fine needle aspiration cytology. Cytojournal. 2016 Apr 20;13:9. PMID:27168758

1018. Zhan C, Jiang T, Yang X, et al. [Clinical characteristics and prognostic factors of lung adenosquamous carcinoma in SEER database between 2010 and 2015]. Zhongguo Fei Ai Za Zhi. 2018 Aug 20;21(8):600–9. Chinese. PMID:30172267

1019. Zhang C, Schmidt LA, Hatanaka K, et al. Evaluation of napsin A, TTF-1, p63, p40, and CK5/6 immunohistochemical stains in pulmonary neuroendocrine tumors. Am J Clin Pathol. 2014 Sep;142(3):320–4. PMID:25125621

1020. Zhang W, Zhang H, Hou Q, et al. Ectopic thyroid microfollicular adenoma in the lung: a case report. Medicine (Baltimore). 2019 Aug;98(35):e16832. PMID:31464909

1021. Zhang X, Kuang Y, Zhang Y, et al. Shifted focus of bronchoalveolar lavage in patients with suspected thoracic malignancy: an analysis of 224 patients. J Thorac Dis. 2016 Nov;8(11):3245–54. PMID:28066604

1022. Zhang Y, Wessman S, Wejde J, et al. Diagnosing synovial sarcoma by fine-needle aspiration cytology and molecular techniques. Cytopathology. 2019 Sep;30(5):504–9. PMID:31161693

1023. Zhang YZ, Brambilla C, Molyneaux PL, et al. Utility of nuclear grading system in epithelioid malignant pleural mesothelioma in biopsy-heavy setting: an external validation study of 563 cases. Am J Surg Pathol. 2020 Mar;44(3):347–56. PMID:32045387

1024. Zhao W, Chen T, Yang Y. Primary extragenital choriocarcinoma in posterior mediastinum in a male adult: a case report. Ann Transl Med. 2019 Nov;7(22):703. PMID:31930104

1025. Zheng G, Ettinger DS, Maleki Z. Utility of the quantitative Ki-67 proliferation index and CD56 together in the cytologic diagnosis of small cell lung carcinoma and other lung neuroendocrine tumors. Acta Cytol. 2013;57(3):281–90. PMID:23635388

1026. Zhou SY, Xue Q, Ying JM, et al. [The clinical and pathological features, biomarker characteristics and prognosis analysis of lung adenosquamous carcinoma]. Zhonghua Zhong Liu Za Zhi. 2019 Jan 23;41(1):50–5. Chinese. PMID:30678417

1027. Zhou Y, Höti N, Ao M, et al. Expression of p16 and p53 in non-small-cell lung cancer: clinicopathological correlation and potential prognostic impact. Biomark Med. 2019 Jun;13(9):761–71. PMID:31157548

1028. Zhu B, Laskin W, Chen Y, et al. NUT midline carcinoma: a neoplasm with diagnostic challenges in cytology. Cytopathology. 2011 Dec;22(6):414–7. PMID:21210877

1029. Zhu F, Liu Z, Hou Y, et al. Primary salivary gland-type lung cancer: clinicopathological analysis of 88 cases from China. J Thorac Oncol. 2013 Dec;8(12):1578–84. PMID:24389442

1030. Zhu L, Jiang L, Yang J, et al. Clinical characteristics and prognosis of patients with lung adenosquamous carcinoma after surgical resection: results from two institutes. J Thorac Dis. 2018 Apr;10(4):2397–402. PMID:29850145

1031. Zhu R, Jia C, Yan J, et al. Primary pulmonary choriocarcinoma in a male that was successfully diagnosed and treated: a case report and review of the literature. Medicine (Baltimore). 2016 Dec;95(52):e5693. PMID:28033262

1032. Zusman-Harach SB, Harach HR, Gibbs AR. Cytological features of non-small cell carcinomas of the lung in fine needle aspirates. J Clin Pathol. 1991 Dec;44(12):997–1002. PMID:1665154

1033. Zwiebel BR, Austin JH, Grimes MM. Bronchial carcinoid tumors: assessment with CT of location and intratumoral calcification in 31 patients. Radiology. 1991 May;179(2):483–6. PMID:2014296

Subject index

Bold page numbers indicate the main discussion(s) of the topic.